Management of Urologic Cancer

Management of Urologic Cancer

Focal Therapy and Tissue Preservation

Edited by Mark P. Schoenberg and Kara L. Watts

Department of Urology, The Montefiore Medical Center & The Albert Einstein College of Medicine, Bronx, NY USA

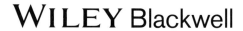

Registered Offices

John Wiley & Sons, Inc., 111 River Street, Hoboken, NJ 07030, USA
John Wiley & Sons Ltd, The Atrium, Southern Gate, Chichester, West Sussex, PO19 8SQ, UK

Editorial Office

9600 Garsington Road, Oxford, OX4 2DQ, UK

For details of our global editorial offices, customer services, and more information about Wiley products visit us at www.wiley.com.

Wiley also publishes its books in a variety of electronic formats and by print-on-demand. Some content that appears in standard print versions of this book may not be available in other formats.

Library of Congress Cataloging-in-Publication Data

Names: Schoenberg, Mark P., editor. | Watts, Kara L., editor.
Title: Management of urologic cancer : focal therapy and tissue preservation / edited by Mark P. Schoenberg and Kara L. Watts.
Description: Hoboken, NJ : Wiley, 2017. | Includes bibliographical references and index. |
Identifiers: LCCN 2017014288 (print) | LCCN 2017014924 (ebook) | ISBN 9781118868096 (pdf) | ISBN 9781118868089 (epub) | ISBN 9781118864623 (cloth)
Subjects: | MESH: Urologic Neoplasms–therapy | Tissue Preservation–methods
Classification: LCC RC280.U74 (ebook) | LCC RC280.U74 (print) | NLM WJ 160 | DDC 616.99/461–dc23
LC record available at https://lccn.loc.gov/2017014288

Cover Design: Wiley
Cover image: © pixologicstudio/Gettyimages

Set in 10/12pt Warnock by SPi Global, Pondicherry, India
Printed in Singapore by C.O.S. Printers Pte Ltd

10 9 8 7 6 5 4 3 2 1

Contents

List of Contributors

Hashim Uddin Ahmed, MD, FRCS, PhD
Division of Surgery & Interventional
Science
University College Hospital,
London, UK

Clare Allen, MBBS, FRCR
Department of Radiology
University College Hospital,
London, UK

Fadi Brimo, MD, FRPC (C)
Department of Pathology
McGill University Health Center
Montreal General Hospital site
Montreal, Quebec, Canada

Arthur L. Burnett, MD, MBA, FACS
Department of Urology
Johns Hopkins Medical Institutions
Baltimore, MD, USA

David Y.T. Chen, MD, FACS
Department of Surgical Oncology
Division of Urologic Oncology
Fox Chase Center–Temple University
Health System
Philadelphia, PA, USA

Victoria Chernyak, MD
Department of Radiology
Albert Einstein College of Medicine
Director of Body MR Imaging
Montefiore Medical Center
Bronx, NY USA

Louise Dickinson, MRCS, PhD
Department of Radiology
University College Hospital,
London, UK

John B. Eifler, MD
Department of Urologic Surgery
Vanderbilt University
Nashville, TN, USA

Elliot K. Fishman, MD
Department of Radiology
John Hopkins University
Baltimore, MD, USA

Francesco Fraioli, MD, FRCR
Institute of Nuclear Medicine
University College Hospital
London, UK

Nilay M. Gandhi, MD
Department of Urology
Johns Hopkins University
Baltimore, MD, USA

Chandan Guha, MBBS, PhD
Department of Radiation Oncology
Montefiore Medical Center
Albert Einstein College of
Medicine
Bronx, NY, USA

Athar Haroon, MBBS, FRCR
Department of Radiology
St Bartholomew's Hospital
London, UK

J. Stephen Jones, MD
Department of Urology
Cleveland Clinic Department of
Regional Urology
Cleveland, OH, USA

Rafi Kabarriti, MD
Department of Radiation Oncology
Montefiore Medical Center
Albert Einstein College of
Medicine
Bronx, NY, USA

Ganesh Kartha, MD
The Glickman Urological and
Kidney Institute
The Cleveland Clinic Foundation
Cleveland, OH, USA

Laurence Klotz, MD, FRCSC
Division of Urology
Sunnybrook Health Sciences Center
University of Toronto
Toronto, Ontario, Canada

Stephan Kruck, MD
Department of Urology
University Hospital Tuebingen
Tuebingen, Germany

Oleksandr N. Kryvenko, MD
Department of Pathology
University of Miami Miller
School of Medicine
Miami, FL, USA

Kyungmouk Steve Lee, MD
Department of Radiology, Division of
Interventional Radiology
New York-Presbyterian Hospital/Weill
Cornell Medical Center
New York, NY, USA

Mark C. Markowski, MD, PhD
Department of Medical Oncology
John Hopkins University
Baltimore, MD, USA

David F. Penson, MD, MPH
Department of Urology
Vanderbilt University Medical Center
Nashville, TN, USA

Kenneth J. Pienta, MD
Department of Medical Oncology
John Hopkins University
Baltimore, MD, USA

Peter A. Pinto, MD
Urologic Oncology Branch
National Cancer Institute
National Institutes of Health
Bethesda, MD, USA

Bradley B. Pua, MD
Department of Radiology, Division of
Interventional Radiology
New York-Presbyterian Hospital/Weill
Cornell Medical Center
New York, NY, USA

Soroush Rais-Bahrami, MD
Departments of Radiology and Urology
University of Alabama at Birmingham
Birmingham, AL, USA

Siva P. Raman, MD
Department of Radiology
John Hopkins University
Baltimore, MD, USA

Pravin K. Rao, MD
Department of Urology
Greater Baltimore Medical Center
Lutherville, MD, USA

Nabeel A. Shakir, MD
Department of Urology
University of Texas Southwestern Medical
Center
Dallas, TX, USA

Mark P. Schoenberg, MD
University Professor & Chair
Department of Urology
The Montefiore Medical Center & The
Albert Einstein College of Medicine
Bronx, NY, USA

Yaalini Shanmugabavan, MD
Division of Surgery & Interventional Science
University College Hospital,
London, UK

Stephen B. Solomon, MD
Interventional Radiology Service
Memorial Sloan-Kettering Cancer Center
New York, NY, USA

Arnulf Stenzl, MD
Department of Urology
University Hospital Tuebingen
Tuebingen, Germany

Joshua M. Stern, MD
Department of Urology
Montefiore Medical Center
Albert Einstein College of Medicine
Bronx, NY, USA

Jeffrey J. Tomaszewski, MD
Division of Urology, Department
of Surgery
MD Anderson Cancer Center at
Cooper, Rowan University School
of Medicine
Camden, NJ, USA

Robert G. Uzzo, MD, FACS
Department of Surgical Oncology
Division of Urologic Oncology
Fox Chase Center–Temple University
Health System
Philadelphia, PA, USA

Kara L. Watts, MD
Assistant Professor
Department of Urology
Montefiore Medical Center
Albert Einstein College
 of Medicine
Bronx, NY, USA

Preface

Two forces have conspired to change the landscape of urologic oncology over the past 30 years. The first is the availability of level-one evidence from authoritative clinical trials [1,2]. Data from randomized experiments have called into question basic assumptions about the blanket application of surgical standards of care for major classes of genito-urinary malignancy. The second is the accelerating pace of discovery in cancer biology. The study of cancer is no longer the exclusive province of the molecular biologist; it now encompasses disciplines as diverse as immuno-oncology, metabolomics, and microbiome science. These new disciplines will doubtless impact the already impressive progress that has been made by integrating molecular data into clinical trial design [3]. The more we know, the more there is to know; and the correlation of observations made in these new fields of inquiry with the natural and treated histories of human disease offers tremendous opportunity for future research. Urologic oncologists find themselves, therefore, on the cusp of a change driven by scientific and technological advance, the public's demand for greater transparency in outcomes reporting, and the disclosure of treatment-related risks and harms coupled with society's ever-present inclination to contain the cost of health care.

In recent years it could be argued that those of us practicing urologic oncology for a living have not fully shouldered a responsibility to ourselves and to our patients. Falling victim to what Tversky and Kahneman called "belief in the law of small numbers," we readily succumbed to the lessons of apprentice-like training, surgical anecdote, and perhaps, as perniciously, to a historical, "heroic" vision of surgical judgment that may have placed the surgeon in the center of the picture instead of the patient [4]. Hamlet's famous mother would likely have chuckled to herself had she witnessed the protests following the recent publication of the U.S. Preventive Services Task Force recommendations regarding prostate-specific antigen testing (https://www.uspreventiveservicestaskforce.org/Page/Document/UpdateSummaryFinal/prostate-cancer-screening) [5,6]. This is by no means intended to disparage the motives of surgeons who, with the best of intentions, applied what was known to what they encountered in practice. No *mea culpa* is required. The fault, if any can be found, lies in human nature, which inclines to overestimate benefit, understate risk, and exaggerate the importance of personal experience. This appears to be so even when compelling data to the contrary are available. Witness the small number of patients with muscle-invasive bladder cancer who are offered neoadjuvant chemotherapy before cystectomy [7].

Having acknowledged some degree of skepticism regarding our contemporary standards of care, we sought to better understand the state of what could arguably be called a new branch of urologic oncology: image-guided, tissue-preserving or focal therapy. This new area of inquiry has deep roots in urologic practice that demand brief mention. Students of medical history are familiar with Philipp Bozzini's introduction of the "lichtleiter" instrument, a tool employing a series of mirrors and candle-illumination that paved the way for modern urologic endoscopy at the beginning of the nineteenth century [8]. Transurethral resection of bladder tumors is a time-honored mainstay of practice that is by definition tissue sparing. In the 1980s, Walsh's modification of Millin's radical prostatectomy (1945) was a tissue-sparing innovation that was initially criticized for fear of incomplete cancer resection [9]. The debate regarding partial nephrectomy continues to this day against the backdrop of a much-refined appreciation of the biology of renal cancer [10]. Ironically, the field has been moving conceptually in the direction of focal therapy for decades. The dilemma we face now is determining how to view the contemporary results from studies of this new approach to cancer. As a corollary, how might we improve our understanding of which patients could benefit from the therapies described in this book?

The authors of the individual chapters were charged with answering a single question: what information can you provide to better inform the reader regarding the impact of tumor ablation on cancer care? Scholars from diverse specialties have contributed to this volume and the answers to the question posed vary accordingly. We sought to be inclusive but make no claim regarding comprehensiveness. This book represents a modest contribution to an ongoing conversation about innovation in urologic oncology; and if we have succeeded only a little in serving the reader, this book will raise many more questions than it could possibly answer.

Mark P. Schoenberg, MD
Kara L. Watts, MD
Bronx, NY

February 2017

References

1 Bill-Axelson A, Holmberg L, Ruutu M, Garmo H, Stark JR, Busch C, et al. Radical prostatectomy versus watchful waiting in early prostate cancer. N Engl J Med. 2011;364:1708–17.

2 Grossman HB, Natale RB, Tangen CM, Speights VO, Vogelzang JO, Trump DL, et al. Neoadjuvant chemotherapy plus cystectomy compared with cystectomy alone for locally advanced bladder cancer. N Engl J Med. 2003;349:859–66.

3 Hyman D, Taylor B, Baselga J. Implementing genome-driven oncology. Cell. 2017;168:584–99.

4 Tversky A, Kahneman, D. Belief in the law of small numbers. Psychological Bulletin. 1971;2:105–10.

5 Shakespeare W. *Hamlet* 1600.

6 PSA screening, 2012, at https://www.uspreventiveservicestaskforce.org/Page/ Document/UpdateSummaryFinal/ prostate-cancer-screening.

7 Aragon-Ching JB, Trump DL. Systemic therapy in muscle-invasive and metastatic bladder cancer: Current trends and future promises. Future Oncol. 2016;12:2049–58.

8 Rathert P, Lutzeyer W, Goddwin WE. Philipp Bozzini (1773–1809) and the Lichtleiter. Urology 1974;3:113–8.

9 Walsh PC. Radical prostatectomy, preservation of sexual function, cancer control. The controversy. Urol Clin North Am. 1987;14:663–73.

10 An JY, Ball MW, Gorin MA, Hong JJ, Johnson MH, Pavlovich CP, et al. Partial vs radical nephrectomy for T1-T2 renal masses in the elderly: Comparison of complications, renal function, and oncologic outcomes. Urology. 2017;100:151–7.

1

Cancer Genetics, Cancer Biology, and Tumor Growth and Metastasis: The Interaction of Cancer and Its Host Environment

Mark C. Markowski, MD, PhD, and Kenneth J. Pienta, MD

Department of Medical Oncology, John Hopkins University, Baltimore, MD, USA

Renal Cell Carcinoma

Premalignant Lesions

Unlike prostate cancer, precursor lesions for renal cell carcinoma (RCC) are not well understood. Renal intraepithelial neoplasia (RIN) and dysplastic changes have been described in the literature [1]. Some of these lesions have common genetic alterations with RCC, share spatial orientation, and have a premalignant appearance, which suggests an evolutionary relationship to carcinoma [2]. Given the sparse data and limited characterization, it is likely that this premalignant state is short lived or that the majority of RCCs occurs de novo. This further suggests that the time from genetic insult to overt carcinoma is rapid, emphasizing the need for early surgical intervention for curative intent.

Molecular Pathogenesis

Almost 100 years ago, Von Hippel and Lindau described a familial pattern of vascularized retinal growths, which was later recognized to be part of an autosomal dominant disorder. These patients were predisposed to develop hemangioblastomas, pheochromocytomas, and clear-cell RCC. In 1993, the *VHL* gene was discovered at 3p25.3, a region that is frequently deleted in RCC. Somatic mutations, promoter methylation, or loss of

heterozygosity of *VHL* is found in up to 90% of sporadic RCCs [3,4]. The VHL protein is best known for its role as the substrate recognition component of an E3 ligase and targeting of hypoxia inducible factors (HIF) for ubiquitination and degradation [5]. In hypoxic environments or in the absence/inactivation of VHL protein, the alpha subunit of HIF heterodimerizes with HIFβ and translocates to the nucleus, and transcribes a number of genes including VEGF, PDGF-β, and TGF-α (Figure 1.1) [6]. The unregulated activation of this pathway is a main driver of angiogenesis, invasion, and metastasis in the majority of sporadic RCCs.

Targeting of the VEGF pathway has been mainstay of treatment for metastatic or unresectable RCC. Small molecule tyrosine kinase inhibitors (TKI) have been successful at disrupting VEGF signaling, resulting in improved patient survival in the metastatic setting. VEGF and PDGFβ can stimulate the proliferation and migration of endothelial cells. The establishment of an enriched blood supply can facilitate the establishment of metastatic niches and lead to disseminated disease. As a result of this high metastatic potential, there is no currently approved neoadjuvant systemic approach for RCC using targeted therapies such as sunitinib or pazopanib. The use of these agents is also not approved in the adjuvant setting after

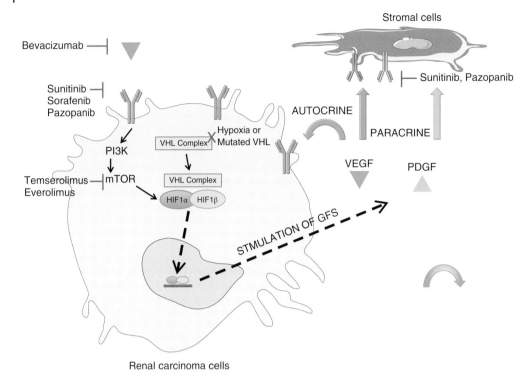

Figure 1.1 Molecular dysregulation of renal cell carcinoma. Under normal hypoxic conditions or in the presence of VHL mutations, HIFα and HIFβ form a heterodimer, translocate to the nucleus and function as a transcription factor. Small molecule tyrosine kinase inhibitors (TKIs), Sunitinib and Pazopanib, or monoclonal antibodies (Bevacizumab) can abrogate VEGF signaling in RCC. TKIs can also attenuate the PI3K/mTOR and MAPK pathways shown. Temsirolimus and everolimus can directly antagonize mTOR signaling, inhibiting growth in certain RCCs. Adapted from Clin Cancer Res. December 15, 2006; 12(24):7215–7220.

nephrectomy. Multiple studies have failed to show a survival benefit of adjuvant TKI use or immunotherapy after definitive surgery underscoring the importance of early intervention with upfront surgery [7].

Loss of chromosome 3p is the most frequent genetic mutation in RCC. In addition to *VHL*, this region also contains the gene, *PBRM1* (3p21). *PBRM1* is a purported "gatekeeper" gene and plays a significant role in DNA repair, replication, and transcription. Somatic mutations have been found in 41% of clear-cell renal carcinomas but may be has high as 50% [8,9]. Loss of the PBRM1 has been correlated with advanced stage, higher-grade disease, and worse patient outcomes [10]. Alterations of chromosome 3p may mark a key genetic event, either inherited or acquired, that drives early tumorigenesis.

Multiple genetic changes have been observed in RCC, including gain of 5q containing *TGFB1* and *CSF1R* and deletion of 14q harboring the tumor suppressor candidate, *NRXN3*.(11) Loss of 14q was associated with higher-grade disease and worse survival [11,12].

mTOR is a serine/threonine kinase that couples with adapter proteins forming two distinct complexes, mTORC1 and mTORC2. mTORC1 activation has been implicated in >50% of RCCs [13]. Interestingly, HIF-1α has been shown to increase the expression of REDD1, a known inhibitor of mTORC1 [14]. Under hypoxic conditions, the stabilization of HIF-1 levels lead to the inhibition of mTOR signaling. This inhibition is dependent on the gene products of *TSC1* (tuberous sclerosis complex 1) and *TSC2* [14].

Mutations in TSC1 and PTEN may abrogate the effect of the HIF-1 signaling axis on mTOR inhibition, resulting in a second and distinct mechanism of carcinogenesis [15].

Everolimus binds to FKBP-12 and inhibits the activity of mTORC1. A Phase III trial that examined the effect of everolimus in patients with metastatic RCC who had progressed on TKI therapy was stopped early when 37% of the total progression events were shown in the everolimus group compared to 65% in the placebo arm [16]. In 2010, the final results of the trial showed a 3-month progression-free survival advantage following treatment with everolimus [17]. Temsirolimus, an intravenous inhibitor of mTORC1, increased overall survival in untreated patients with metastatic RCC and poor prognostic features [18]. Similar to TKI therapy, there is no role for mTOR inhibitors in the treatment of localized RCC.

The discovery of TKIs has revolutionized the treatment of metastatic disease and improved overall survival. Surgery remains the main treatment for localized disease. With the development of next-generation TKIs, targeted therapy may complement a surgical approach for early-stage disease.

Bladder Cancer

Bladder cancer is the fourth-most common neoplasm in males, consisting predominantly of urothelial carcinoma. The pathological stage of the tumor distinguishes between nonmuscle-invasive disease and muscle-invasive disease. Use of "molecular grading" may also aid conventional staging parameters and further define muscle- versus nonmuscle-invasive disease. Common alterations in cell-cycle regulation and growth pathways of bladder cancers are described next.

Cell-Cycle Regulation

Alterations in cell-cycle regulation pathways were found in approximately 90% of all muscle-invasive bladder cancers [19]. In this study, the Cancer Genome Atlas Research Network (CGARN) found that *TP53* mutations were found in 49% of cancers. Other studies have found that mutations in *TP53* were associated with recurrence of nonmuscle-invasive bladder cancer as well as disease progression and poor prognosis [20,21]. There are conflicting data regarding the utility of p53 alteration when used to direct the administration of neoadjuvant therapy [22–24]. Although a common event in carcinogenesis, using p53 alterations as a sole biomarker to dictate treatment is of unclear clinical significance.

Studies have also incorporated other cell-cycle regulators in conjunction with p53 to better risk stratify patients. Garcia del Muro *et al.* examined the relationship of p53 and p21 overexpression to survival [25]. P53 regulates p21 expression, a cyclin-dependent kinase inhibitor, which can arrest cell growth by inhibiting Rb phosphorylation. Patients with T2-T4a, N0 disease received neoadjuvant chemotherapy followed by either radiation or surgery, depending on residual disease status. Patients harboring tumors that overexpressed p53 and p21 had a worse overall survival compared to patients with normal expression levels. A retrospective study showed that patients with pT1 disease treated with radical cystectomy were 24 and 27 times more likely to have disease relapse and cancer-specific death if alterations were found in p53, p27, and Ki-67 expression [26]. The combination of increased p53 and pRB expression with alterations in p21 levels resulted in an 8% five-year survival rate after cystectomy in another study [27].

Other genes and proteins involved in mediating p53 signaling have also been implicated in promoting bladder carcinogenesis. Loss of chromosome 9 is thought to be an early event occurring in more than 50% of all cases [28]. *CDK2NA/ARF* maps to 9p21, a region commonly lost in bladder cancer. This region encodes p16^{ink4A} and p14^{ARF}, respectively [29]. Cycle D1 can complex with CDK4, which results in the phosphorylation of Rb and release of E2F, allowing for progression of the cycle. In the absence of mutation, p16 can form a binary complex with CDK4 antagonizing the effect of cyclin D1 and preventing the cell from progressing into S phase [30]. Frequent deletion of p16^{ink4A} and the resulting loss of p16 in bladder cancer allow the function of Cyclin D1 to go unchecked. Loss of p14 allows MDM2, the E3 ubiquitin ligase, to downregulate p53 protein levels further destabilizing cell-cycle regulation [31]. In one study, homozygous and heterozygous deletions in *CDK2NA/ARF* have been reported to occur in 14% and 12% of bladder cancers, respectively [32]. More recently, recurrent focal deletions in *CDK2NA/ARF* were found in 47% of tumors [19].

FGFR3 and Receptor Tyrosine Kinases

Fibroblast growth factor receptor 3 is part of a family of receptor tyrosine kinases that have been implicated in angiogenesis, apoptosis, and chemotaxis [33]. Inherited mutations in *FGFR3* have been well studied because of resulting achondroplasia and skeletal dysplasia [34]. Acquired mutation of *FGFR3* is a common event in low-grade and nonmuscle-invasive bladders cancers [35,36]. FGFR3 mutation has also been associated with a low recurrence rate in nonmuscle-invasive bladder cancers treated with transurethral resection of bladder tumor (TURBT) and, in conjunction of normal MIB-1 expression, may be a better predictor of outcome than pathological staging [37,38]. The role of *FGFR3* mutation in muscle-invasive disease is less well established.

FGFR3 can activate multiple downstream pathways including the Ras/Raf/MEK/ERK and PI3K/AKT signaling axis (Figure 1.2). *HRAS* has been shown to be frequently mutated in bladder cancer and is known to be activated by FGFR3 through adaptor proteins [39]. Activation of the resulting MAPK pathway may serve as a potential target for therapy. Small molecular inhibitors of FGFR3 have shown promise in preclinical studies [40]. However, mutation in downstream mediators may convey early resistance and

limit therapeutic benefit. Targeting the c-RAF/MEK/ERK pathway could complement FGFR inhibition or be considered as monotherapy with growth inhibition shown in xenograft models [41].

The PI3K/AKT pathway is also known to be active in bladder cancer with activating mutations found in 17% of cases [19]. In this study, AKT was overexpressed in 12% of patients, TSC1 truncated in 6%, and PTEN mutated in 2% of specimens. PI3K and AKT have known small molecular inhibitors currently being used in clinical trials, but no data is available with respect to bladder cancer. mTOR inhibitors, such as everolimus, have shown modest clinical benefit in metastatic transitional cell carcinoma [42].

EGFR, ERBB2 (HER2), ERBB3, and ERBB4 have also been shown to be overexpressed in bladder cancer [43–45]. A Phase II trial showed potential clinical benefit of cituximab in combination with paclitaxel in patients with metastatic urothelial cancer [46]. Lapatinib, a dual kinase inhibitor of EGFR and HER2, did not meet its primary end point for treatment as a single agent for recurrent transitional cell carcinoma [47].

The identification of well-studied signaling pathways that are altered in bladder carcinogenesis is vital to understanding disease development and progression. The role of targeted therapy in the neoadjuvant or adjuvant setting remains unknown. Most clinical trials looking at the effect of small molecular inhibitors in the metastatic setting are currently of unclear benefit. Currently, these altered pathways can be used to better characterize more indolent from aggressive disease within the known categories of muscle-invasive or nonmuscle-invasive disease via a process called *molecular grading* or *staging.*

Molecular Grading

Several groups have identified molecular profiles to help predict recurrence and overall survival. *TP53* mutations have been associated with muscle-invasive disease, whereas

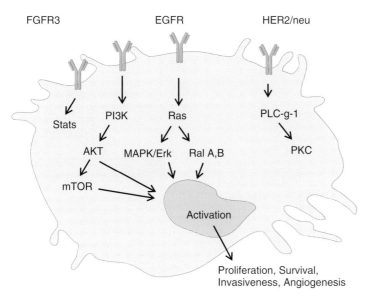

Figure 1.2 Activated signaling pathways in bladder cancer. Mutations and overexpression of FGFR3, EGFR, and HER2 result in activation of downstream pathways shown and drive cell cycle progression, growth, and angiogenesis. PI3K, MAPK, and mTOR inhibitors are clinically available and may attenuate downstream signaling. Adapted from Thomas CY, and Theodorescu D. "Molecular Pathogenesis of Urothelial Carcinoma and the Development of Novel Therapeutic Strategies." In Lee CT, and Wood DP. *Bladder Cancer: Diagnosis, Therapeutics, and Management.* New York, NY: Humana Press, 2010.

FGFR3-activating mutations are thought to result in lower stage/grade tumors (Figure 1.3) [45]. Lindgren *et al.* developed a molecular signature defining two molecular subtypes of tumors within both low/high grade as well as invasive versus noninvasive categories [48]. *TP53/MDM2* alterations were seen in the more aggressive MS2 subtype. The MS1 group was defined by *FGFR3/ PIK3CA* mutated tumors and conveyed a better prognosis across grade and stage. Sjodahl *et al.* defined five molecular subclasses of urothelial cell carcinoma: urobasal A, genomically unstable, urobasal B, SCC-like, and heterogeneous infiltrated [49]. Urobasal A was characterized by high FGFR3 and TP63 expression as well as a normal pattern of cytokeratin expression and conveyed the best prognosis. Genomically unstable tumors had *TP53* mutations, ERBB2 expression, and decreased cytokeratin staining, all of which portended a worse prognosis. Urobasal B shared FGFR3 overexpression and *TP53* mutation with several alterations

in cytokeratin expression to suggest an evolution from urobasal A. Other groups have shown increased expression in lysosomal cysteine proteases, matrix metalloproteinases, and genes involved in angiogenesis in muscle-invasive tumors [50]. Choi *et al.* designated three major clusters for bladder tumors: basal, luminal, and P53-like [51]. The basal phenotype had overall shorter survival and was characterized by p63 activation, squamous cell differentiation as well as the presence of EMT biomarkers. Luminal type showed a similar pattern of expression to luminal breast cancers, including the activation of ER pathways, ERBB2 expression, and activating *FGFR3* mutations, which respond more favorably to therapy. *TP53* mutations were distributed equally among all three classes, but the P53-like group had "normal" expression of P53 regulated genes but still conveyed a resistance to chemotherapy.

These findings lay the groundwork for using "molecular staging" of bladder cancers

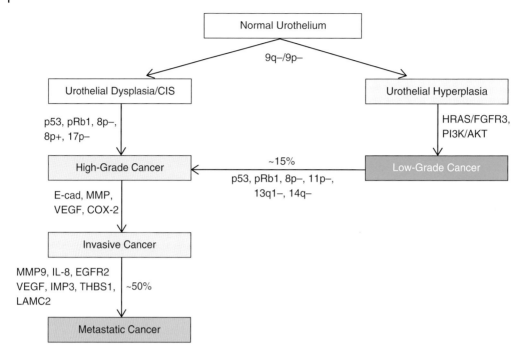

Figure 1.3 Molecular pathogenesis of bladder cancer. Clear patterns of dysregulation are observed in low-grade (LG) urothelial cancer (UCa) versus high-grade (HG) and invasive disease. LG UCa have a high rate of recurrence and can progress to HG UCa in 15% of cases, which may lead to invasive and metastatic disease. Adapted from Nat Rev Urol. 2011 Dec 13;9(1):41–51.

to better define high- and low-risk groups within invasive and noninvasive tumors. This may provide a clearer basis for recommendations regarding surveillance cystoscopies and early intervention in certain nonmuscle-invasive cancers. More research needs to be done to define the "invasiveness" of bladder tumors. Alterations in P53 may lead to a more aggressive phenotype through an unclear mechanism, whereas FGFR3 mutation may facilitate growth without the necessary dysregulation for invasion and eventually metastasis.

Prostate Cancer

Epidemiology

Prostate cancer is the most-common epithelial cancer in males with a lifetime risk of more than 15% for developing the disease. Despite the high incidence of the disease in

the United States, only 4% of prostate cancers are metastatic at the time of diagnosis. The large majority of new cases are confined to the prostate or regional lymph nodes, which confers a favorable prognosis. The SEER database (2003–2009) estimates the 5-year relative survival for newly diagnosed prostate cancer to be above 99%. Based on epidemiology alone, these data suggest that many prostate cancers have an indolent phenotype.

On autopsy, prostate cancer was incidentally found in 34.6% of U.S. Caucasian men older than the age of 50 [52]. Younger men in their 40s (34%) and 30s (27%) also had a considerable likelihood of harboring foci of prostate cancer [53]. The high prevalence of clinically insignificant disease in young individuals underscores the notion that many cases of prostate cancer do not need to be treated. Precancerous lesions such as prostatic intraepithelial neoplasia (PIN) and proliferative inflammatory atrophy (PIA) were also identified in these men. PIN lesions contain proliferating epithelial cells characterized by an enlarged nucleus and prominent nucleoli found within a ductal structure [54]. High-grade PIN (HGPIN) is more common in the aging prostate and contains similar genetic and molecular alterations to that of carcinoma [55]. Although atrophic in appearance, PIA lesions have high levels of Bcl-2, increased Ki-67, and reduced levels of cell-cycle inhibitors [56]. A chronic inflammatory infiltrate is commonly found associated with these lesions and has been implicated in carcinogenesis. PIA is found adjacent to or in close proximity to HGPIN in 46% of samples analyzed in one study, which may suggest an evolutionary relationship between the two [57]. The progression from normal epithelium to precursor lesions and eventual prostate cancer may take years or even decades. In many of these men, their disease will remain subclinical and untreated without consequence. The difficulty for the urology and oncology communities is to identify the aggressive, lethal forms of the disease. Decades of research have been dedicated to studying the tumor biology of precursor lesions, hormone sensitive PCa, castration resistant PCa, and metastatic disease in the hope of identifying those patients who will require treatment.

Molecular Pathogenesis: Inflammation and Genomic and Protein Alterations

Nelson *et al.* studied and characterized the molecular pathogenesis of prostate cancer [58]. Similar to the findings in colon cancer [59], prostate cancer progresses from normal epithelium to carcinoma through a series of common molecular alterations (Figure 1.4). Inherited mutations and early somatic changes have been discovered in genes mediating the body's inflammatory response.

A study of prostate cancer families identified a region of chromosome 1 (1q24-25) involved in cancer susceptibility [60]. Germline mutations in *RNASEL/HPC1* (1q25) cosegrated with prostate cancer within these families. *RNASEL/HPC1* encodes

RNAseI, an interferon regulated endoribonuclease, which degrades both cellular and viral RNA [61]. Casey *et al.* noted that an Arg462Gln variant was implicated in 13% of prostate cancers [62]. Impaired apoptosis has resulted from mutations in RNAsel and is a proposed mechanism for tumorigenesis [63]. Macrophage scavenger receptor 1 (MSR1) has also been implicated in hereditary prostate cancer and has a role in the innate immune response [64]. This gene maps to chromosome 8p22, a region that undergoes loss of heterozygosity in 69% in cases of prostate cancer [65]. A mutation in the receptor may impair the ability of the cell to remove reactive oxygen species leading to increased level of oxidative DNA damage [66]. NKX3.1, located at 8p21, is an androgen-regulated, prostate-specific homeodomain protein essential for normal prostate development and thought to be a key tumor suppressor in prostate carcinogenesis [67,68]. NKX3.1 levels are decreased in proliferative inflammatory atrophy and downregulated in response to inflammatory cytokines [69,70]. Decreased levels of NKX3.1 have been shown to increase growth, decrease apoptosis, and affect DNA repair [71,72]. Moreover, the loss of NKX3.1 correlates with disease progression [73]. *GSTP1* undergoes somatic inactivation via promoter methylation in approximately 90% of prostate cancers [74,75]. This "caretaker" gene encodes a glutathione S-transferase that is responsible for neutralizing electrophilic carcinogens and reactive oxygen species [76]. Loss of GSTπ protein expression was seen in more than 90% of prostate cancer specimens in one study [74]. It is thought that GSTπ has a key role in maintaining genetic integrity. Many of the inherited mutations/deletions as well as acquired somatic changes implicated in prostate carcinogenesis, involve genes regulating inflammation, oxidative DNA damage, and cellular immunity.

The ultimate tumor-sparing approach to prostate cancer would be chemoprevention. The preceding data generated significant interest in antioxidants and nonsteroidal anti-inflammatory drugs (NSAIDs) as potential

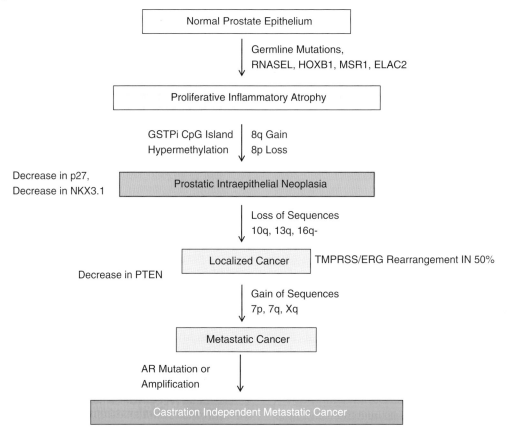

Figure 1.4 Pathogenesis of prostate cancer. Several common genetic insults have been observed throughout the progression of normal epithelium to malignancy. Inherited and somatic mutations are found in key genes regulating the immune response. Loss of the tumor suppressor genes, *NKX3.1* and *PTEN*, are early events in tumorigenesis predisposing the epithelium to malignant change. Loss of response to androgen withdrawal can occur later in disease development. Adapted from N Engl J Med. 2003 Jul 24;349(4):366–81.

agents to reduce cancer incidence. Several meta-analysis studies have not definitively shown any benefit of NSAIDs to protect against prostate cancer [77]. Unfortunately, the side-effect profiles of these drugs preclude their long-term daily use, particularly without compelling evidence of therapeutic benefit. Antioxidants such as selenium and vitamin E are common over-the-counter supplements. The SELECT trial sought to examine the effect of selenium alone, vitamin E alone, or the combination of both on prostate cancer incidence. The initial data, released in 2009, showed no benefit in any of the trial arms [78]. However, after longer follow-up, the arm using vitamin E

alone had a statistically significant increase in the amount of prostate cancer compared with the placebo group [79]. This data was discouraging, particularly given the strong interest in inflammation-induced carcinogenesis. Although it is widely accepted that intraprostatic, chronic inflammation is a risk factor for development of prostate cancer, a novel means to reduce cancer incidence by taking advantage of this mechanism remains unknown.

Amplification of chromosome 8q, which contains the gene, *c-MYC* (8q24), is a known finding in both HGPIN and carcinoma. Increased copy numbers of *c-MYC* and 8q correlate with increasing Gleason score, disease progression, and poor prognosis [80–82]. MYC is a known oncoprotein upregulated in a variety of cancers and regulates cell proliferation, protein synthesis, and metabolism. Both mRNA and protein levels of c-MYC are elevated in prostate cancer as well as PIN, which suggests a key role of the protein in tumorigenesis [83]. Gain of MYC expression in murine models resulted in both PIN and adenocarcinoma formation recapitulating human prostate cancer [84].

Both amplification of 8q24 and c-MYC overexpression has been shown to predict biochemical recurrence after prostatectomy [85]. Fluorescence in situ hybridization (FISH) detection of 8q copy number may be a useful strategy to better risk stratify low-grade tumors. One study using RNA interference showed that MYC might be a downstream target of AR signaling [86]. Additionally, MYC has been shown to be a mediator of ligand-independent AR signaling, suggesting a mechanism for castration resistance [87]. The development of an effective inhibitor of MYC function may have clinical use to treat early hormone refractory prostate cancer. For now, MYC is a useful marker for disease progression and tumor aggressiveness.

PTEN is a known tumor-suppressor gene that encodes a phosphatase, which can target both protein and lipid substrates. By inhibiting the PI3k-Akt pathway, PTEN is thought to have a key role in inhibiting cellular growth. The gene undergoes somatic mutation during prostate cancer progression and reduced protein expression is observed in higher grade and advanced disease [88,89]. In mouse models, *Nkx3.1* loss cooperates with *Pten* loss to form murine PIN and invasive adenocarcinoma of the prostate [90,91]. NKX3.1 can upregulate IGFBP3 leading to decreased AKT phosphorylation and cell growth [72]. In the presence of decreased levels of NKX3.1, loss of PTEN activity may lead to unregulated activity of AKT and downstream targets such as p27. *CDKN1B* encodes p27, a cyclin-dependent kinase inhibitor. Decreased levels of p27 has been

shown to be a negative predictor of survival in organ-confined PCa treated with radical prostatectomy [92]. Inhibition of the androgen receptor has been shown to increase AKT signaling, which suggests a novel mechanism for resistance to androgen resistance [93]. Androgen ablation in conjunction with abrogation of the AKT signaling axis may be a potential therapeutic intervention for high-risk, localized prostate cancer. The Eastern Cooperative Oncology Group (ECOG) is studying the effect of AKT inhibition in combination bicalutamide in patients with biochemical recurrence. The results of this Phase II study are pending.

In 2005, *ERG* was discovered to be overexpressed in prostate cancer specimens [94]. Using cancer outlier profile analysis (COPA), ERG and ETV1, both members of the ETS transcription factor family, were noted to be outliers in prostate cancer [95]. Further analysis showed that both genes were found as fusion products with the 5′ untranslated region of the androgen responsive *TMPRSS2* gene. More than 20 members of the ETS family have been found in gene rearrangements with ERG being the most-common and implicated in approximately 50% of prostate cancers [96]. Interestingly, the TMPRSS2-ERG fusion has not been found in normal prostate epithelium but has been shown in HGPIN [97]. This finding suggests a key role for this fusion product in carcinogenesis. The prognostic significance of the gene fusion is less clear. Although higher levels of ETS transcription factor expression were found in cancers with a lower Gleason score, a population cohort study found an association between the presence of the TMPRSS2:ERG fusion and prostate cancer-specific death in patients managed with watchful waiting [98,99]. In 2012, a cohort of 1,180 men treated with radical prostatectomy found no significant association between TMPRSS2:ERG and biochemical recurrence or mortality [100]. There remains conflicting evidence regarding the prognostic implication of the gene fusion and how best to use this information. However, the presence of the fusion at early stages of disease may aid with more accurate and earlier diagnosis particularly when combined with prostate-specific antigen (PSA) screening [101].

Gene Expression and Molecular-Modeling Concepts

The link between high PSA, Gleason score, and clinical staging with PCA outcomes is well established. Yet within each category, there is a large degree of heterogeneity resulting in uncertainty about which cancers will remain clinically irrelevant or aggressive and fatal. As research techniques have become more sophisticated, a better understanding of the genetic and molecular dysregulation has resulted. The clarification of tumor biology may serve to complement the conventional risk stratification criteria for treatment.

Several studies have examined the gene expression profiles within prostate cancers at different stages of both development and progression. Clarifying the mechanism of how prostate cancers are initiated and eventually evolve may explain how some cancers can be managed with a tissue-sparing approach compared with definitive resection.

Microarray expression profiling became popularized in the late 1990s and early 2000s. This technique allowed researchers to survey the differential expression of a large number of genes. Common molecular changes in prostate cancer were already known including overexpression of c-MYC and loss of p27 and PTEN. Several groups investigated the gene expression profiles of tumor compared to normal prostate tissue [102,103]. These early studies validated the technique and identified a number of genes differentially expressed in malignant tissue. Singh *et al.* compared microdissected tumor cells to normal prostate and sought to identify a high-risk signature that could be correlated with outcome [104]. A 5-gene signature that included, IGFBP3, PDGFRb, and Chromogranin A was predictive of disease-free survival. Traditional markers of aggressiveness, PSA, and Gleason score did not significantly correlate with disease-free survival in this study. In 2003, Best *et al.* analyzed high- and moderate-grade tumors to identify a different 21-gene signature to predict high-grade cancers (Gleason 9-10 vs. 5-7) [105]. This signature was not tested to predict clinical outcome and showed little commonality with prior studies. Biochemical recurrence was also predicted based on microarray analysis, but little overlap was noted in comparison to the Singh data [106].

A consensus pattern defining high-risk disease has remained elusive. It is this heterogeneity that has limited attempts to define a meaningful molecular signature that may be used in the clinical setting to guide therapy. LaPointe *et al.* made the observation that low-grade tumors had a profile closer to normal prostate epithelium, perhaps suggestive of a more differentiated state [106]. Genes involved in cellular invasion and angiogenesis defined higher grade cancers. Because there is not a defining gene "signature" across multiple studies, a potential use of microarray analysis may be to identify themes of molecular changes.

Tomlins *et al.* used "molecular concepts," which are defined as a set of biologically connected genes to characterize prostate carcinogenesis [107]. This approach seeks to identify patterns of dysregulation rather than changes in individual genes. In their study, more than 14,000 molecular concepts were analyzed to define progression signatures from benign epithelium through metastatic disease (Figure 1.5). Interestingly, Tomlins *et al.* found only subtle differences in gene expression between low- and high-grade tumors as in LaPointe *et al.* No clear pattern of differential gene expression was identified. Using molecular concept mapping analysis, the group found a strong enrichment of decreased androgen signaling in high-grade tumors. Genes known to be upregulated in

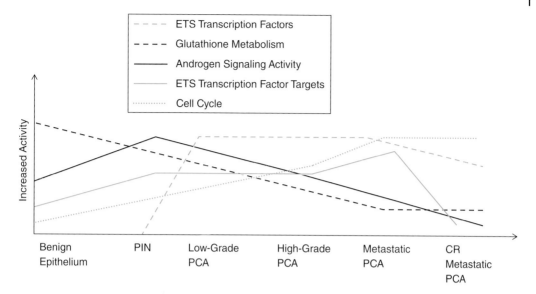

Figure 1.5 Molecular concept mapping of prostate cancer. The relative expression of molecular concepts are mapped according to prostate cancer progression from benign epithelium to hormone naïve (HN) and hormone refractory (HR) metastatic disease. Seven of the highest enriched concepts are shown. Adapted from Nat Genet. 2007 Jan;39(1):41–51.

the presence of androgens had lower levels of expression with more advanced disease. This trend was most significant in metastatic disease and may highlight the selection of cell populations that can survive with low levels of androgen signaling. Also noted throughout disease progression was an increase in ETS target genes, protein biosynthesis, and amplification of MYC, which are known markers of advanced disease.

The studies using microarray and, later, molecular concept mapping, highlight the evolutionary changes in prostate cancer. Teasing out the key regulator genes and proteins that define both low- and high-risk disease has been difficult. What is clear is that prostate cancer remains largely an indolent disease. Several alterations in gene expression, mutation, and copy number are required to progress from normal epithelium to prostate cancer, which can take decades to occur.

As shown in Tomlins *et al.* decreases in androgen signaling may be a hallmark of higher risk disease and eventually metastasis. The dedifferentiation that defines higher Gleason scores may reflect the ability of the tumor to progress with less reliance on the androgen signaling axis. Perhaps, the efficiency of the tumor to use alternative pathways for survival may be a key determinant for further disease progression. Such an example may involve MYC, which also becomes amplified in progression of disease as well as correlating with higher Gleason score. Moreover, the transformation to androgen independence may be reflective of changes in sugar metabolism or the ability to metabolize sex hormones [108]. As tumors become less responsive to hormonal therapies, new targeted therapies are needed to further prolong survival and delay chemotherapy. Molecular concept mapping has identified novel pathways that may be key to further understanding androgen independence and lead to clinically relevant interventions.

References

1 Van Poppel H, Nilsson S, Algaba F, Bergerheim U, Dal Cin P, Fleming S, *et al.* Precancerous lesions in the kidney. Scand J Urol Nephrol Suppl. 2000 (205):136–65.

2 Kirkali Z, Yorukoglu K. Premalignant lesions in the kidney. ScientificWorldJournal. 2001 Dec 7;1:855–67.

3 Gossage L, Eisen T. Alterations in VHL as potential biomarkers in renal-cell carcinoma. Nat Rev Clin Oncol. 2010 May; 7(5):277–88.

4 Nordstrom-O'Brien M, van der Luijt RB, van Rooijen E, van den Ouweland AM, Majoor-Krakauer DF, Lolkema MP, *et al.* Genetic analysis of von Hippel-Lindau disease. Hum Mutat. 2010 May; 31(5):521–37.

5 Kaelin WG, Jr. The von Hippel-Lindau tumour suppressor protein: O2 sensing and cancer. Nat Rev Caner. 2008 Nov; 8(11):865–73.

6 Audenet F, Yates DR, Cancel-Tassin G, Cussenot O, Roupret M. Genetic pathways involved in carcinogenesis of clear cell renal cell carcinoma: Genomics towards personalized medicine. BJU Int. 2012 Jun; 109(12):1864–70.

7 Smaldone MC, Fung C, Uzzo RG, Haas NB. Adjuvant and neoadjuvant therapies in high-risk renal cell carcinoma. Hematol Oncol Clin North Am. 2011 Aug; 25(4):765–91.

8 Duns G, Hofstra RM, Sietzema JG, Hollema H, van Duivenbode I, Kuik A, *et al.* Targeted exome sequencing in clear cell renal cell carcinoma tumors suggests aberrant chromatin regulation as a crucial step in ccRCC development. Hum Mutat. 2012 Jul;33(7):1059–62.

9 Varela I, Tarpey P, Raine K, Huang D, Ong CK, Stephens P, *et al.* Exome sequencing identifies frequent mutation of the SWI/SNF complex gene PBRM1 in renal carcinoma. Nature. 2011 Jan 27;469(7331):539–42.

10 Pawlowski R, Muhl SM, Sulser T, Krek W, Moch H, Schraml P. Loss of PBRM1 expression is associated with renal cell carcinoma progression. Int J Cancer. 2013 Jan 15;132(2):E11–7.

11 Rydzanicz M, Wrzesinski T, Bluyssen HA, Wesoly J. Genomics and epigenomics of clear cell renal cell carcinoma: Recent developments and potential applications. Cancer Lett. 2013 Dec 1;341(2):111–26.

12 Yoshimoto T, Matsuura K, Karnan S, Tagawa H, Nakada C, Tanigawa M, *et al.* High-resolution analysis of DNA copy number alterations and gene expression in renal clear cell carcinoma. J Pathol. 2007 Dec;213(4):392–401.

13 Robb VA, Karbowniczek M, Klein-Szanto AJ, Henske EP. Activation of the mTOR signaling pathway in renal clear cell carcinoma. J Urol. 2007 Jan;177(1):346–52.

14 Brugarolas J, Lei K, Hurley RL, Manning BD, Reiling JH, Hafen E, *et al.* Regulation of mTOR function in response to hypoxia by REDD1 and the TSC1/TSC2 tumor suppressor complex. Genes Dev. 2004 Dec 1;18(23):2893–904.

15 Kucejova B, Pena-Llopis S, Yamasaki T, Sivanand S, Tran TA, Alexander S, *et al.* Interplay between pVHL and mTORC1 pathways in clear-cell renal cell carcinoma. Mole Cancer Res. 2011 Sep;9(9):1255–65.

16 Motzer RJ, Escudier B, Oudard S, Hutson TE, Porta C, Bracarda S, *et al.* Efficacy of everolimus in advanced renal cell carcinoma: A double-blind, randomised, placebo-controlled phase III trial. Lancet. 2008 Aug 9;372(9637):449–56.

17 Motzer RJ, Escudier B, Oudard S, Hutson TE, Porta C, Bracarda S, *et al.* Phase 3 trial of everolimus for metastatic renal cell carcinoma: Final results and analysis of prognostic factors. Cancer. 2010 Sep 15; 116(18):4256–65.

18 Hudes G, Carducci M, Tomczak P, Dutcher J, Figlin R, Kapoor A, *et al.* Temsirolimus, interferon alfa, or both for advanced renal-cell carcinoma. N Engl J Med. 2007 May 31;356(22):2271–81.

19 Cancer Genome Atlas Research Network. Comprehensive molecular characterization

of urothelial bladder carcinoma. Nature. 2014 Mar 20;507(7492):315–22.

20 Sarkis A, Zhang Z, Cordoncardo C, Melamed J, Dalbagni G, Sheinfeld J, *et al.* P53 nuclear overexpression and disease progression in ta-bladder carcinoma. Int J Oncol. 1993 Aug;3(2):355–60.

21 Sarkis AS, Dalbagni G, Cordon-Cardo C, Zhang ZF, Sheinfeld J, Fair WR, *et al.* Nuclear overexpression of p53 protein in transitional cell bladder carcinoma: A marker for disease progression. J Natl Cancer Inst. 1993 Jan 6;85(1):53–59.

22 Siu LL, Banerjee D, Khurana RJ, Pan X, Pflueger R, Tannock IF, *et al.* The prognostic role of p53, metallothionein, P-glycoprotein, and MIB-1 in muscle-invasive urothelial transitional cell carcinoma. Clin Cancer Res. 1998 Mar; 4(3):559–65.

23 Kakehi Y, Ozdemir E, Habuchi T, Yamabe H, Hashimura T, Katsura Y, *et al.* Absence of p53 overexpression and favorable response to cisplatin-based neoadjuvant chemotherapy in urothelial carcinomas. Jpn J Cancer Res. 1998 Feb;89(2):214–20.

24 Stadler WM, Lerner SP, Groshen S, Stein JP, Shi SR, Raghavan D, *et al.* Phase III study of molecularly targeted adjuvant therapy in locally advanced urothelial cancer of the bladder based on p53 status. J Clin Oncol. 2011 Sep 1;29(25):3443–9.

25 Garcia del Muro X, Condom E, Vigues F, Castellsague X, Figueras A, Munoz J, *et al.* p53 and p21 Expression levels predict organ preservation and survival in invasive bladder carcinoma treated with a combined-modality approach. Cancer. 2004 May 1;100(9):1859–67.

26 Shariat SF, Bolenz C, Godoy G, Fradet Y, Ashfaq R, Karakiewicz PI, *et al.* Predictive value of combined immunohistochemical markers in patients with pT1 urothelial carcinoma at radical cystectomy. J Urol. 2009 Jul;182(1):78–84.

27 Chatterjee SJ, Datar R, Youssefzadeh D, George B, Goebell PJ, Stein JP, *et al.* Combined effects of p53, p21, and pRb expression in the progression of bladder

transitional cell carcinoma. J Clin Oncol. 2004 Mar 15;22(6):1007–13.

28 Tsai YC, Nichols PW, Hiti AL, Williams Z, Skinner DG, Jones PA. Allelic losses of chromosomes 9, 11, and 17 in human bladder cancer. Cancer Res. 1990 Jan 1;50(1):44–7.

29 Devlin J, Keen AJ, Knowles MA. Homozygous deletion mapping at 9p21 in bladder carcinoma defines a critical region within 2cM of IFNA. Oncogene. 1994 Sep; 9(9):2757–60.

30 Liggett WH, Jr., Sidransky D. Role of the p16 tumor suppressor gene in cancer. J Clin Oncol. 1998 Mar;16(3):1197–206.

31 Alarcon-Vargas D, Ronai Z. p53-Mdm2—the affair that never ends. Carcinogenesis. 2002 Apr;23(4):541–7.

32 Berggren P, Kumar R, Sakano S, Hemminki L, Wada T, Steineck G, *et al.* Detecting homozygous deletions in the CDKN2A(p16(INK4a))/ARF(p14(ARF)) gene in urinary bladder cancer using real-time quantitative PCR. Clin Cancer Res. 2003 Jan;9(1):235–42.

33 Basilico C, Moscatelli D. The FGF family of growth factors and oncogenes. Adv Cancer Res. 1992;59:115–65.

34 Vajo Z, Francomano CA, Wilkin DJ. The molecular and genetic basis of fibroblast growth factor receptor 3 disorders: The achondroplasia family of skeletal dysplasias, Muenke craniosynostosis, and Crouzon syndrome with acanthosis nigricans. Endocr Rev. 2000 Feb;21(1):23–39.

35 Billerey C, Chopin D, Aubriot-Lorton MH, Ricol D, Gil Diez de Medina S, Van Rhijn B, *et al.* Frequent FGFR3 mutations in papillary non-invasive bladder (pTa) tumors. Am J Pathol. 2001 Jun; 158(6):1955–9.

36 Sibley K, Cuthbert-Heavens D, Knowles MA. Loss of heterozygosity at 4p16.3 and mutation of FGFR3 in transitional cell carcinoma. Oncogene. 2001 Feb 8; 20(6):686–91.

37 van Rhijn BW, Vis AN, van der Kwast TH, Kirkels WJ, Radvanyi F, Ooms EC, *et al.* Molecular grading of urothelial cell carcinoma with fibroblast growth factor

receptor 3 and MIB-1 is superior to pathologic grade for the prediction of clinical outcome. J Clin Oncol. 2003 May 15;21(10):1912–21.

38 van Rhijn BW, Lurkin I, Radvanyi F, Kirkels WJ, van der Kwast TH, Zwarthoff EC. The fibroblast growth factor receptor 3 (FGFR3) mutation is a strong indicator of superficial bladder cancer with low recurrence rate. Cancer Res. 2001 Feb 15; 61(4):1265–8.

39 Czerniak B, Cohen GL, Etkind P, Deitch D, Simmons H, Herz F, *et al.* Concurrent mutations of coding and regulatory sequences of the Ha-ras gene in urinary bladder carcinomas. Hum Pathol. 1992 Nov;23(11):1199–204.

40 Lamont FR, Tomlinson DC, Cooper PA, Shnyder SD, Chester JD, Knowles MA. Small molecule FGF receptor inhibitors block FGFR-dependent urothelial carcinoma growth in vitro and in vivo. Br J Cancer. 2011 Jan 4;104(1):75–82.

41 Cirone P, Andresen CJ, Eswaraka JR, Lappin PB, Bagi CM. Patient-derived xenografts reveal limits to PI3K/mTOR- and MEK-mediated inhibition of bladder cancer. Cancer Chemother Pharmacol. 2014 Mar;73(3):525–38.

42 Seront E, Rottey S, Sautois B, Kerger J, D'Hondt LA, Verschaeve V, *et al.* Phase II study of everolimus in patients with locally advanced or metastatic transitional cell carcinoma of the urothelial tract: Clinical activity, molecular response, and biomarkers. Ann Oncol. 2012 Oct; 23(10):2663–70.

43 Coogan CL, Estrada CR, Kapur S, Bloom KJ. HER-2/neu protein overexpression and gene amplification in human transitional cell carcinoma of the bladder. Urology. 2004 Apr;63(4):786–90.

44 Wagner U, Sauter G, Moch H, Novotna H, Epper R, Mihatsch MJ, *et al.* Patterns of p53, erbB-2, and EGF-r expression in premalignant lesions of the urinary bladder. Hum Pathol. 1995 Sep; 26(9):970–8.

45 Wu XR. Urothelial tumorigenesis: A tale of divergent pathways. Nat Rev Cancer. 2005 Sep;5(9):713–25.

46 Wong YN, Litwin S, Vaughn D, Cohen S, Plimack ER, Lee J, *et al.* Phase II trial of cetuximab with or without paclitaxel in patients with advanced urothelial tract carcinoma. J Clin Oncol. 2012 Oct 1; 30(28):3545–51.

47 Wulfing C, Machiels JP, Richel DJ, Grimm MO, Treiber U, De Groot MR, *et al.* A single-arm, multicenter, open-label phase 2 study of lapatinib as the second-line treatment of patients with locally advanced or metastatic transitional cell carcinoma. Cancer. 2009 Jul 1;115(13):2881–90.

48 Lindgren D, Frigyesi A, Gudjonsson S, Sjodahl G, Hallden C, Chebil G, *et al.* Combined gene expression and genomic profiling define two intrinsic molecular subtypes of urothelial carcinoma and gene signatures for molecular grading and outcome. Cancer Res. 2010 May 1; 70(9):3463–72.

49 Sjodahl G, Lauss M, Lovgren K, Chebil G, Gudjonsson S, Veerla S, *et al.* A molecular taxonomy for urothelial carcinoma. Clin Cancer Res. 2012 Jun 15;18(12):3377–86.

50 Blaveri E, Simko JP, Korkola JE, Brewer JL, Baehner F, Mehta K, *et al.* Bladder cancer outcome and subtype classification by gene expression. Clin Cancer Res. 2005 Jun 1;11(11):4044–55.

51 Choi W, Porten S, Kim S, Willis D, Plimack ER, Hoffman-Censits J, *et al.* Identification of distinct basal and luminal subtypes of muscle-invasive bladder cancer with different sensitivities to frontline chemotherapy. Cancer Ce... 2014 Feb 10; 25(2):152–65.

52 Yatani R, Chigusa I, Akazaki K, Stemmermann GN, Welsh RA, Correa P. Geographic pathology of latent prostatic carcinoma. Int J Cancer. 1982 Jun 15; 29(6):611–6.

53 Sakr WA, Haas GP, Cassin BF, Pontes JE, Crissman JD. The frequency of carcinoma and intraepithelial neoplasia of the prostate

in young male patients. J Urol. 1993
Aug;150(2 Pt 1):379–85.

54 Bostwick DG, Brawer MK. Prostatic
intra-epithelial neoplasia and early invasion
in prostate cancer. Cancer. 1987 Feb
15;59(4):788–94.

55 Brawer MK. Prostatic intraepithelial
neoplasia: An overview. Rev Urol. 2005;
7 Suppl 3:S11–8.

56 De Marzo AM, Marchi VL, Epstein JI,
Nelson WG. Proliferative inflammatory
atrophy of the prostate: Implications for
prostatic carcinogenesis. Am J Pathol. 1999
Dec;155(6):1985–92.

57 Putzi MJ, De Marzo AM. Morphologic
transitions between proliferative
inflammatory atrophy and high-grade
prostatic intraepithelial neoplasia. Urology.
2000 Nov 1;56(5):828–32.

58 Nelson WG, De Marzo AM, Isaacs WB.
Prostate cancer. New Engl J Med.
2003 Jul 24;349(4):366–81.

59 Fearon ER, Hamilton SR, Vogelstein B.
Clonal analysis of human colorectal
tumors. Science. 1987 Oct 9;
238(4824):193–7.

60 Smith JR, Freije D, Carpten JD,
Gronberg H, Xu J, Isaacs SD, *et al.*
Major susceptibility locus for prostate
cancer on chromosome 1 suggested by
a genome-wide search. Science.
1996 Nov 22;274(5291):1371–4.

61 Castelli JC, Hassel BA, Maran A, Paranjape J,
Hewitt JA, Li XL, *et al.* The role of 2'-5'
oligoadenylate-activated ribonuclease L in
apoptosis. Cell Death Differ. 1998 Apr;
5(4):313–20.

62 Casey G, Neville PJ, Plummer SJ, Xiang Y,
Krumroy LM, Klein EA, *et al.* RNASEL
Arg462Gln variant is implicated in up to
13% of prostate cancer cases. Nat Genet.
2002 Dec;32(4):581–3.

63 Xiang Y, Wang Z, Murakami J, Plummer S,
Klein EA, Carpten JD, *et al.* Effects of
RNase L mutations associated with
prostate cancer on apoptosis induced by
2',5'-oligoadenylates. Cancer Res.
2003 Oct 15;63(20):6795–801.

64 Platt N, Gordon S. Is the class A
macrophage scavenger receptor (SR-A)
multifunctional? The mouse's tale. J Clin
Invest. 2001 Sep;108(5):649–54.

65 Bova GS, Carter BS, Bussemakers MJ,
Emi M, Fujiwara Y, Kyprianou N, *et al.*
Homozygous deletion and frequent allelic
loss of chromosome 8p22 loci in human
prostate cancer. Cancer Res. 1993 Sep 1;
53(17):3869–73.

66 Xu J, Zheng SL, Komiya A, Mychaleckyj JC,
Isaacs SD, Hu JJ, *et al.* Germline mutations
and sequence variants of the macrophage
scavenger receptor 1 gene are associated
with prostate cancer risk. Nature Genet.
2002 Oct;32(2):321–5.

67 Bhatia-Gaur R, Donjacour AA, Sciavolino
PJ, Kim M, Desai N, Young P, *et al.* Roles
for Nkx3.1 in prostate development and
cancer. Genes Dev. 1999 Apr 15;
13(8):966–77.

68 He WW, Sciavolino PJ, Wing J, Augustus
M, Hudson P, Meissner PS, *et al.* A novel
human prostate-specific, androgen-
regulated homeobox gene (NKX3.1) that
maps to 8p21, a region frequently deleted
in prostate cancer. Genomics. 1997 Jul 1;
43(1):69–77.

69 Bethel CR, Faith D, Li X, Guan B, Hicks JL,
Lan F, *et al.* Decreased NKX3.1 protein
expression in focal prostatic atrophy,
prostatic intraepithelial neoplasia, and
adenocarcinoma: Association with gleason
score and chromosome 8p deletion. Cancer
Res. 2006 Nov 15;66(22):10683–90.

70 Markowski MC, Bowen C, Gelmann EP.
Inflammatory cytokines induce
phosphorylation and ubiquitination of
prostate suppressor protein NKX3.1.
Cancer Res. 2008 Sep 1;68(17):6896–901.

71 Bowen C, Gelmann EP. NKX3.1 activates
cellular response to DNA damage. Cancer
Res. 2010 Apr 15;70(8):3089–97.

72 Muhlbradt E, Asatiani E, Ortner E,
Wang A, Gelmann EP. NKX3.1 activates
expression of insulin-like growth factor
binding protein-3 to mediate insulin-like
growth factor-I signaling and cell

proliferation. Cancer Res. 2009 Mar 15; 69(6):2615–22.

73 Bowen C, Bubendorf L, Voeller HJ, Slack R, Willi N, Sauter G, *et al.* Loss of NKX3.1 expression in human prostate cancers correlates with tumor progression. Cancer Res. 2000 Nov 1;60(21):6111–5.

74 Lee WH, Morton RA, Epstein JI, Brooks JD, Campbell PA, Bova GS, *et al.* Cytidine methylation of regulatory sequences near the pi-class glutathione S-transferase gene accompanies human prostatic carcinogenesis. Proc Natl Acad Sci USA. 1994 Nov 22;91(24):11733–7.

75 Nakayama M, Gonzalgo ML, Yegnasubramanian S, Lin X, De Marzo AM, Nelson WG. GSTP1 CpG island hypermethylation as a molecular biomarker for prostate cancer. J Cell Biochem. 2004 Feb 15;91(3):540–52.

76 Armstrong RN. Structure, catalytic mechanism, and evolution of the glutathione transferases. Chem Res Toxicol. 1997 Jan;10(1):2–18.

77 Stock D, Groome PA, Siemens DR. Inflammation and prostate cancer: A future target for prevention and therapy? Urol Clin North Am. 2008 Feb;35(1): 117–30; vii.

78 Lippman SM, Klein EA, Goodman PJ, Lucia MS, Thompson IM, Ford LG, *et al.* Effect of selenium and vitamin E on risk of prostate cancer and other cancers: The Selenium and Vitamin E Cancer Prevention Trial (SELECT). JAMA. 2009 Jan 7;301(1):39–51.

79 Klein EA, Thompson IM, Jr., Tangen CM, Crowley JJ, Lucia MS, Goodman PJ, *et al.* Vitamin E and the risk of prostate cancer: The Selenium and Vitamin E Cancer Prevention Trial (SELECT). JAMA. 2011 Oct 12;306(14):1549–56.

80 Sato K, Qian J, Slezak JM, Lieber MM, Bostwick DG, Bergstralh EJ, *et al.* Clinical significance of alterations of chromosome 8 in high-grade, advanced, nonmetastatic prostate carcinoma. J Natl Cancer Inst. 1999 Sep 15; 91(18):1574–80.

81 Ribeiro FR, Henrique R, Martins AT, Jeronimo C, Teixeira MR. Relative copy number gain of MYC in diagnostic needle biopsies is an independent prognostic factor for prostate cancer patients. Eur Urol. 2007 Jul;52(1):116–25.

82 Jenkins RB, Qian J, Lieber MM, Bostwick DG. Detection of c-myc oncogene amplification and chromosomal anomalies in metastatic prostatic carcinoma by fluorescence in situ hybridization. Cancer Res. 1997 Feb 1; 57(3):524–31.

83 Gurel B, Iwata T, Koh CM, Jenkins RB, Lan F, Van Dang C, *et al.* Nuclear MYC protein overexpression is an early alteration in human prostate carcinogenesis. Mod Pathol. 2008 Sep;21(9):1156–67.

84 Ellwood-Yen K, Graeber TG, Wongvipat J, Iruela-Arispe ML, Zhang J, Matusik R, *et al.* Myc-driven murine prostate cancer shares molecular features with human prostate tumors. Cancer Cell. 2003 Sep; 4(3):223–38.

85 Fromont G, Godet J, Peyret A, Irani J, Celhay O, Rozet F, *et al.* 8q24 amplification is associated with Myc expression and prostate cancer progression and is an independent predictor of recurrence after radical prostatectomy. Hum Pathol. 2013 Aug;44(8):1617–23.

86 Bernard D, Pourtier-Manzanedo A, Gil J, Beach DH. Myc confers androgen-independent prostate cancer cell growth. J Clin Invest. 2003 Dec;112(11):1724–31.

87 Gao L, Schwartzman J, Gibbs A, Lisac R, Kleinschmidt R, Wilmot B, *et al.* Androgen receptor promotes ligand-independent prostate cancer progression through c-Myc upregulation. PLoS One. 2013;8(5):e63563.

88 Cairns P, Okami K, Halachmi S, Halachmi N, Esteller M, Herman JG, *et al.* Frequent inactivation of PTEN/MMAC1 in primary prostate cancer. Cancer Re. 1997 Nov 15; 57(22):4997–5000.

89 McMenamin ME, Soung P, Perera S, Kaplan I, Loda M, Sellers WR. Loss of PTEN expression in paraffin-embedded primary prostate cancer correlates with

high Gleason score and advanced stage. Cancer Res. 1999 Sep 1;59(17):4291–6.

90 Kim MJ, Cardiff RD, Desai N, Banach-Petrosky WA, Parsons R, Shen MM, *et al.* Cooperativity of Nkx3.1 and Pten loss of function in a mouse model of prostate carcinogenesis. Proc Natl Acad Scie USA. 2002 Mar 5;99(5):2884–9.

91 Abate-Shen C, Banach-Petrosky WA, Sun X, Economides KD, Desai N, Gregg JP, *et al.* Nkx3.1; Pten mutant mice develop invasive prostate adenocarcinoma and lymph node metastases. Cancer Res. 2003 Jul 15; 63(14):3886–90.

92 Yang RM, Naitoh J, Murphy M, Wang HJ, Phillipson J, deKernion JB, *et al.* Low p27 expression predicts poor disease-free survival in patients with prostate cancer. J Urol. 1998 Mar;159(3):941–5.

93 Cohen MB, Rokhlin OW. Mechanisms of prostate cancer cell survival after inhibition of AR expression. J Cell Biochem. 2009 Feb 15;106(3):363–71.

94 Petrovics G, Liu A, Shaheduzzaman S, Furusato B, Sun C, Chen Y, *et al.* Frequent overexpression of ETS-related gene-1 (ERG1) in prostate cancer transcriptome. Oncogene. 2005 May 26;24(23):3847–52.

95 Tomlins SA, Rhodes DR, Perner S, Dhanasekaran SM, Mehra R, Sun XW, *et al.* Recurrent fusion of TMPRSS2 and ETS transcription factor genes in prostate cancer. Science. 2005 Oct 28; 310(5748):644–8.

96 Soller MJ, Isaksson M, Elfving P, Soller W, Lundgren R, Panagopoulos I. Confirmation of the high frequency of the TMPRSS2/ERG fusion gene in prostate cancer. Genes, Chromosomes Cancer. 2006 Jul; 45(7):717–9.

97 Mosquera JM, Perner S, Genega EM, Sanda M, Hofer MD, Mertz KD, *et al.* Characterization of TMPRSS2-ERG fusion high-grade prostatic intraepithelial neoplasia and potential clinical implications. Clin Cancer Res. 2008 Jun 1; 14(11):3380–5.

98 Ghadersohi A, Sharma S, Zhang S, Azrak RG, Wilding GE, Manjili MH, *et al.* Prostate-derived Ets transcription factor (PDEF) is a potential prognostic marker in patients with prostate cancer. Prostate. 2011 Aug 1;71(11):1178–88.

99 Demichelis F, Fall K, Perner S, Andren O, Schmidt F, Setlur SR, *et al.* TMPRSS2:ERG gene fusion associated with lethal prostate cancer in a watchful waiting cohort. Oncogene. 2007 Jul 5; 26(31):4596–9.

100 Pettersson A, Graff RE, Bauer SR, Pitt MJ, Lis RT, Stack EC, *et al.* The TMPRSS2:ERG rearrangement, ERG expression, and prostate cancer outcomes: A cohort study and meta-analysis. Cancer Epidemiol, Biomarkers Prev. 2012 Sep;21(9):1497–509.

101 Tomlins SA, Aubin SM, Siddiqui J, Lonigro RJ, Sefton-Miller L, Miick S, *et al.* Urine TMPRSS2:ERG fusion transcript stratifies prostate cancer risk in men with elevated serum PSA. Sci Transl Med. 2011 Aug 3;3(94):94ra72.

102 Chetcuti A, Margan S, Mann S, Russell P, Handelsman D, Rogers J, *et al.* Identification of differentially expressed genes in organ-confined prostate cancer by gene expression array. Prostate. 2001 May 1;47(2):132–40.

103 Dhanasekaran SM, Barrette TR, Ghosh D, Shah R, Varambally S, Kurachi K, *et al.* Delineation of prognostic biomarkers in prostate cancer. Nature. 2001 Aug 23; 412(6849):822–6.

104 Singh D, Febbo PG, Ross K, Jackson DG, Manola J, Ladd C, *et al.* Gene expression correlates of clinical prostate cancer behavior. Cancer Cell. 2002 Mar; 1(2):203–9.

105 Best CJ, Leiva IM, Chuaqui RF, Gillespie JW, Duray PH, Murgai M, *et al.* Molecular differentiation of high- and moderate-grade human prostate cancer by cDNA microarray analysis. Diagn Mol Pathol. 2003 Jun;12(2):63–70.

106 Lapointe J, Li C, Higgins JP, van de Rijn M, Bair E, Montgomery K, *et al.* Gene expression profiling identifies clinically relevant subtypes of prostate cancer. Proc

Natl Acad Sci USA. 2004 Jan 20;101(3): 811–6.

107 Tomlins SA, Mehra R, Rhodes DR, Cao X, Wang L, Dhanasekaran SM, *et al.* Integrative molecular concept modeling of prostate cancer progression. Nat Genet. 2007 Jan;39(1):41–51.

108 Kaushik AK, Vareed SK, Basu S, Putluri V, Putluri N, Panzitt K, *et al.* Metabolomic profiling identifies biochemical pathways associated with castration-resistant prostate cancer. J Proteome Res. 2013 Dec 31.

2

Pathological Basis of Tumor Characterization: Cytopathology, Surgical Pathology, and How Histo-Morphology Informs Treatment Decision Making

Oleksandr N. Kryvenko, MD,[1] and Fadi Brimo, MD, FRPC (C)[2]

[1] Department of Pathology, University of Miami Miller School of Medicine, Miami, FL, USA
[2] Department of Pathology, McGill University Health Center, Montreal General Hospital site, Montreal, Quebec, Canada

The Prostate

Although often simply referred to as *prostate cancer*, malignant tumors of the prostate represent a wide spectrum of morphological features with a clinical behavior ranging from generally indolent to metastatic and fatal. The most common and widely studied type generally referred to as prostate cancer is acinar adenocarcinoma, which is treated based on preoperative clinico-pathological parameters, the most important being biopsy Gleason score (GS), number of positive cores and extent of core involvement, serum prostate-specific antigen (PSA) levels, age, and comorbidity. With accumulated experience, it has become clear that the main challenge in treating prostate cancer is to avoid overtreatment of insignificant cancer (organ-confined disease with GS ≤6 and tumor volume <0.5 cm^3), while being able to identify cases that warrant definitive therapy [1]. Selecting patients for active surveillance or active intervention of some type requires a full understanding of the Gleason grading system and its implications with regard to tumor multifocality.

In the last 10 years, the Gleason grading system has undergone significant changes related to defining new histological variants and refinement of the morphological criteria of different Gleason grades [2]. Using the contemporary system, cribriform glands are not accepted as pattern 3, and ill-defined nonfused glands are considered pattern 4 (Figure 2.1a,b). This has resulted in upward shift of Gleason grading, making a cancer with Gleason score of 6 a pure homogeneous group with a uniformly excellent prognosis. A recent study analyzing more than 14,000 prostatectomies from four institutions demonstrated that none of the cases with a final GS of 6 had positive lymph nodes, while the presence of pattern 4, even as a tertiary pattern, was associated with the presence of lymph nodes metastases [3].

Gleason grading is generally applied to the acinar variant of adenocarcinoma with some of its subtypes tightly linked to corresponding grades such as the signet cell ring-like variant, which is equivalent to grade 5. In comparison, some variants have a variable behavior and are assigned a grade solely based on the underlying architecture. As an example, the mucinous carcinoma is graded as 3 or 4 depending on underlying architecture (Figure 2.1c), whereas pseudo-hyperplastic and atrophic variants are more commonly assigned grade 3. Similarly, the presence of extensive intracytoplasmic vacuoles (Figure 2.1d) or Paneth-cell like changes should be disregarded when assigning a grade because they may be misinterpreted as patterns 4 or 5, which is not consistently

Management of Urologic Cancer: Focal Therapy and Tissue Preservation, First Edition.
Edited by Mark P. Schoenberg and Kara L. Watts.
© 2017 John Wiley & Sons Ltd. Published 2017 by John Wiley & Sons Ltd.

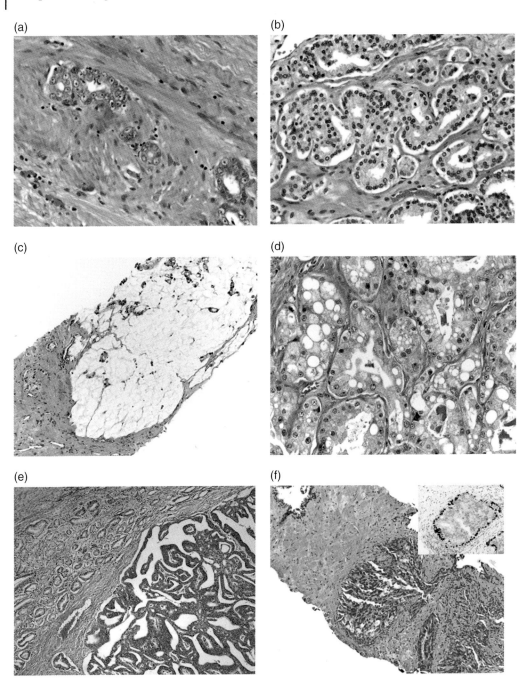

Figure 2.1 (a) Individual well-formed glands of Gleason pattern 3. (b) Fused glands of Gleason pattern 4. (c) Mucinous prostatic adenocarcinoma in prostate biopsy. Separate malignant glands in mucin pool should be graded as Gleason score 3 + 3 = 6. (d) Gleason score 3 + 3 = 6 prostatic adenocarcinoma with multiple intracytoplasmic vacuoles which should be not included in grading. (e) Prostatic duct adenocarcinoma (right-hand side) and acinar prostatic carcinoma (left-hand side) in the same specimen. (f) Intraductal spread of prostatic carcinoma in biopsy specimen. Presence of basal cells demonstrated by p63 immunostain (*inset*).

reflective of their biologic behavior. Nonacinar variants such as prostatic duct adenocarcinoma (Figure 2.1e) and small cell carcinoma are not assigned a grade but are clinically equivalent to patterns 4 and 5, respectively. Intraductal carcinoma (Figure 2.1f) is the perfect illustration of a noninvasive lesion that should be recognized by pathologists and urologists because it indicates the presence of an associated higher-grade cancer even when not sampled by the biopsy (GS ≥7).

In 1994, Epstein *et al.* suggested criteria for appropriately selecting patients for inclusion in active surveillance protocols; nonpalpable disease (T1c), biopsy GS ≤6, involvement of two ore less cores, 50% maximal core involvement, and PSA density <0.15 [1]. These recommendations were based on relatively limited biopsy material (the median number of cores per biopsy set was five). In addition, the population studied for this report was predominantly Caucasian. Refinements of the originally suggested criteria have led to modest improvements in the robust negative predictive value of this approach [4]. Although the Epstein criteria provide excellent guidance with regard to initial risk stratification, several factors related to biopsy technique have contributed to disease misclassification and warrant mention.

Large anterior dominant tumor nodules were often not sampled because of the deficiency of template 12-core biopsy technique to access the transitional and anterior zones (Figure 2.2a). In addition, posterolateral small-volume tumor nodules of GS ≥7 could be missed using 12-core template biopsy (Figure 2.2b). In addition to these known limitations of template biopsy strategies, prediction of clinically insignificant disease has been a challenge in specific populations of patients. For example, standard criteria are significantly less successful in identifying AA candidates of active surveillance for reasons that may have an underlying biological basis. Anterior dominant tumor nodules may be seen in 28.5–28.7% of Caucasian and 44–50.6% of African American patients [4,5].

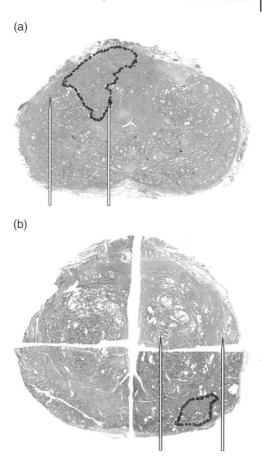

(a)

(b)

Figure 2.2 (a) Anterior dominant tumor nodule only partially sampled by a biopsy leading to either undergrading or inaccurate volume estimation. (b) Small volume high-grade posterolateral tumor volume not sampled by template biopsy.

Multifocality has long been known to be a characteristic feature of prostate cancer. The analysis of radical prostatectomy specimens has revealed multifocality in 50–87% of cases [6,7]. Multifocal cancer was often believed to result from a field effect with multifocal primary disease, and only limited data show this to be the result of intra-organal dissemination of one primary tumor to different areas within the gland [8,9]. Previous reports suggested that multifocal prostate cancer is associated with higher grade, stage, and recurrence rate. In the most recent work on the subject, Huang *et al.* analyzed consecutive radical prostatectomies and concluded that there was no significant difference in grade, stage, total tumor volume, and status of surgical margins in unifocal versus multifocal disease [6]. In cases with final GS of 6, multifocality was seen in 70% of cases with approximately two-thirds of these having bilateral disease [10]. Multifocality was mostly restricted to two or three separate tumor nodules with four or more nodules only rarely seen.

Tumor multifocality carries significant grading implications. Separate tumor nodules need to be assigned individual grades rather than combining all patterns to create a composite Gleason score. The concept of the dominant/index tumor nodule was developed by the Stanford pathology group and reflects the importance of identifying the prognostically meaningful tumor nodule, which usually combines the largest volume, the most advanced pathological stage, and the highest grade [6,11]. In 11.3% of multifocal cancers, the largest volume and highest stage and grade do not occur within the same nodule [6]. This fact has significant treatment implications in rapidly emerging sampling techniques guided by magnetic resonance imaging (MRI) because biopsies targeting a larger lower-grade tumor nodule may not sample a smaller higher-grade prognostically meaningful lesion. In addition, because only two positive cores are allowed for active surveillance, the theoretical risk of hitting three or more separate insignificant tumor nodules may falsely misclassify the patient as having significant disease. This being said, testing a variation of the Epstein surveillance criteria allowing three or more positive cores in template extended biopsy resulted in a noticeable increase of misclassifying significant cancers as amenable to active surveillance without appreciably increasing the pool of men correctly classified as having insignificant disease [4]. The true value of subclassifying pathological stage T2 is highly questionable because it is largely linked to tumor multifocality rather than the grade and stage of each tumor nodule, which are the real prognosis determinants (Figure 2.3). In our practice we report the location and grade of each

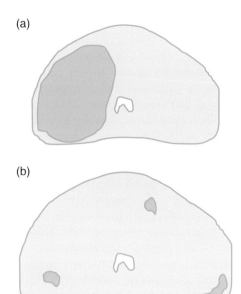

(a)

(b)

Figure 2.3 (a) pT2b tumor defined by unilateral disease involving >50% of a lobe. (b) pT2c tumor defined by bilateral disease. Despite higher stage in image b, the cancer in image a is of greater potential clinical significance because of a large tumor volume.

tumor nodule and we semi-quantitatively estimate tumor involvement of the gland as a percentage [4,12].

Unlike active surveillance, there are no standard criteria for enrollment of patients in focal therapy programs. The International Task Force on Prostate Cancer and the Focal Lesion Paradigm suggested that selection criteria include a minimum of 12 cores sampling and absence of any Gleason pattern 4 or 5 in addition to other histological, clinical, and imaging criteria [13]. Some experts have suggested that patients with limited pattern 4 cancer may be candidates for focal intervention [14]. Independent of the Gleason grade, the main limitation of focal therapy stems from the high incidence of multifocal and bilateral disease, and the inconsistent association between size of the tumor nodule and the grade and stage of cancer, potentially leaving some high-grade/high-stage cancer contralateral to the treated side unsampled and untreated.

The Kidney

The kidney is composed of two separate intimately related systems, the renal parenchyma, which performs excretory and endocrine functions, and the collecting system, which transports urine and is lined by urothelial cells. In this section, we will focus on epithelial and stromal tumors arising from the renal parenchyma. Renal urothelial tumors will be discussed in the corresponding section.

Following the publication of the latest World Health Organization (WHO) classification of genitourinary tumors in 2004, there was a significant number of clinical, morphological, immunohistochemical, and molecular discoveries that have significantly enhanced the knowledge in the field of renal tumors. In 2013, the members of the International Society of Urologic Pathology (ISUP) held a consensus conference analyzing, categorizing, and summarizing the available data of renal neoplasms. This resulted in the development of the ISUP Vancouver Classification of Renal Neoplasia (Table 2.1). There was a consensus that published literature was sufficient to recognize five new epithelial tumor types as distinct neoplasms. Additionally, three rare carcinomas (thyroid-like follicular renal cell carcinoma [RCC], succinate dehydrogenase B deficiency-associated RCC, and ALK translocation RCC) were recognized as provisional entities. In addition, because no recurrence or metastases were documented in more than 200 cases of what was called "multilocular cystic clear cell RCC," the decision was made to substitute the term *carcinoma* with *low malignant potential* in those tumors [15].

With the exception of papillary adenoma, metanephric adenoma, and oncocytoma, most renal epithelial tumors are considered malignant. Clear-cell, papillary, and chromophobe RCC, and collecting duct carcinoma constitute the majority of sporadic RCCs. Although the latter is an aggressive tumor in which focal therapy is seldom, if ever, considered, the first three carcinomas presented in

Table 2.1 ISUP Classification of Renal Cell Tumors.

Benign
  Papillary adenoma
  Oncocytoma

Borderline
  Multilocular cystic clear-cell renal cell
    neoplasm of low malignant potential[a]

Malignant
  Clear-cell RCC
  Papillary RCC
  Chromophobe RCC
  Hybrid oncocytic chromophobe tumor
  Carcinoma of the collecting ducts of Bellini
  Renal medullary carcinoma
  Carcinoma associated with neuroblastoma
  Mucinous tubular and spindle cell carcinoma
  MiTF family translocation RCC[b]
    Xp11 translocation RCC
    T(6;11) RCC
  Tubulocystic RCC[b]
  Acquired cystic disease associated renal cell
    carcinoma[b]
  Clear-cell tubulopapillary RCC[b]
  Hereditary leiomyomatosis renal cell carcinoma
    syndrome-associated RCC[b]
  RCC, unclassified

[a] terminology change; [b] new entities
ISUP, International Society of Urologic Pathology.

the order of decreasing clinical aggressiveness may be considered for such therapy [16,17]. In this context, biopsy of renal masses was shown to accurately subtype 86–96% of tumors and to provide an accurate grading of 63–76% of cases in contemporary series [12]. Although clear-cell, chromophobe, and papillary RCCs can be diagnosed on biopsy without much difficulty in most cases, several histological caveats should be taken in consideration.

First, the distinction of clear-cell RCC from the recently described clear-cell papillary RCC, which may show overlapping features in small samples, is important clinically because the latter has a consistently indolent course. Second, papillary RCC type 1 and papillary adenoma are indistinguishable microscopically because they share the same morphology and immunoprofile, with the size of the lesion (0.5-cm cutoff) being the only differentiating finding in localized disease. We address this issue by adding a comment to the pathology report emphasizing the need for clinical correlation with tumor size and adequacy of sampling. Finally, the eosinophilic variant of chromophobe RCC can have and hybrid tumors do have areas indistinguishable from oncocytoma, which in addition to some overlapping immunophenotypic features make the distinction difficult in some cases. In terms of grading, the previously used Fuhrman's grading system was supplanted by the ISUP grading system that relies solely on nucleolar features. Although grading chromophobe RCC is not prognostic and is therefore not used, nucleolar grade is effectively applied to both clear-cell and papillary RCCs (Figure 2.4). High-grade tumors are usually not considered for focal therapy because they are associated with more aggressive local and systemic tumor characteristics in addition to a higher incidence of sarcomatoid, plasmacytoid, and rhabdoid changes that may not be sampled by a biopsy core [18]. Some of the newly described entities such as tubulocystic RCC and acquired cystic kidney disease (ACKD)-associated RCC typically have prominent nucleoli, but they are associated with an indolent course.

Size is also an important criterion for considering focal therapy because it is closely linked to pathological stage. In a comprehensive work by Bonsib, 85% of clear-cell RCCs <4 cm were limited to the kidney, in comparison to 32% of tumors between 4.1 and 7 cm, and only 3% of those >7 cm [16]. Extrarenal extension, particularly renal sinus fat invasion, is one of the most important RCC prognostic factors, and its increased likelihood with the size is an indication for definitive and more radical surgical approaches. Overall, multifocal disease is seen in approximately 5% of nephrectomies performed in the sporadic setting with the highest rates reported in papillary RCC (10–16%) in comparison to 4% in chromophobe and 2% in clear-cell RCC [19]. These rates increase significantly in the settings of familial RCC syndromes or end-stage renal disease (ESRD) as will be discussed.

(a)

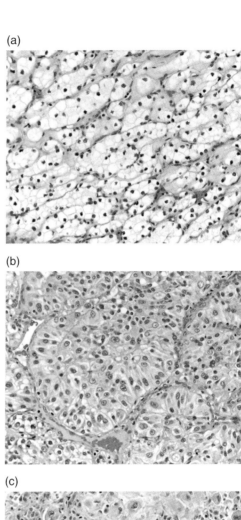

(b)

(c)

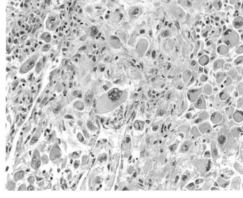

Figure 2.4 (a) Grade 1 clear-cell RCC with small monomorphic nuclear and absence of nucleoli. (b) Grade 3 clear-cell RCC with larger irregular nucleoli and prominent nucleoli. Higher grade clear-cell RCC often has eosinophilic cytoplasm. (c) Grade 4 RCC with bizarre nuclei and rhabdoid change.

In ESRD with hemodialysis, the likelihood of developing renal epithelial neoplasms is increased 100-fold compared to a nonaffected kidney. This is applicable to both carcinomas analogous to those developing in healthy kidneys and entities appearing to be specific to ESRD. In the setting of ESRD, the likelihood of primary multifocal tumors is also increased. Carcinomas not specific to ESRD show comparable behavior in end-stage and nonaffected kidneys. Before the description of entities specific to ESRD, most studies reported papillary RCC as the most common neoplasm developing in the end-stage kidney [20]. However, more recent investigations discovered that carcinomas with focal papillary architecture mimicking papillary RCC are more common than true papillary RCCs. Clear-cell tubulo-papillary RCC was originally believed to be specific for ESRD, but later reports demonstrated that most cases occur in the sporadic setting [20]. With more than 200 reported cases with limited follow-up, no metastasis or recurrence was described [21]. Therefore, the term *carcinoma* may be changed in the future if aggressive behavior is not documented with extended follow-up.

Another tumor developing in the setting of ESRD was originally described by Sule *et al.* who noted a peculiar association of carcinoma with calcium oxalate crystal and labeled it as ACKD-associated RCC [22]. In the subsequent report Tickoo *et al.*, the authors concluded that this tumor is the most common cancer developing in the end-stage kidney [20]. This cancer is preceded by the development of cysts, often multifocal, lined by atypical epithelium, yet not forming solid masses, and containing intraluminal oxalate crystals (Figure 2.5) [23]. This carcinoma is also characterized by the presence of prominent nucleoli (ISUP grade 3), which are not reflective of its indolent course. Whether their small size and favorable outcome is related to earlier detection because of regular imaging with ESRD is not entirely clear.

A recent analysis of ESRD nephrectomies in five large tertiary care institutions reported

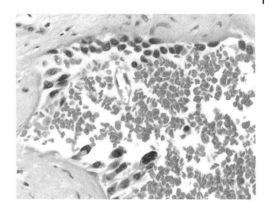

Figure 2.5 Hemorrhagic cyst lined by atypical epithelium with intraluminal oxalate crystal (polarized). This should be classified as ACKD-associated RCC precursor.

a new association of anastomosing hemangioma and ESRD that may arise in patients with or without ACKD [20]. Hemangiomas are usually centered in the renal medulla and may extend into the renal sinus fat. Intravascular growth pattern often accompanies the latter. Multiple hemangiomas may develop unilaterally or bilaterally (Figure 2.6). Radiologically, anastomosing hemangiomas are heterogeneously enhancing masses that may be difficult to distinguish from RCC [22]. This new association is important because malignancy, excluding some indolent cutaneous cancers, is one of the contraindications for renal transplant. Thus, a thorough diagnostic work-up including renal biopsy should be performed in patients with ESRD with a newly diagnosed renal mass waiting for renal transplant; however, in a biopsy specimen, it may be difficult to distinguish renal hemangioma from low-grade clear-cell RCC with extensive degeneration and myxoid change, which leave a rich vascular network with rare bland neoplastic cells mimicking hemangioma [23].

Table 2.2 summarizes the most important familial adult RCC syndromes. Most of the commonly encountered syndromes are inherited in an autosomal dominant fashion. When two or more oncocytic tumors are present in one patient (unilateral or bilateral),

(a) (b)

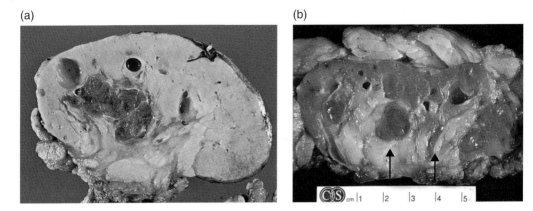

Figure 2.6 (a) Grossly apparent extension of anastomosing hemangioma into renal sinus fat and renal vein. (b) Multiple hemangiomas of different size scattered throughout the kidney and in the renal sinus fat (*arrows*). The latter hemangiomas had intravascular growth pattern. (a) Courtesy of Dr. Anna-Luise A. Katzenstein, SUNY Upstate Medical University, Syracuse, NY; (b) Courtesy of Dr. Mahul Amin, Cedar Sinai, Los Angeles, CA.

Table 2.2 Familiar Renal Cell Carcinoma (RCC) Syndromes.

Syndrome	Inheritance Pattern	Mean Age	Disease Genes	Tumor Morphology
Von Hippel-Lindau	AD	~35	Von Hippel-Lindau	Clear-cell RCC
Hereditary papillary RCC	AD	~60	c-Met	Papillary RCC type 1
Hereditary leiomyomatosis RCC	AD	~40	Fumarate hydratase	Papillary RCC type 2
Birt-Hogg-Dubé syndrome	AD	~60	Folliculin	Oncocytoma Chromophobe RCC Hybrid tumor Clear-cell RCC Papillary RCC
Tuberous sclerosis complex (TSC)	AD	~35	Hamartin Tuberin	Angiomyolipoma Oncocytoma RCC (different types)

AD, autosomal dominant.

the possibility of syndromic association is raised and recommendation for genetic counseling should be made. In the presence of multiple oncocytic tumors, oncocytosis and Birt-Hogg-Dubé syndrome are the most common underlying conditions. Although the former is limited to the kidney, the latter commonly presents to clinical attention because of multiple fibrofolliculomas, a skin tumor typical of the syndrome. Patients may also present with pneumothorax because of pulmonary cysts. The clinical behavior of the tumors is less aggressive in this setting, and when bilateral tumors are seen, a nephron-sparing approach should be considered [24]. In patient with Von Hippel-Lindau syndrome, renal tumors are mostly limited to clear-cell RCC. Although clear-cell RCC is more aggressive than papillary and chromophobe RCC, strategies for preserving the kidney are recommended in patients with Von Hippel-Lindau syndrome with treatment initiated for lesions larger than 3 cm.

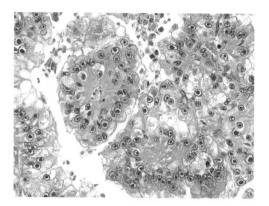

Figure 2.7 Type 2 papillary RCC developing in hereditary leiomyomatosis associated RCC syndrome. Note prominent nucleoli and perinucleolar halo not typically seen in other settings. Courtesy of Dr. Jonathan Epstein, Johns Hopkins Hospital, Baltimore, MD.

Table 2.3 The WHO/ISUP 2004 Classification of Urothelial Neoplasia.

Flat	Papillary
Hyperplasia	Papilloma
Dysplasia (low-grade)	Papillary neoplasm of low malignant potential (PNLMP)
Carcinoma in situ (high-grade)	
	Low-grade papillary carcinoma
	High-grade papillary carcinoma

ISUP, International Society of Urologic Pathology; WHO, World Health Organization.

With other inherited cancer syndromes, the incidence of aggressive clinical behavior of renal tumors is low. However, a notable exception is the hereditary leiomyomatosis associated RCC, in which renal tumors were commonly misdiagnosed in the past as type 2 papillary RCC because of the prominent papillary architecture and the presence of abundant deeply eosinophilic cytoplasm. Those tumors have aggressive clinical behavior with approximately 50% of cases presenting with or developing lymph node or distant metastasis. The characteristic morphological feature of those tumors, irrespective of architecture, is the presence of "viral inclusion-like" prominent nucleoli with peri-nucleolar halos (Figure 2.7). Although diagnosis cannot be established based on morphology alone, recognition of this tumor can initiate testing of fumarate hydratase gene mutations.

The Urothelium

The urothelium lines a number of hollow organs including the minor calices and extends to the urethra. Although most of urothelial lesions develop in the urinary bladder, similar lesions may be seen throughout the entire system lined by urothelium. Hence, the current discussion is applicable to all the urothelium-lined organs because the spectrum of disease and clinical behavior are comparable for urothelial neoplasia regardless of the location. In the United States, urothelial carcinoma (UCa) constitutes more than 90% of neoplasia of the urinary bladder followed by adenocarcinoma and, rarely, squamous cell carcinoma. The WHO/ISUP 2004 classification distinguishes flat and papillary noninvasive urothelial lesions (Table 2.3) [25]. The major distinction of this classification is the dichotomy into low- and high-grade lesions in contrast to the less reproducible WHO 1973 grading system, which included grades 1, 2, and 3 categories. In the United States, the WHO/ISUP 2004 classification is largely followed, whereas the three-tiered system is still used in Europe [26]. In the flat lesions category, hyperplasia and dysplasia are infrequently seen as the primary manifestation of the disease but are rather detected either in patients followed for UCa or in association with concurrent symptomatic papillary urothelial neoplasm. Urothelial carcinoma in situ (CIS) is a flat and multifocal lesion usually not amenable to complete cystoscopic excision. CIS is one of the precursors of invasive UCa with a variable natural course. It appears that recurrence and survival rates are better in patients with CIS when compared to those presenting with high-grade noninvasive papillary neoplasms [27]. Pathologically, most cases of CIS are easily recognized because of the presence of sever atypia not explained by other non-neoplastic causes (Figure 2.8a). In some cases of CIS, severe discohesion and extensive shedding into the urine may result in a totally denuded urothelial mucosa with underlying congested vessels (Figure 2.8b). Pathologists are encouraged to comment on this finding and its potential association with CIS, which should be ruled out by a repeat biopsy. Such association increases in the event of a concurrent "positive" urine cytology result.

Papillary lesions are more likely to be symptomatic in comparison to flat lesions, even when benign, because of fragmentation of the papillae causing gross hematuria. Benign urothelial papilloma has no risk of progression into carcinoma and is only capable of local recurrence in less than 5% of cases. Papillary urothelial neoplasm of low malignant potential has no cytologic atypia and is distinguished from papilloma by higher number of urothelial cell layers. It has a significantly higher incidence of recurrence (up to 45%) and may progress to a higher grade lesion in 10% or less of the cases.

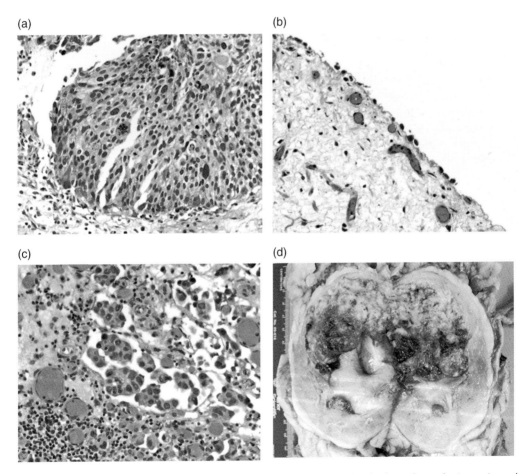

(a)

(b)

(c)

(d)

Figure 2.8 (a) Urothelial carcinoma in situ with marked architectural disarray, high-grade cytologic atypia, and atypical mitotic figure. (b) Denuded urothelial mucosa with congested vessels in a patient with UCa diagnosed in urine cytology. Occasional atypical cells are seen along the basement membrane. (c) Micropapillary invasive urothelial carcinoma. Presence of multiple papillae without fibrovascular cores in the same lacuna is the diagnostic feature. (d) Multifocal noninvasive high-grade UCa discontinuously involving upper and lower portions of the renal pelvis.

Low-grade papillary UCa has scattered cytologic atypia and usually absent or rare mitotic figures. Although the likelihood of its progression to a higher grade lesion is still less than 10%, the incidence of recurrence may reach 70%. High-grade papillary UCa is distinguished by high cytological grade, similar to that seen in CIS, and its high likelihood to progress to invasive UCa. Papillary lesions are commonly associated with adjacent flat neoplasm of the same grade, so called "shoulder" lesions. For this reason to diagnose a CIS in the biopsy of papillary carcinoma, it should be a separate biopsy of a spacially remote flat lesion.

With invasive UCa, the stage rather than grade determines treatment and prognosis. Although clinically noninvasive UCa (both CIS and papillary) and UCa invading into lamina propria (pT1) are commonly referred to as *superficial* bladder cancer and are treated similarly, pathologically these are two different diseases. The latter has already distinguished itself by aggressive/invasive behavior, and if left untreated, will inevitably progress to muscle-invasive disease. Some variants of invasive UCa (e.g., plasmacytoid and micropapillary) are notorious for aggressive behavior and resistance to standard therapy (Figure 2.8c). Some centers have advocated radical cystectomy in treating invasive micropapillary UCa even in the absence of muscularis propria invasion, but this has not become routine practice yet [28].

Around 70% of newly diagnosed papillary UCas are multifocal (Figure 2.8d). Multifocality is a risk factor for recurrence and progression [29]. Although in some cases, multiple primary tumors may develop as a result of a "field effect" [30], it has been shown that it often represents an intraluminal seeding and intra-epithelial migration of malignant cells resulting in multifocal proliferation of the same malignant cell clone [31]. This is one of the rationales for treating patients with bacillus Calmette-Guérin (BCG) or chemotherapy refractory "superficial bladder cancer" with radical rather than partial cystectomy. Multifocality is also present in upper-tract lesions, and we often see patients with a history of upper-tract high-grade UCa treated with nephroureterectomy who present after extended period of time with recurring high-grade disease in the bladder (incidence up to 44% at a 5-year interval) [32]. Partial cystectomy is rarely considered as treatment modality for patients with high-grade UCa who fail intravesical BCG or chemotherapy because many of these will develop intravesicla recurrence [33]. This is reflected in the overall trend in the United States of decreasing frequency of partial cystectomy, which is often reserved for older patients and those with high risk of perioperative complications [34]. At the same time, there is a minor subset of patients presenting with solitary tumors in whom complete transurethral resection of bladder tumor (TURBT) of the lesion may be curative [35]. There are no validated ancillary methods in contemporary practice to predict which high-grade noninvasive cancers will become invasive and which invasive cancers are likely to be lethal. Some genetic alterations, particularly in cell cycle regulatory genes (e.g., FGFR3, p53, and retinoblastoma), show promising results to help further molecularly classify the disease [36,37]. Rare UCa in the pediatric population has different genomic alterations, has less aggressive disease, and is amenable to more conservative therapy [38].

The Testis

Among urologic organs, testicular tumors are the least common. In general, older men are more likely to present with secondary involvement by lymphoma/leukemia or metastasis, and malignant soft-tissue paratesticular neoplasms are more common in young children. Adolescents and young adults are the group in whom primary testicular neoplasms are mostly seen and include two large categories: germ cell tumors (GCT) and sex cord/stromal tumors, the former being by far more common.

Contrarily, only the tumors in the latter category could be subjected to partial orchiectomy. Benign paratesticular tumors (adenomatoid tumor) and vestiges are seen with the same incidence (e.g., appendix testis is the most common cause of acute testicular pain) and are amenable to local excision because they are mostly unifocal and do not involve the testicular parenchyma.

The distinctive feature of GCTs is their association with the malignant precursor—intratubular germ cell neoplasia (ITGCN)—which is multifocal and cannot be detected grossly, excluding the possibility of partial orchietcomy in those tumors (Figure 2.9). The exception is spermatocystic seminoma, a tumor unassociated with ITGCN and incapable of metastasis, and therefore cured by surgery. Clinical behavior of teratoma depends on patient's age rather the tumor's composition because both the mature and immature elements are indolent in pre-puberty and potentially malignant in post-puberty. Epidermoid cyst, a variant of teratoma with uniformly benign clinical course, is unassociated with ITGCN and is composed of a unilocular cyst lined by keratinizing squamous epithelium without skin adnexa. It may be suspected on preoperative imaging and treated with excision after intraoperative frozen section confirmation. With the exception of spermatocytic seminoma and epidermoid cyst, focal therapy is usually not considered for GCT because of

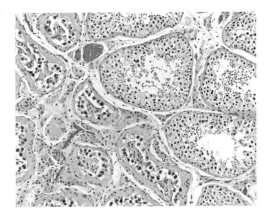

Figure 2.9 A contrast of intratubular germ cell neoplasia (ITGCN) with thickened basement membranes and absent spermatogenesis on the left and normal seminiferous tubules on the right with preserved spermatogenesis.

the tumor's multifocality and its association with ITGCN. In addition, these tumors are fragile and seeding may occur if GCT ruptures in the operative field.

Sex cord/stromal tumors are generally benign and may have some atypical histological features like infiltrative growth pattern not warranting a malignant diagnosis [33,35]. They are less common than GCTs and serum tumor markers are usually not elevated. Whenever there is any clinical suspicion of a benign testicular tumor, intraoperative frozen section consultation should be sought before partial orchiectomy is considered [35].

References

1 Epstein JI, Walsh PC, Carmichael M, Brendler CB. Pathologic and clinical findings to predict tumor extent of nonpalpable (stage T1c) prostate cancer. JAMA. 1994 Feb 2;271(5):368–74.

2 Epstein JI, Allsbrook WC, Jr., Amin MB, Egevad LL. The 2005 International Society of Urological Pathology (ISUP) Consensus Conference on Gleason Grading of Prostatic Carcinoma. Am J Surg Pathol. 2005 Sep;29(9):1228–42.

3 Ross HM, Kryvenko ON, Cowan JE, Simko JP, Wheeler TM, Epstein JI. Do adenocarcinomas of the prostate with Gleason score (GS) </=6 have the potential to metastasize to lymph nodes? Am J Surg Pahtol. 2012 Sep;36(9):13461609641452.

4 Kryvenko ON, Carter HB, Trock BJ, Epstein JI. Biopsy criteria for determining appropriateness for active surveillance in the modern era. Urology. 2014 Apr; 83(4):869–74.

5 Sundi D, Kryvenko ON, Carter HB, Ross AE, Epstein JI, Schaeffer EM. Pathological examination of radical prostatectomy specimens in men with very low risk disease at biopsy reveals distinct zonal distribution of cancer in black American men. J Urol. 2014 Jan;191(1):60–67.

6 Huang CC, Deng FM, Kong MX, Ren Q, Melamed J, Zhou M. Re-evaluating the concept of "dominant/index tumor nodule" in multifocal prostate cancer. Virchows Archiv. 2014 Mar 12.

7 Djavan B, Susani M, Bursa B, Basharkhah A, Simak R, Marberger M. Predictability and significance of multifocal prostate cancer in the radical prostatectomy specimen. Tech Urol. 1999 Sep; 5(3):139–42.

8 Kryvenko ON, Gupta NS, Virani N, Schultz D, Gomez J, Amin A, *et al.* Gleason score 7 adenocarcinoma of the prostate with lymph node metastases: Analysis of 184 radical prostatectomy specimens. Arch Pathol Lab Med. 2013 May;137(5):610–7.

9 Andreoiu M, Cheng L. Multifocal prostate cancer: Biologic, prognostic, and therapeutic implications. Hum Pathol. 2010 Jun;41(6):781–93.

10 Swanson GP, Epstein JI, Chul SH, Kryvenko ON. Pathologic characteristics of low risk prostate cancer based on totally embedded prostatectomy specimens. Prostate. 2015 Mar 1; 75(4):424–9.

11 McNeal JE, Price HM, Redwine EA, Freiha FS, Stamey TA. Stage A versus stage B adenocarcinoma of the prostate: Morphological comparison and biological significance. J Urol. 1988 Jan;139(1):61–5.

12 van der Kwast TH, Amin MB, Billis A, Epstein JI, Griffiths D, Humphrey PA, *et al.* International Society of Urological Pathology (ISUP) Consensus Conference on Handling and Staging of Radical Prostatectomy Specimens. Working group 2: T2 substaging and prostate cancer volume. Mod Pathol. 2011 Jan;24(1):16–25.

13 Eggener SE, Scardino PT, Carroll PR, Zelefsky MJ, Sartor O, Hricak H, *et al.* Focal therapy for localized prostate cancer: A critical appraisal of rationale and modalities. J Urol. 2007 Dec;178(6): 2260–7.

14 de la Rosette J, Ahmed H, Barentsz J, Johansen TB, Brausi M, Emberton M, *et al.* Focal therapy in prostate cancer-report from a consensus panel. J Endourol. May;24(5):775–80.

15 Suzigan S, Lopez-Beltran A, Montironi R, Drut R, Romero A, Hayashi T, *et al.* Multilocular cystic renal cell carcinoma: A report of 45 cases of a kidney tumor of low malignant potential. American journal of clinical pathology. 2006 Feb;125(2):217–22.

16 Bonsib SM. T2 clear cell renal cell carcinoma is a rare entity: A study of 120 clear cell renal cell carcinomas. J Urol. 2005 Oct;174 (4 Pt 1):1199–202; discussion 202.

17 Cheville JC, Lohse CM, Zincke H, Weaver AL, Blute ML. Comparisons of outcome and prognostic features among histologic subtypes of renal cell carcinoma. Am J Surg Pathol. 2003 May;27(5):612–24.

18 Gokden N, Nappi O, Swanson PE, Pfeifer JD, Vollmer RT, Wick MR, *et al.* Renal cell carcinoma with rhabdoid features. Am J Sur Pathol. 2000 Oct;24(10):1329–38.

19 Richstone L, Scherr DS, Reuter VR, Snyder ME, Rabbani F, Kattan MW, *et al.* Multifocal renal cortical tumors: Frequency, associated clinicopathological features and impact on survival. The Journal of urology. 2004 Feb;171(2 Pt 1):615–20.

20 Kryvenko ON, Haley SL, Smith SC, Shen SS, Paluru S, Gupta NS, *et al.* Hemangiomas in kidneys with end-stage renal disease: A novel clinicopathological association. Histopathology. 2014 Sep; 65(3):309–18.

21 Srigley JR, Delahunt B, Eble JN, Egevad L, Epstein JI, Grignon D, *et al.* The International Society of Urological Pathology (ISUP) Vancouver Classification of Renal Neoplasia. Am J Surg Pathol. 2013 Oct;37(10):1469–89.

22 Kryvenko ON, Gupta NS, Meier FA, Lee MW, Epstein JI. Anastomosing hemangioma of the genitourinary system: Eight cases in the kidney and ovary with

immunohistochemical and ultrastructural analysis. Am J Clin Pathol. 2011 Sep; 136(3):450–7.

23 Kryvenko ON, Roquero L, Gupta NS, Lee MW, Epstein JI. Low-grade clear cell renal cell carcinoma mimicking hemangioma of the kidney: A series of 4 cases. Arch Pathol Lab Med. 2013 Feb;137(2):251–4.

24 Kryvenko ON, Jorda M, Argani P, Epstein JI. Diagnostic approach to eosinophilic renal neoplasms. Arch Pathol Lab Med. 2014 Nov; 138(11):1531–41.

25 Eble JN, Epstein JI, Sesterhenn IA. Pathology and genetics of tumors of the urinary system and male genital organs. Lyon, France: IARC Press, 2004.

26 Babjuk M, Burger M, Zigeuner R, Shariat SF, van Rhijn BW, Comperat E, *et al.* EAU guidelines on non-muscle-invasive urothelial carcinoma of the bladder: Update 2013. Eur Urol. 2013 Oct; 64(4):639–53.

27 Orozco RE, Martin AA, Murphy WM. Carcinoma in situ of the urinary bladder. Clues to host involvement in human carcinogenesis. Cancer. 1994 Jul 1; 74(1):115–22.

28 Kamat AM, Dinney CP, Gee JR, Grossman HB, Siefker-Radtke AO, Tamboli P, *et al.* Micropapillary bladder cancer: A review of the University of Texas M. D. Anderson Cancer Center experience with 100 consecutive patients. Cancer. 2007 Jul 1; 110(1):62–7.

29 Kiemeney LA, Witjes JA, Heijbroek RP, Verbeek AL, Debruyne FM. Predictability of recurrent and progressive disease in individual patients with primary superficial bladder cancer. J Urol. 1993 Jul; 150(1):60–4.

30 Jones TD, Wang M, Eble JN, MacLennan GT, Lopez-Beltran A, Zhang S, *et al.* Molecular evidence supporting field effect in urothelial carcinogenesis. Clin Cancer Res. 2005 Sep 15;11(18):6512–9.

31 Hafner C, Knuechel R, Stoehr R, Hartmann A. Clonality of multifocal urothelial carcinomas: 10 years of molecular genetic studies. Int J Cancer. 2002 Sep 1;101(1):1–6.

32 Ishioka J, Saito K, Kijima T, Nakanishi Y, Yoshida S, Yokoyama M, *et al.* Risk stratification for bladder recurrence of upper urinary tract urothelial carcinoma after radical nephroureterectomy. BJU Int. 2015 May; 115(5):705–12

33 Knoedler JJ, Boorjian SA, Kim SP, Weight CJ, Thapa P, Tarrell RF, *et al.* Does partial cystectomy compromise oncologic outcomes for patients with bladder cancer compared to radical cystectomy? A matched case-control analysis. J Urol. 2012 Oct;188(4):1115–9.

34 Faiena I, Dombrovskiy V, Koprowski C, Singer EA, Jang TL, Weiss RE. Performance of partial cystectomy in the United States from 2001 to 2010: Trends and comparative outcomes. Can J Urol. 2014 Dec;21(6):7520–7.

35 Maarouf AM, Khalil S, Salem EA, ElAdl M, Nawar N, Zaiton F. Bladder preservation multimodality therapy as an alternative to radical cystectomy for treatment of muscle invasive bladder cancer. BJU Int. 2011 May; 107(10):1605–10.

36 Shariat SF, Chromecki TF, Cha EK, Karakiewicz PI, Sun M, Fradet Y, *et al.* Risk stratification of organ confined bladder cancer after radical cystectomy using cell cycle related biomarkers. J Urol. 2012 Feb;187(2):457–62.

37 Mitra AP, Jorda M, Cote RJ. Pathological possibilities and pitfalls in detecting aggressive bladder cancer. Curr Opin Urol. 2012 Sep;22(5):397–404.

38 Williamson SR, Wang M, Montironi R, Eble JN, Lopez-Beltran A, Zhang S, *et al.* Molecular characteristics of urothelial neoplasms in children and young adults: A subset of tumors from young patients harbors chromosomal abnormalities but not FGFR3 or TP53 gene mutations. Mod Pathol. 2014 Nov;27(11):1540–8.

3

The Immunobiology of Tumor Ablation

Rafi Kabarriti, MD, and Chandan Guha, MBBS, PhD

Department of Radiation Oncology, Montefiore Medical Center, Albert Einstein College of Medicine, Bronx, NY, USA

Manipulating the Immune System to Fight Cancer

An emerging tool in the oncologist's armamentarium is cancer immunotherapy, which refers to treatment strategies that induce the patient's own immune system to attack tumor cells. One of the earliest attempts to recruit the immune system against cancer occurred in 1891 when William Coley in New York attempted intratumoral injections of live or inactivated *Streptococcus pyogenes* and *Serratia marcescens* bacteria in in patients with advanced cancer to reproduce the spontaneous remissions of sarcomas observed in patients with rare forms and who had developed erysipelas [1]. The hypothesis was that "Coley's toxins" could stimulate antibacterial phagocytes to kill bystander tumor cells. Over the next 40 to 50 years, many attempts were made to induce a systemic cancer immune response with only sporadic successes that were difficult to reproduce. One major exception was the use of intravesical injection of live bacillus Calmette-Guérin (BCG) after surgical resection for superficial bladder cancer, which resulted in an overall survival benefit [2]. An early observation implicating involvement of the immune system in eliminating tumor cells came in the 1940s when evidence demonstrated that mice could be immunized against chemically induced tumors [3] and subsequent evidence demonstrating that it was the CD8+ cytotoxic T cells recognizing tumor-specific antigens that was primarily responsible for this immunity [4]. The tumor-specific antigens can be presented to cytotoxic T cells by MHC class I molecules on tumor cells and antigen-presenting cells (APCs). Since then, we have made significant progress in our understanding of the different mechanisms in which the immune system can selectively recognize tumor cells and ways in which cancers evade the immune system.

Tumors can make tumor-specific antigens that are recognized by the cytotoxic T cells through a variety of different mechanisms. Some potential ways of making these antigens to appear as foreign antigens that can be recognized by the immune system include the mutation of self-proteins, expression of new proteins encoded by viral oncogenes, inappropriate presentation of self-proteins, or overexpression of self-proteins, which changes the density of peptide presentation. However, despite the presence of tumor-specific antigens, tumors have also developed multiple mechanisms to escape immune recognition. For a cytotoxic T cell to become activated, it requires a second co-stimulatory signal from an APC. Some tumors lose one or more MHC molecules, and most tumors do not express co-stimulatory proteins.

Management of Urologic Cancer: Focal Therapy and Tissue Preservation, First Edition.
Edited by Mark P. Schoenberg and Kara L. Watts.
© 2017 John Wiley & Sons Ltd. Published 2017 by John Wiley & Sons Ltd.

There are also a number of suppressive signals that tumors have evolved to block the activation of the cytotoxic T cells. Some of these immune checkpoints include PD-1 and CTLA-4. There are additional cells that produce inhibitory signals and include T regulatory cells (Tregs), myeloid derived suppressor cells, and the tumor-associated macrophages [5]. In addition to all these components, there are a variety of soluble factors, including cytokines and toll-like receptor agonists, that play an important role in both stimulating and inhibiting immunity.

Since the US Food and Drug Administration (FDA) approved a dendritic cell-based vaccine, Sipuleucel-T (Provenge, APC8015, Dendreon Corp, WA, USA) for the treatment of prostate cancer, significant effort has been directed toward the development of new immunotherapeutic strategies for the treatment of prostate cancer. Provenge conferred a modest survival advantage in men with metastatic castration-resistant prostate cancer (CRPC) [6]. In line with this, multiple prostate-specific antigen (PSA)–based immunotherapeutic strategies, including DNA vaccines, recombinant viruses, *Listeria*-based vaccines, and dendritic cells (DCs), have been shown to effectively induce PSA-specific T cell responses in preclinical studies [7,8].

Can We Take Advantage of Ablative Therapies to Activate the Immune System?

Ablative therapies, such as high-intensity focused ultrasound (HIFU), cryotherapy, radiofrequency ablation (RFA), focal radiation therapy using stereotactic body radiation therapy (SBRT) or brachytherapy, and photodynamic therapy, have been shown to be safe, noninvasive, image-guided therapies for local tumor ablation. The immunomodulatory effect of these therapies is intriguing. All forms of ablative therapies allow for the

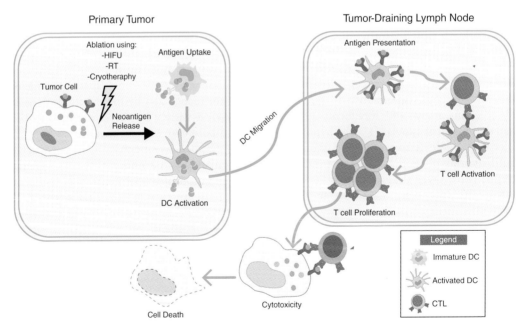

Figure 3.1 Ablative therapies including HIFU, RT, and cryotherapy allow for the release of tumor-specific antigens that are then be taken up by antigen-presenting cells. The antigen-presenting cells then migrate to the draining lymph nodes where they can activate CD4+ T helper cells as well as cytotoxic CD8+ T cells that could potentially kill tumor cells both at the primary and metastatic sites. DC, dendritic cell; HIFU, high-intensity focused ultrasound; RT, radiation therapy.

release of tumor-specific antigens, which are then taken up by APCs. The APCs then migrate to the draining lymph nodes where they can activate CD4+ T helper cells as well as cytotoxic CD8+ T cells that could potentially kill tumor cells both at the primary and metastatic sites (Figure 3.1). The use of these ablative therapies alone is not sufficient to induce a sustainable immune response, and there is a need to combine this with other immunotherapies. Although these ablative therapies allow for the release of tumor antigens through tumor breakdown with antigen shedding and release of tumor-infiltrating lymphocytes, tumors secrete immunosuppressive signals to promote tolerance and facilitate immune escape. Therefore, it is necessary to boost the immune system to take advantage of the released tumor antigens to generate a sustained immune response.

Immunomodulatory Properties of HIFU

HIFU uses sonic waves generated by a spherical transducer to create a sharply delineated target area of energy at the focal point. The concentrated ultrasound energy can generate temperatures exceeding 80°C, resulting in tissue destruction by thermal, mechanical, and cavitation effects, to produce a clearly demarcated region of coagulative necrosis surrounded by normal tissue on microscopic examination [9,10]. HIFU has been used in clinical therapies because of its noninvasiveness, safety, and precise targeting when coupled with image guidance [9]. For example, HIFU can noninvasively target and destroy specific prostatic areas with high precision while sparing the normal tissues along its path. This has made HIFU highly suited for focal therapy and allows for repeat focal treatments.

Systemic treatments, such as chemotherapy and immunotherapy, are favorable options to be used in combination with localized HIFU treatment to gain both local and systemic control of tumor. A number of clinical investigators have reported anecdotal evidence of tumor immunomodulation after treatment with HIFU. A pilot clinical study on 16 patients with solid malignancies (osteosarcoma, hepatocelluar carcinoma, or renal cell carcinoma) revealed a significant increase in the population of CD4+ T lymphocytes and the ratio of CD4+/CD8+ in the patients' circulation 7 to 10 days after ablative HIFU treatment [11]. Further clinical studies on 48 patients with breast cancer showed increased lymphocyte infiltration in the treated tumor after HIFU [12]. The lymphocytes infiltrated along the margins of the ablated regions and were enriched with cells expressing an activated phenotype, including FasL, granzyme, and perforin. In murine models with colon adenocarcinoma and melanoma, HIFU treatment stimulated DC proliferation and maturation and induced DC infiltration in tumor tissues with an increase in tumor-specific interferon (IFN-)γ–secreting cells in lymphoid organs [13,14]. The systemic protective effects of HIFU was demonstrated in a murine model of melanoma with a decrease in metastases after the primary tumor was treated with HIFU, 2 days prior to resection [15], suggesting that HIFU induced a tumor-specific protective immunity. HIFU-ablated tumor cells could also serve as a source of tumor antigens for DC-based tumor vaccine, where autologous DC are purified and expanded ex vivo, followed by incubation with HIFU-treated tumor cells to stimulate uptake of tumor antigens by DCs. Upon injection of autologous DCs loaded with HIFU-treated tumor cells a systemic anti-tumor immune response is induced in mice [16,17].

The mechanism of immunomodulatory effects of ablative HIFU is unclear. Studies from local ablative therapies, such as radiation therapy [18–21] and RFA [22], revealed that in situ tumor ablation can generate a source of tumor antigens that are released in situ from dying tumor cells and can be engulfed by APC, such as DCs to generate a systemic T-cell mediated tumor-specific immune response. Chakravarty *et al.* demonstrated that administration of Flt3L to stimulate proliferation of DCs in combination with an ablative dose of a single fraction of local tumor irradiation induces long-term protective anti-tumor immunity, reduces lung metastases. and improves survival with long-term cures in a murine model of Lewis lung adenocarcinoma [18,19]. This report indicated that an autologous in situ tumor vaccine could be generated by amplifying DCs in the blood and enabling antigen uptake from the tumor microenvironment that has been treated with a locally ablative therapy. Since this publication, multiple groups have confirmed the potential of tumor immunomodulation by combining various immunotherapeutic approaches with locally ablative therapies [23–27]. Since the tumor microenvironment is usually immunosuppressive [28], induction of a protective anti-tumor immunity is limited after primary tumor ablation alone.

Most of the studies on HIFU-induced immune response are limited and have not definitely proven that the immune response is directed against tumor antigen. In addition, the magnitude of ablation-induced immune response is generally weak and whether it could fully protect patients from tumor metastases is still uncertain. Therefore, combining ablative HIFU with a relevant systemic therapy is still considered the most efficient way to achieve a beneficial clinical outcome. Although various immunotherapeutic agents are available to amplify the immune effects of HIFU, optimization of the immunomodulatory properties of ultrasound relative to the sonic energy and the potential complexity and unpredictable adverse events of combination therapies determining clinical outcome should be investigated for effective clinical application.

Immunomodulatory Properties of Cryotherapy

Cellular death from cryotherapy results from shifts in osmotic fluids, physical disruption of cell membranes and organelles by the ice crystals within the ice ball, and by causing vascular compromise through thrombosis of small vessels [29,30]. Histologically, this leads to a central area of coagulative necrosis surrounded by an area of sublethal tissue injury [30,31]. Upon thawing, dying tumor cells within the ice ball release intact tumor-specific antigens as well as proinflammatory cytokines, nuclear proteins, and HMGB1, which is a molecule that acts as a ligand for toll-like receptor (TLR) 4 and promotes antitumor immunity [32,33]. The proinflammatory cytokines and danger signals recruit the DCs to the ablation site, which can then efficiently take up the released tumor-specific antigens and induce the DC maturation [22]. These activated DCs display the tumor antigens in the MHC molecules and travel to the nearest lymph node to activate cytotoxic CD8+ T cells and CD4+ T helper cells, which can then mount an immune response against the tumor [22,32].

One of the first pieces of evidence implicating recruitment of the immune system following cryotherapy came in 1970 when patients with metastatic prostate cancer treated with cryotherapy were observed to have a decrease in their metastatic burden [34]. Since then, experiments in animal models confirmed the induction of systemic anti-tumor immune response by tumor cryoablation. Using a rat model of myosarcoma and carcinosarcoma, Blackwood and Cooper showed that cryotherapy resulted in regression of an untreated tumor and the treated animals failed to develop transplantable tumors when challenged with a second tumor [35]. Bagley *et al.* demonstrated that it was the lymphocytes that mediated the cytotoxicity following cryotherapy [36]. More recently, Den Brok *et al.* showed that cryotherapy doubled the number of antigen-loaded DCs and increased the number of mature DCs in tumor-draining lymph nodes [37]. Using a murine model of kidney cancer, cryotherapy resulted in infiltration of macrophages, neutrophils, and lymphocytes into perivascular and intravascular spaces and parenchyma of tumors. Immunologically, there was a shift from Th1 to Th2 response with a reduction in IFN-γ and an increase in IL-4, resulting in stimulation of antitumor immune response [38].

Despite the evidence confirming the recruitment of the immune system following cryotherapy, its use alone in the clinic is not enough to overcome the strong immunotolerance that tumors evolve. Therefore, there is a need to add a second immunotherapy to increase the immune response and overcome the immunotolerance. Some potential ways include the addition of immune checkpoints or inhibition of Tregs [32]. For example, the addition of CTLA-4 to cryotherapy produced systemic immunity and tumor rejection in a TRAMP C2 mouse prostate cancer model [39]. Animals treated with both therapies had slower growth and sometimes even rejection of a secondary tumor. The secondary tumors were highly infiltrated by CD4+ T cells and CD8+ T cells, and there was a significant increase in the ratio of intratumoral T effector cells to CD4 + FoxP3+ Tregs [39]. Another study combining cryotherapy with cyclophosphamide to inhibit Tregs resulted in a potent, systemic antitumor immunity in animals with established metastatic disease and 50% of the animals with metastatic disease were cured with the combination therapy [40].

Immunomodulatory Properties of Radiation Therapy

Preclinical studies and a clinical trial with a prostate cancer vaccine have demonstrated that radiation therapy (RT) and immunotherapy can be combined to enhance their mutual efficacies [41–43]. Unlike surgery, RT does not deplete the patient of tumor-specific antigens and allows for the induction of an effective immune response. Irradiated tumor cells are slowly cleared over time by APCs and tissue resident macrophages resulting in tumor-antigen processing and presentation [44]. Irradiation induces immunogenic cell death, which involves changes in the composition of the cell surface as well as the release of soluble mediators to stimulate the presentation of tumor antigens to T cells [33,45]. For example, irradiation of a colon carcinoma cell line CT26, leads to the translocation of cytosolic calreticulin to the cell membrane and provides a phagocytosis signal to DCs [46]. Irradiation also induces the secretion of HMGB1 by tumor cells, and this acts as a ligand for TLR 4, which subsequently leads to DC recruitment and activation [33]. As for its direct action on tumor cells, RT increases the cell surface expression of MHC class I molecules and amplifies the diversity of peptide antigen presentation by tumor cells [47]. It also increases the expression of Fas/CD95, which leads to an increased susceptibility of tumor cells to cytotoxic T lymphocyte (CTL) mediated cell killing [48]. Further, the level of IFN-γ in the tumor microenvironment and IFN-γ–inducible genes is increased following RT, and this leads to the inhibition of cellular proliferation, angiogenesis, an increase in caspase mediated cell killing, and an increase in MHC class I expression on nonirradiated tumor cells [49]. RT also affects the tumor vasculature leading to an increase in the expression of endothelial adhesion molecules: VCAM-1, ICAM-1, P-selectin, and E-selectin [50]. These observations suggest that a combination of RT and immunotherapy will have greater potential in improving the chances of success for the treatment of cancer when compared to monotherapy. RT has been tested in combination with DNA-based vaccines as well as using viral vectors, and these combinations lead to an increase in CTL infiltration into the tumors. Additionally, epitope spreading has been observed with RT combinations, as evidenced by the generation of CTLs directed toward other tumor-associated antigens than just the vaccine target antigen [51].

References

1 Mellman I, Coukos G, Dranoff G. Cancer immunotherapy comes of age. Nature. 2011;480(7378):480–9.

2 Herr HW, Morales A. History of bacillus Calmette-Guerin and bladder cancer: An immunotherapy success story. J Urol. 2008;179(1):53–6.

3 Gross L. Intradermal immunization of C3H mice against a sarcoma that originated in an animal of the same line. Cancer Res. 1943;3(5):326–33.

4 Jaffee EM, Pardoll DM. Murine tumor antigens: Is it worth the search? Curr Opin Immunol. 1996;8(5):622–7.

5 Schweizer MT, Drake CG. Immunotherapy for prostate cancer: Recent developments and future challenges. Cancer Metastasis Rev. 2014;33(2–3):641–55.

6 Kantoff PW, Higano CS, Shore ND, Berger ER, Small EJ, Penson DF, *et al.* Sipuleucel-T immunotherapy for castration-resistant prostate cancer. N Engl J Med. 2010;363(5):411–22.

7 Hodge JW, Schlom J, Donohue SJ, Tomaszewski JE, Wheeler CW, Levine BS, *et al.* A recombinant vaccinia virus expressing human prostate-specific antigen (PSA): Safety and immunogenicity in a non-human primate. Int J Cancer. 1995;63(2):231–7.

8 Shahabi V, Reyes-Reyes M, Wallecha A, Rivera S, Paterson Y, Maciag P. Development of a Listeria monocytogenes based vaccine against prostate cancer. Cancer Immunol Immunother. 2008;57(9):1301–13.

9 Kennedy JE. High-intensity focused ultrasound in the treatment of solid tumours. Nat Rev Cancer. 2005;5(4):321–7.

10 Jang HJ, Lee JY, Lee DH, Kim WH, Hwang JH. Current and future clinical applications of high-intensity focused ultrasound (HIFU) for pancreatic cancer. Gut Liver.4(Suppl. 1):S57–S61.

11 Wu F, Wang ZB, Lu P, Xu ZL, Chen WZ, Zhu H, *et al.* Activated anti-tumor immunity in cancer patients after high intensity focused ultrasound ablation. Ultrasound Med Biol. 2004;30(9):1217–22.

12 Lu P, Zhu XQ, Xu ZL, Zhou Q, Zhang J, Wu F. Increased infiltration of activated tumor-infiltrating lymphocytes after high intensity focused ultrasound ablation of human breast cancer. Surgery. 2009;145(3):286–93.

13 Hu Z, Yang XY, Liu Y, Sankin GN, Pua EC, Morse MA, *et al.* Investigation of HIFU-induced anti-tumor immunity in a murine tumor model. J Transl Med. 2007;5:34.

14 Liu F, Hu Z, Qiu L, Hui C, Li C, Zhong P, *et al.* Boosting high-intensity focused ultrasound-induced anti-tumor immunity using a sparse-scan strategy that can more effectively promote dendritic cell maturation. J Transl Med.8:7.

15 Xing Y, Lu X, Pua EC, Zhong P. The effect of high intensity focused ultrasound treatment on metastases in a murine melanoma model. Biochem Biophys Res Commun. 2008;375(4):645–50.

16 Deng J, Zhang Y, Feng J, Wu F. Dendritic cells loaded with ultrasound-ablated tumour induce in vivo specific antitumour immune responses. Ultrasound Med Biol. 2010;36(3):441–8.

17 Zhang Y, Deng J, Feng J, Wu F. Enhancement of antitumor vaccine in ablated hepatocellular carcinoma by high-intensity focused ultrasound. World J Gastroenterol. 2010;16(28):3584–91.

18 Chakravarty PK, Alfieri A, Thomas EK, Beri V, Tanaka KE, Vikram B, *et al.* Flt3-ligand administration after radiation therapy prolongs survival in a murine model of metastatic lung cancer. Cancer Res. 1999;59(24):6028–32.

19 Chakravarty PK, Guha C, Alfieri A, Beri V, Niazova Z, Deb NJ, *et al.* Flt3L therapy following localized tumor irradiation generates long-term protective immune response in metastatic lung cancer: Its implication in designing a vaccination strategy. Oncology. 2006;70(4):245–54.

20 Demaria S, Kawashima N, Yang AM, Devitt ML, Babb JS, Allison JP, *et al.* Immune-mediated inhibition of metastases

after treatment with local radiation and CTLA-4 blockade in a mouse model of breast cancer. Clin Cancer Res. 2005; 11(2 Pt 1):728–34.

21 Demaria S, Santori FR, Ng B, Liebes L, Formenti SC, Vukmanovic S. Select forms of tumor cell apoptosis induce dendritic cell maturation. J Leukoc Biol. 2005;77(3):361–8.

22 den Brok MH, Sutmuller RP, van der Voort R, Bennink EJ, Figdor CG, Ruers TJ, *et al.* In situ tumor ablation creates an antigen source for the generation of antitumor immunity. Cancer Res. 2004;64(11): 4024–9.

23 Hodge JW, Guha C, Neefjes J, Gulley JL. Synergizing radiation therapy and immunotherapy for curing incurable cancers. Opportunities and challenges. Oncology. 2008;22(9):1064–70; discussion 75, 80–1, 84.

24 Ferrara TA, Hodge JW, Gulley JL. Combining radiation and immunotherapy for synergistic antitumor therapy. Curr Opin Mol Ther. 2009;11(1):37–42.

25 Saito K, Araki K, Reddy N, Guang W, O'Malley BW, Jr., Li D. Enhanced local dendritic cell activity and tumor-specific immunoresponse in combined radiofrequency ablation and interleukin-2 for the treatment of human head and neck cancer in a murine orthotopic model. Head Neck. 2011; Mar; 33(3):350–67

26 Habibi M, Kmieciak M, Graham L, Morales JK, Bear HD, Manjili MH. Radiofrequency thermal ablation of breast tumors combined with intralesional administration of IL-7 and IL-15 augments anti-tumor immune responses and inhibits tumor development and metastasis. Breast Cancer Res Treat. 2009;114(3):423–31.

27 Fagnoni FF, Zerbini A, Pelosi G, Missale G. Combination of radiofrequency ablation and immunotherapy. Front Biosci. 2008;13:369–81.

28 Zou W. Immunosuppressive networks in the tumour environment and their therapeutic relevance. Nat Rev Cancer. 2005;5(4):263–74.

29 Baust JG, Gage AA. The molecular basis of cryosurgery. BJU Int. 2005;95(9):1187–91.

30 Sabel MS. Cryo-immunology: A review of the literature and proposed mechanisms for stimulatory versus suppressive immune responses. Cryobiology. 2009;58(1):1–11.

31 Bishoff JT, Chen RB, Lee BR, Chan DY, Huso D, Rodriguez R, *et al.* Laparoscopic renal cryoablation: Acute and long-term clinical, radiographic, and pathologic effects in an animal model and application in a clinical trial. J Endourol 1999;13(4):233–9.

32 Sidana A. Cancer immunotherapy using tumor cryoablation. Immunotherapy. 2014;6(1):85–93.

33 Apetoh L, Ghiringhelli F, Tesniere A, Obeid M, Ortiz C, Criollo A, *et al.* Toll-like receptor 4-dependent contribution of the immune system to anticancer chemotherapy and radiotherapy. Nat Med. 2007;13(9):1050–9.

34 Soanes WA, Ablin RJ, Gonder MJ. Remission of metastatic lesions following cryosurgery in prostatic cancer: Immunologic considerations. J Urol. 1970;104(1):154–9.

35 Blackwood CE, Cooper IS. Response of experimental tumor systems to cryosurgery. Cryobiology. 1972;9(6):508–15.

36 Bagley DH, Faraci RP, Marrone JC, Beazley RM. Lymphocyte mediated cytotoxicity after cryosurgery of a murine sarcoma. J Surg Res. 1974;17(6):404–6.

37 den Brok MH, Sutmuller RP, Nierkens S, Bennink EJ, Frielink C, Toonen LW, *et al.* Efficient loading of dendritic cells following cryo and radiofrequency ablation in combination with immune modulation induces anti-tumour immunity. Br J Cancer. 2006; 95(7):896–905.

38 Matin SF, Sharma P, Gill IS, Tannenbaum C, Hobart MG, Novick AC, *et al.* Immunological response to renal cryoablation in an in vivo orthotopic renal cell carcinoma murine model. J Urol. 2010;183(1):333–8.

39 Waitz R, Solomon SB, Petre EN, Trumble AE, Fasso M, Norton L, *et al.* Potent induction of tumor immunity by combining tumor cryoablation with anti-CTLA-4 therapy. Cancer Res. 2012;72(2):430–9.

40 Levy MY, Sidana A, Chowdhury WH, Solomon SB, Drake CG, Rodriguez R, *et al.* Cyclophosphamide unmasks an antimetastatic effect of local tumor cryoablation. J Pharmacol Exp Ther. 2009;330(2):596–601.

41 Demaria S, Bhardwaj N, McBride WH, Formenti SC. Combining radiotherapy and immunotherapy: A revived partnership. Int J Radiat Oncol Biol Phys. 2005;63(3):655–66.

42 Hodge JW, Guha C, Neefjes J, Gulley JL. Synergizing radiation therapy and immunotherapy for curing incurable cancers. Opportunities and challenges. Oncology (Williston Park). 2008;22(9):1064–70; discussion 75, 80–1, 84.

43 Kantoff PW, Schuetz TJ, Blumenstein BA, Glode LM, Bilhartz DL, Wyand M, *et al.* Overall survival analysis of a phase II randomized controlled trial of a Poxviral-based PSA-targeted immunotherapy in metastatic castration-resistant prostate cancer. J Clin Oncol. 2010;28(7):1099–105.

44 Sauter B, Albert ML, Francisco L, Larsson M, Somersan S, Bhardwaj N. Consequences of cell death: Exposure to necrotic tumor cells, but not primary tissue cells or apoptotic cells, induces the maturation of immunostimulatory dendritic cells. J Exp Med. 2000;191(3):423–34.

45 Kroemer G, Galluzzi L, Kepp O, Zitvogel L. Immunogenic cell death in cancer therapy. Annu Rev Immunol. 2013;31:51–72.

46 Obeid M, Tesniere A, Ghiringhelli F, Fimia GM, Apetoh L, Perfettini JL, *et al.* Calreticulin exposure dictates the immunogenicity of cancer cell death. Nat Med. 2007;13(1):54–61.

47 Reits EA, Hodge JW, Herberts CA, Groothuis TA, Chakraborty M, Wansley EK, *et al.* Radiation modulates the peptide repertoire, enhances MHC class I expression, and induces successful antitumor immunotherapy. J Exp Med. 2006;203(5):1259–71.

48 Chakraborty M, Abrams SI, Camphausen K, Liu K, Scott T, Coleman CN, *et al.* Irradiation of tumor cells up-regulates Fas and enhances CTL lytic activity and CTL adoptive immunotherapy. J Immunol. 2003;170(12):6338–47.

49 Burnette BC, Liang H, Lee Y, Chlewicki L, Khodarev NN, Weichselbaum RR, *et al.* The efficacy of radiotherapy relies upon induction of type i interferon-dependent innate and adaptive immunity. Cancer Res. 2011;71(7):2488–96.

50 Lugade AA, Sorensen EW, Gerber SA, Moran JP, Frelinger JG, Lord EM. Radiation-induced IFN-gamma production within the tumor microenvironment influences antitumor immunity. J Immunol. 2008;180(5):3132–9.

51 Chakraborty M, Abrams SI, Coleman CN, Camphausen K, Schlom J, Hodge JW. External beam radiation of tumors alters phenotype of tumor cells to render them susceptible to vaccine-mediated T-cell killing. Cancer Res. 2004;64(12):4328–37.

4

Computed Tomography of Urologic Malignancies: The Role of MDCT in Renal Cell Carcinoma and Transitional Cell Carcinoma

Siva P. Raman, MD, and Elliot K. Fishman, MD

Department of Radiology, John Hopkins University, Baltimore, MD, USA

Introduction

There have been tremendous advancements in multidetector computed tomography (MDCT) scanner technology over the last 10 years, allowing dramatic improvements in both spatial and temporal resolution. As a result, it is now possible to perform studies nearly devoid of motion or respiratory artifacts and to consistently acquire images at peak enhancement. Accordingly, despite the development and advancement of radiologic modalities such as magnetic resonance imaging (MRI), positron emission tomography (PET), and other molecular imaging techniques, MDCT has maintained its primacy in the diagnosis and staging of urologic malignancies, most importantly renal cell carcinoma (RCC) and transitional cell carcinoma (TCC). Although other modalities may have an ancillary role to play in the imaging of these malignancies, MDCT remains the first-line imaging tool for lesion identification, characterization, and staging.

However, the diagnosis and staging of these two urologic malignancies is not merely a function of scanner technology, but it also requires a detailed understanding of proper protocol design, as well as an appreciation of the spectrum of different appearances these malignancies can take. This chapter will begin with a discussion of proper MDCT protocol design for the evaluation of the urinary tract, followed by a detailed discussion of the imaging characteristics of each of these two urologic tumors and several other tumors in the differential diagnosis.

MDCT Protocol Design

When constructing a MDCT protocol for the evaluation of a patient with a suspected urologic malignancy, the goal is twofold: maximize the enhancement and conspicuity of any potential solid RCC and maximally distend the intrarenal collecting systems, ureters, and bladder to improve the conspicuity of TCCs. Given that a sizeable percentage of patients with both TCC and RCC will present with macroscopic hematuria, and that the radiologist may not be prospectively aware which tumor is more likely, any MDCT protocol must be designed to optimize diagnosis of *both* tumors. Of course, although any imaging protocol must be comprehensive enough to diagnose both categories of tumors, our increasing awareness of the dangers of MDCT-related ionizing radiation make it necessary to acquire only the imaging phases that *are absolutely necessary* so as to avoid unnecessary radiation dose to the patient.

Management of Urologic Cancer: Focal Therapy and Tissue Preservation, First Edition.
Edited by Mark P. Schoenberg and Kara L. Watts.
© 2017 John Wiley & Sons Ltd. Published 2017 by John Wiley & Sons Ltd.

Prior to the administration of contrast, a set of noncontrast images is typically acquired through the upper abdomen, focused only on the kidneys, Given that the most common cause of hematuria in daily practice is nephrolithiasis, the noncontrast images maximize stone detection (because of the lack of contrast in the renal parenchyma). Just as importantly, when confronted with an indeterminate renal lesion, the noncontrast images serve as an invaluable baseline, allowing the radiologist to determine whether a mass is intrinsically hyperdense (i.e., hyperdense or hemorrhagic cyst), or alternatively, is truly an enhancing solid renal mass. Because of radiation dose concerns, there is little reason to needlessly extend these noncontrast images beyond the upper abdomen.

Arterial phase images are then acquired through the entirety of the abdomen and pelvis, typically at 30–40 seconds following the rapid injection of intravenous contrast (100–120 mL of either Omnipaque 350 or Visipaque-320). This set of images is absolutely the most critical for detection of most RCCs, particularly the clear-cell variant because hypervascular lesions tend to be most conspicuous on the early phase images. Moreover, given that many TCCs also tend to show some degree of hypervascularity on early phase imaging, the arterial phase can be valuable for diagnosing subtle ureteral and bladder lesions, which may end up obscured by surrounding excreted contrast on the delayed phase images. Notably, the arterial phase images should extend through the *entirety* of the abdomen and pelvis, allowing imaging through the ureter and bladder, both of which should be filled with unopacified urine (rather than contrast) in this phase of imaging. Accordingly, it can sometimes be easier to identify subtle urothelial thickening or filling defects on the arterial phase images (because of the juxtaposition of an avidly enhancing tumor with the low-density urine), rather than the delayed phase, even though the delayed phase images have traditionally been considered the most important phase for TCC detection.

In patients older than age 50, a separate set of venous phase images are often acquired at roughly 60–70 seconds after the injection of intravenous contrast. Although the arterial phase images (and the delayed phase images as well) are certainly much more sensitive for the majority of renal masses, there are rare occasions when a renal mass is more conspicuous on the venous phase images, and the addition of this phase does increase sensitivity for subtle lesions. Moreover, the venous phase is the best imaging phase for the evaluation of the parenchymal organs of the upper abdomen, maximizing sensitivity for liver metastases or locoregional lymphadenopathy, while also allowing evaluation of the renal veins and inferior vena cava (IVC) in cases of RCC with tumor thrombus. Although we typically include venous phase images in older patients (older than 40 years of age) at our institution, this phase is typically not acquired when imaging younger patients presenting with hematuria. In younger patients, the added benefit of this phase is likely outweighed by the increased radiation dose, particularly in light of this demographic group's markedly lower risk of malignancy.

Finally, any renal mass protocol must include delayed excretory phase images, which not only provide opacification of the upper urinary tract (allowing the identification of urothelial filling defects and thickening that might herald the presence of a TCC), but also serve as another quite sensitive phase for the detection of RCC. Many RCCs (particularly clear-cell variants) are hypervascular and "wash-out" on the delayed phase, appearing conspicuously hypodense on the delayed phase images (nicely juxtaposed against the uniform nephrographic phase enhancement of the kidney in the delayed phase). Moreover, small subtle hypervascular RCCs in the arterial phase can be easy to overlook if they are located at the corticomedullary junction, but they are often easier to perceive in the delayed phase. At our institution, delayed phase images are typically acquired at 4 minutes after contrast injection. Acquiring these images earlier often results in suboptimal opacification of the urinary tract, but waiting longer can result in the pooling of dense contrast in the collecting system, thus potentially obscuring pathology as a result of beam-hardening or streak artifact.

It should be noted that there are several different protocols available for the acquisition of excretory phase images, each of which has its own benefits and downsides in terms of image quality and radiation dose: *Single-bolus technique* is by far the most commonly used protocol in radiology practices across the country and is the simplest to implement. A single full dose of intravenous contrast (typically 100–120 mL of Omnipaque-350 or Visipaque-320) is administered, followed by the acquisition of separate arterial, venous, and delayed phases. This technique maximizes opacification and distension of the collecting systems and ureters, thus increasing sensitivity for TCC. Moreover, because separate arterial, venous, and delayed phases are acquired, RCC sensitivity is also maximized. Of course, given that this protocol involves the acquisition of three separate contrast phases, the radiation dose will consequently be higher. At our institution, we have chosen this protocol for daily use because we believe that the slightly higher radiation dose to the patient is outweighed by the improved sensitivity and image quality of this method [1]. The *split-bolus technique* was designed to reduce the radiation dose associated with the traditional single-bolus technique by reducing the number of acquired postcontrast phases. In this method, the administered contrast dose is *split* into two, with 50 mL of contrast injected initially, followed by a second contrast bolus of 80 mL administered 5 minutes later, with the subsequent acquisition of combined nephrographic and delayed images at 7 minutes. By combining two phases into one, this protocol does, in fact, reduce radiation dose considerably. However, it should be noted that only 50 mL (out of the total of 130 mL administered) is

excreted into the collecting system at the time of image acquisition at 7 minutes, resulting in considerably less distension of the collecting system and ureters (particularly the distal ureters), potentially reducing sensitivity for TCC. In addition, by reducing the number of acquired phases, sensitivity for RCC is also likely to be less robust [2,3]. The *triple bolus technique* rarely, if ever, is used in practice and involves splitting the contrast dose into three separate boluses, with the acquisition of a single combined corticomedullary-nephrographic-excretory phase (usually at roughly 8–9 minutes). By combining three phases into one, this method substantially decreases radiation dose to the patient. However, this method provides *very* poor opacification of the collecting systems and ureters, and the lack of discrete arterial, venous, and delayed phases potentially reduces sensitivity for RCC as well [4,5].

The design of a proper MDCT protocol can also vary depending on the utilization of a number of other ancillary techniques, each of which is designed to maximize distension of the upper urinary tract.

- *Abdominal compression*: This method entails placing a compression band across the upper abdomen, thereby "trapping" the contrast in the intrarenal collecting systems and upper ureters, thus increasing distension. Accordingly, the use of an abdominal compression band necessitates acquisition of a separate set of excretory phase images once the band has been released to distend the mid and distal ureters. This method can be painful and cumbersome in patients who have undergone prior surgery, may be contraindicated in patients with abdominal pathology, and can be difficult to use in patients who are obese. Moreover, at least one study by Caoli *et al.* found no significant improvement in distension with the use of a compression band [6].
- *Intravenous diuretics*: A small dose of IV LASIX (usually as little as 10 mg) has been

shown to substantially improve distension of the collecting system. Moreover, LASIX can also dilute the contrast in the collecting system and potentially improve lesion conspicuity by reducing beam-hardening artifacts. Nevertheless, these benefits must be weighed against the need for nursing and physician staff to take into account allergies, blood pressure fluctuations, and a patient's underlying renal function, and the routine administration of LASIX can potentially interfere with daily workflow [7].

- *Prone positioning* was once thought to improve upper urinary tract opacification, but studies have shown that supine positioning may actually be superior, without the pain and discomfort that can be associated with lying in the prone position for several minutes.

- *Oral hydration*: Similar to intravenous LASIX, oral hydration improves distension and opacification of the collecting system and ureters, while also diluting the contrast within the collecting system and reducing beam hardening and streak artifacts. In addition, if the patient is instructed not to urinate before the study, oral hydration can result in increased distension of bladder, potentially improving identification of bladder lesions. A study by Kawamoto *et al.* showed that oral hydration (with only 500 mL of water) was essentially equivalent to intravenous LASIX and a number of other ancillary techniques (without any disruption to daily workflow) [8]. Accordingly, at our own institution, we rely solely on oral hydration and have moved away from using the other ancillary techniques previously described [9].

Three-Dimensional Reconstructions

Although the interpretation of MDCT data sets has traditionally been contingent solely on a review of the source axial images and coronal/sagittal multiplanar reformats, three-dimensional (3D) reconstruction techniques have proven to be increasingly important for lesion detection and characterization in the urinary tract, as well as providing preoperative guidance for surgeons. At our institution, source axial images are acquired at 0.75-mm collimation and are subsequently reconstructed into axial 3-mm images for routine image review, while coronal and sagittal multiplanar reformations are automatically reconstructed directly at the computed tomography (CT) scanner console. The source axial images are then sent to an independent workstation, where two sets of 3D reconstructions are created: *Maximum intensity projection (MIP)* imaging entails the selection of the highest attenuation voxels in a data set and their projection into a two-dimensional image. MIP reconstructions have proven valuable for illustrating the high attenuation vasculature and also nicely demonstrate the opacified collecting systems and ureters on the delayed excretory phase images. Subtle asymmetric collecting system distension, obstruction or destruction of a calyx by tumor, sites of transition or stricturing in the urinary tract, and subtle urothelial filling defects can all be much easier to perceive using this reconstruction technique. *Volume rendered (VR)* imaging is a more complex technique that involves assigning a color and transparency to each voxel in a data set depending on its attenuation and relationship to other adjacent voxels, and then projecting this information into a true 3D display. VR images can accentuate subtle sites of urothelial thickening or abnormal enhancement that may not be readily visible on the source axial images and can also accentuate subtle renal mass lesions [10]. Moreover, VR images maintain the true 3D relationships of the kidneys and its vasculature to surrounding organs/structures and are thus ideal in the preoperative planning of almost any invasive procedure.

Neoplasms of the Intrarenal Collecting Systems, Ureters, and Bladder

Transitional Cell Carcinoma

Urothelial malignancies make up the vast majority of neoplasms involving the intrarenal collecting system, ureters, and bladder, with more than 90% of these malignancies representing TCCs. In rare cases, squamous cell carcinomas and adenocarcinomas can also arise from the urothelium. In the vast majority of cases, these tumors occur in men older than age 60, with other risk factors including smoking, analgesic use, phenacetin, radiation, aniline dyes, and a variety of other chemical carcinogens [9,11]. Regardless of their location, TCCs have a strong tendency for multiplicity, metachronous lesions, and recurrence, features that must be kept in mind when interpreting studies with a potential TCC. The presence of a single lesion must, by necessity, result in a careful appraisal for other lesions. The most common presentation for patients with a TCC, regardless of location, is gross hematuria, and any patient with this history must undergo MDCT for evaluation of the upper urinary tract, as well as cystoscopy for evaluation of the bladder. Notably, microscopic hematuria confers a much lesser risk of malignancy and is present in many patients who are asymptomatic. Thus, the decision to perform MDCT or cystoscopy in this population is a matter of more debate and is largely contingent on individual patient risk factors.

When evaluating the intrarenal collecting systems and ureters for a potential TCC, a combination of direct and indirect signs must be used to surmise the presence of a tumor. Clearly, the presence of a discrete urothelial filling defect or mass is strongly suspicious for the presence of a malignancy, although such a finding is relatively rare (Figures 4.1 and 4.2). Small lesions, in particular, can be quite difficult to prospectively identify because beam-hardening artifact from contrast in the collecting system can

obscure subtle filling defects. Urothelial thickening is the other major direct finding that should suggest the presence of a tumor. Notably, when confronted with bilateral, diffuse urothelial thickening, this is much more likely to be either infectious or inflammatory in nature. Alternatively, focal urothelial thickening, regardless of its location, is suspicious for malignancy and should prompt further evaluation. Urothelial thickening, in particular, can sometimes be easier to detect on the arterial phase images because beam-hardening artifact from intraluminal contrast can obscure subtle sites of thickening [12–18].

Although both of these direct signs (urothelial thickening, filling defect) are important, a variety of secondary signs can be equally valuable, particularly when confronted by small lesions that are not readily visible. In particular, careful attention should be paid to any sites of asymmetric collecting system distension, whether it is asymmetric hydronephrosis, hydroureter, or even focal distension of a calyx. In such cases, the distended segments of the collecting system should be followed to the site of transition or change in caliber, and an obstructing lesion should be searched for at this site. Another important secondary sign is urothelial hyperenhancement.

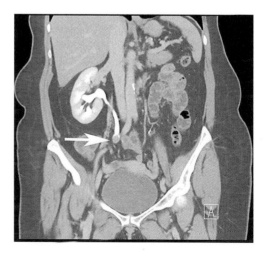

Figure 4.1 Coronal MDCT image in the excretory phase demonstrates an obstructing transitional cell carcinoma (*arrow*) in the right mid ureter resulting in upstream hydronephrosis and hydroureter.

(a)

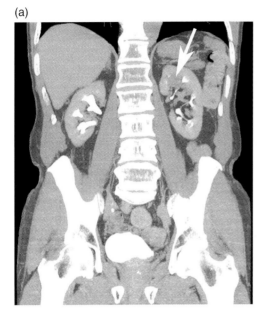

(b)

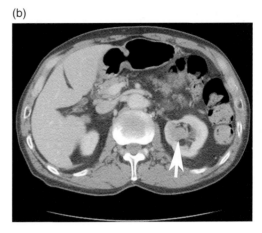

Figure 4.2 Axial (a) and coronal (b) MDCT images demonstrate a subtle mass (*arrow*) in the upper pole kidney, representing a transitional cell carcinoma.

Although TCCs have not traditionally been thought of as hypervascular tumors, they do tend to be fairly avidly enhancing on the arterial phase images. Whereas diffuse hyperenhancement is often on the basis of infection, instrumentation, or urothelial inflammation, focal hyperenhancement should always be considered abnormal and should prompt careful evaluation for a tumor. Finally, TCCs, regardless of location, have a tendency to calcify, and any calcification along the urothelium should raise concern, particularly when seen in association with focal urothelial thickening or nodularity.

Interestingly, although MDCT has primarily been seen as a tool for evaluating the upper urinary tract, MDCT is better than commonly thought for evaluation of the bladder. While no one would argue that cystoscopy should be displaced as the primary diagnostic test for identification of bladder tumors, MDCT can perform reasonably well, particularly when proper CT urography technique is used (i.e., good distension of the bladder with multiphase imaging). Several studies have shown reasonably good results for MDCT,

including a study by Turney *et al.* that compared MDCT with cystoscopy in a group of patients with hematuria and found a sensitivity and specificity for MDCT of 93% and 99%, respectively [19–21]. Of course, the sensitivity and specificity of MDCT in such patients is highly contingent on the protocols and techniques used, but such studies do emphasize that the radiologist might be able to diagnose a sizeable percentage of bladder tumors if careful attention is paid to the bladder in every case. Moreover, in our own experience, bladder cancers are not infrequently identified incidentally on MDCT, and such cases will undoubtedly be missed if subtle findings are not appreciated [22].

The imaging findings of a TCC in the bladder are not dissimilar to those in the upper urinary tract, with the most reliable findings including a focal nodule/mass or focal urothelial thickening (Figures 4.3–4.5) [23,24]. In our experience, although the delayed images have traditionally been considered the most important for detection of lesions in the bladder, subtle or small lesions can easily be missed in this phase

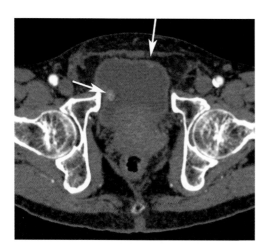

Figure 4.3 Axial arterial phase MDCT demonstrates two tiny hyperenhancing nodules (*arrows*) in the bladder, representing small bladder transitional cell carcinomas.

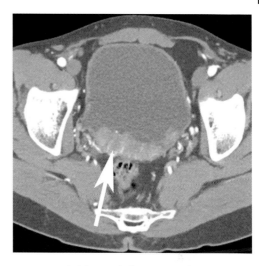

Figure 4.4 Axial arterial phase MDCT demonstrates a markedly hypervascular mass (*arrow*) in the posterior bladder, representing a large transitional cell carcinoma.

(a)

(b)

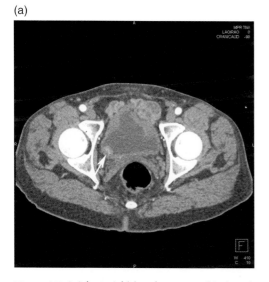

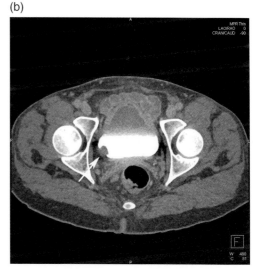

Figure 4.5 Axial arterial (a) and excretory (b) phase images demonstrate a small transitional cell carcinoma (*arrow*) in the posterior aspect of the right bladder.

because of obscuration by surrounding dense contrast. As a result, the arterial phase images can often be more helpful, particularly as bladder TCCs, like TCCs in the upper urinary tract, tend to avidly enhance on the arterial phase images. Kim *et al.* found that bladder tumors tended to show peak enhancement (up to 105 Hounsfield units) early, at roughly 60 seconds, before slowly "washing out" over time [25,26]. Accordingly, if the bladder if effectively distended with good oral hydration before the study (and the patient is instructed to avoid urination until the study is completed), the arterial phase images should be the primary focus when searching for a bladder TCC. Similarly, a careful search should be made for calcification (which should be distinguished from nondependent bladder stones), and such calcifications are much easier to identify (particularly in the dependent portion of the bladder) when the bladder is not filled with radiodense contrast material.

Other Less Common Tumors of the Collecting Systems, Ureters, and Bladder

- *Lymphoma:* Lymphoma can rarely involve the intrarenal collecting system and the ureters, often infiltrating along the margins of the urothelium. Like lymphoma elsewhere in the body, these tend to be "soft" tumors that result in little mass effect or obstruction. Accordingly, although these lesions can superficially mimic TCCs in their appearance, they will conspicuously not result in hydronephrosis or hydroureter. Moreover, lymphoma of the collecting system is usually associated with significant lymphadenopathy elsewhere in the abdomen.
- *Metastases:* Metastatic disease to the collecting systems or bladder is quite rare and based on the MDCT appearance alone, is usually not readily distinguishable from

a primary TCC. The most common tumors to metastasize to the collecting systems include breast cancer, gastrointestinal tract malignancies, prostate cancer, and cervical cancer (Figure 4.6). In such cases, the patient's history of a primary malignancy should be the key to suggesting the correct diagnosis.

- *Leiomyoma:* Benign tumors of the bladder, leiomyomas are intramural lesions arising from the smooth muscle layer of the urothelium. Although they can arise anywhere along the course of the urinary tract, they are most common in the bladder. They are almost always smoothly marginated and will often be mildly hyperenhancing on the arterial phase images because of their smooth muscle component. For all practical purposes, these lesions are not reliably distinguishable from a TCC based on the MDCT appearance alone.
- *Extra-adrenal pheochomocytoma or paraganglioma:* Rare tumors with a characteristic clinical presentation (i.e., episodic hypertension during micturition), paragangliomas of the bladder have a unique appearance on MDCT. These lesions tend to be intramural in location, with a smoothly marginated contour, and most importantly, are profoundly hypervascular on arterial

(a)

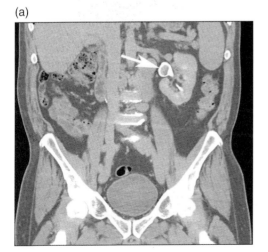

(b)

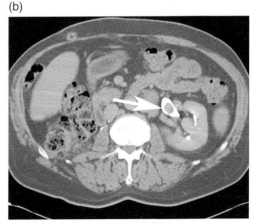

Figure 4.6 Coronal (a) and axial (b) excretory phase images demonstrate a nodular filling defect (*arrow*) in the renal pelvis. This was found to represent a metastasis from the patient's known renal cell carcinoma.

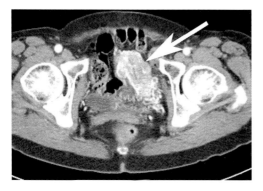

Figure 4.7 Axial arterial phase image demonstrates a profoundly hypervascular mass (*arrow*) in the left anterior bladder, found to represent a paraganglioma.

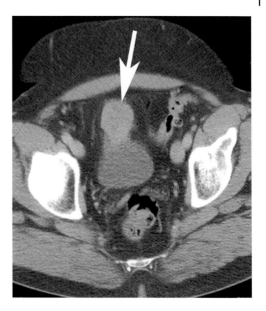

Figure 4.8 Axial MDCT image demonstrates a urachal adenocarcinoma (*arrow*) arising from near the bladder dome anteriorly.

phase imaging, routinely demonstrating Hounsfield attenuation values over 100, much higher than TCCs (Figure 4.7). When confronted with a characteristic clinical history or a patient with suggestive biochemical abnormalities, a lesion with such an appearance should be strongly suggestive of this diagnosis.

- *Adenocarcinoma of the urachus:* Adenocarcinomas of the bladder are quite rare, accounting for less than 1% of all bladder tumors, and of these, up to 40% arise from the urachus. These tumors characteristically arise in the midline near the dome of the bladder, in the expected location of the urachus, which runs from the bladder to the umbilicus (Figure 4.8). These lesions have a unique predisposition for peripheral calcification, often with solid and cystic components.

Solid Renal Parenchymal Lesions

Renal Cell Carcinoma

The identification of a solid, enhancing renal mass requires a MDCT examination with noncontrast imaging and at least one postcontrast phase (arterial, venous, or delayed). In practice, however, the inclusion of multiple postcontrast phases improves lesion detection and sensitivity because any given solid renal mass may be more or less conspicuous on a given phase. Most RCCs (the majority of which are clear-cell RCCs) tend to be maximally conspicuous on the arterial and delayed phase images, although it is not uncommon to intermittently be confronted with a tumor only visible on the venous or delayed images. The inclusion of noncontrast images is critical because measurement of Hounsfield attenuation values within a lesion to quantify enhancement may be necessary in equivocal cases, where a hyperdense or hemorrhagic cyst cannot be differentiated from a hypoenhancing solid renal mass (such as a papillary or chromophobe RCC) by visual analysis alone. In general, any lesion which enhances more than 20 Hounsfield units is considered to be solid, whereas lesions enhancing less than 10 Hounsfield units can be confidently characterized as benign. Lesions showing changes in Hounsfield attenuation of 10–20 Hounsfield units are considered equivocal, perhaps deserving of follow-up, although the vast majority of such lesions are benign.

Once a renal mass is identified and determined to be solid, both enhancement characteristics and lesion morphology may help differentiate the different subtypes of RCC, namely clear-cell RCC (the most common), papillary RCC, and chromophobe RCC. From an enhancement perspective, clear-cell RCCs tend to be avidly hypervascular, with Hounsfield attenuation values usually over 100 in the arterial phase, high tumor-to-cortex enhancement ratios, and rapid washout in the delayed phase (>40%; Figure 4.9) [27–30]. Accordingly, given this avid vascularity, it is not surprising that most clear-cell RCCs are most conspicuous in the arterial phase of imaging. Papillary RCCs, alternatively, are relatively *hypovascular*, with different authors reporting Hounsfield attenuation values of 75 or less in the corticomedullary phase, low tumor-to-cortex enhancement ratios, and a lack of washout in the delayed phase (Figure 4.10). This relative lack of enhancement or washout presents a unique challenge on MDCT because not only are these tumors relatively less conspicuous in any phase of imaging, but they are also not uncommonly mistaken for hyperdense cysts (particularly on routine scans where only one phase of imaging is acquired). Finally, chromophobe RCCs, the least common of the three major variants, tend to show enhancement and attenuation values somewhere in between the clear-cell and papillary variants, with intermediate tumor-to-cortex values and mild washout (roughly 30%; Figure 4.11) [27–32]. Morphologically, all three subtypes can demonstrate calcification, although calcification is most common in the clear-cell subtype. Clear-cells RCCs, particularly when larger, tend to be relatively heterogeneous, especially with more aggressive subtypes, whereas papillary RCCs tend to be more homogeneous in appearance. Chromophobe RCCs most often are homogeneous but also have a unique predisposition for developing a central scar [33–38]. Overall, although these individual morphologic and enhancement characteristics of each tumor type may be *suggestive* of a histologic diagnosis, there is a great deal of overlap, and accurate prospective diagnosis based on imaging features alone is *not possible* at this point in time.

Oncocytoma

Renal oncocytomas represent 3–7% of all renal masses and are benign lesions that arise from the collecting duct epithelium. Unfortunately, there is no reliable means on MDCT (or any other imaging modality) to confidently distinguish oncocytomas from clear-cell RCCs. Although oncocytomas do have a tendency to demonstrate homogenous enhancement with a central stellate scar, as

(a)

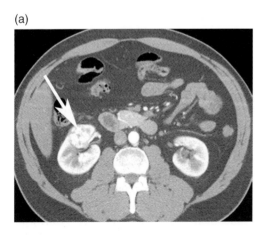

(b)

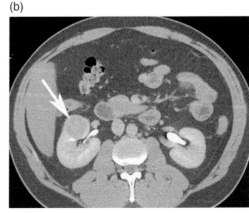

Figure 4.9 Axial arterial (a) and excretory (b) phase images demonstrate a markedly hypervascular mass in the right kidney which washes out on the delayed images, in keeping with a clear-cell renal cell carcinoma.

(a)

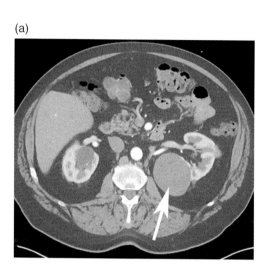

(b)

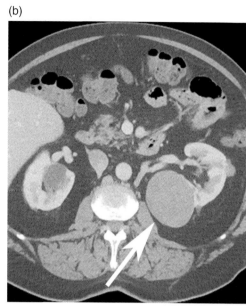

Figure 4.10 Axial arterial (a) and venous (b) phase images demonstrate a left sided renal mass (*arrow*), which demonstrates no significant change in enhancement between the two phases, and which enhanced only 25 Hounsfield units compared to the noncontrast images (not shown). This was found to be a papillary renal cell carcinoma.

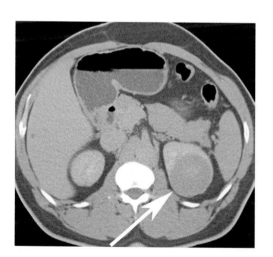

Figure 4.11 Axial MDCT image demonstrates a homogenous, hypovascular renal mass (*arrow*) found to represent a chromophobe renal cell carcinoma.

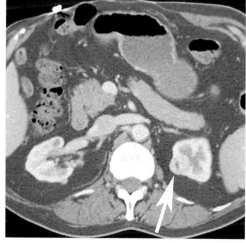

Figure 4.12 Axial arterial phase MDCT demonstrates small hypervascular mass (*arrow*) with a central scar in the left kidney found to represent a small oncocytoma.

opposed to the more heterogeneous enhancement of clear-cell RCCs, there is too much overlap for any morphologic feature to be a useful discriminator (Figures 4.12–4.14) [39].

Enhancement characteristics may be mildly useful, with a recent study by Raman *et al.* suggesting that clear-cell RCCs demonstrated slightly greater degrees of enhancement on

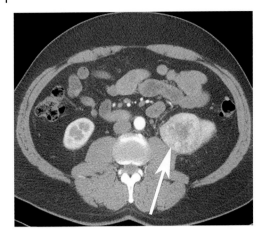

Figure 4.13 Axial arterial phase MDCT demonstrates a hypervascular mass (*arrow*) with a central scar in the left kidney found to represent a oncocytoma.

which a renal mass shows two discrete regions of enhancement, one of which shows greater enhancement in the corticomedullary phase and the other of which shows greater enhancement on the excretory phase [39,41–43]. The reliability of this finding has been debated in a number of articles, and its wider applicability in daily practice is debatable at best.

Angiomyolipomas

Renal angiomyolipomas (AMLs) are the most common type of benign renal mass, and the vast majority of these benign lesions can be easily identified by the presence of macroscopic fat (typically −10 to −40 Hounsfield units). Although most AMLs will demonstrate some amount of internal fat on MDCT, 4.5% of all AMLs do not demonstrate any appreciable fat on imaging (so called "lipid-poor angiomyolipomas") and consist of predominantly muscle and vascular components. Several attempts have been made to differentiate RCCs from lipid-poor AMLs, including histogram analysis of individual pixels within the lesion to search for microscopic fat, and morphologic analyses, which have suggested AMLs are more likely to have an "angular interface" with the renal cortex, a "hypodense rim" at the margins of the mass,

both the corticomedullary and excretory phases compared to oncocytomas, but the differences in enhancement were too small to reliably discriminate the two tumor types with any confidence [40]. In general, oncocytomas, like clear-cell RCCs, are hypervascular tumors that tend to be most conspicuous in the arterial phase of imaging. Some studies have suggested that oncocytomas may be more likely than other renal tumor types to demonstrate "segmental enhancement inversion," a phenomenon in

(a)

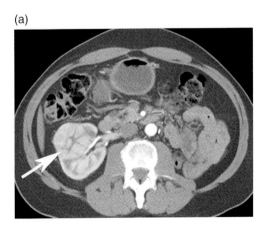

(b)

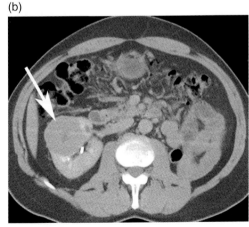

Figure 4.14 Axial arterial (b) and excretory (b) phase MDCT images demonstrate a hypervascular mass (*arrow*) with a central scar in the right kidney and rapid washout out on the delayed image, found to represent a oncocytoma.

(a)

(b)

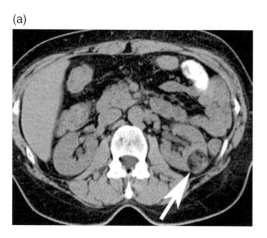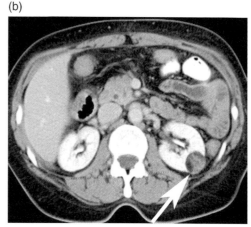

Figure 4.15 Axial noncontrast (a) and post-contrast (b) demonstrate a fat-containing angiomyolipoma (*arrow*) in the left kidney.

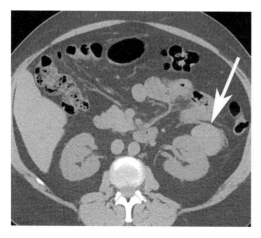

Figure 4.16 Axial noncontrast MDCT image demonstrates a hyperdense (Hounsfield attenuation of 40) mass (*arrow*) arising from the left kidney, found to represent a lipid-poor angiomyolipoma.

and be hyperdense on noncontrast imaging (Hounsfield attenuation >38.5) [44]. None of these are highly specific signs, however, and the ability of MDCT to accurately character lipid-poor AMLs is still quite limited (Figures 4.15–4.17).

Evaluation of Small Renal Masses

Largely as a result of dramatic improvements in MDCT scanner technology over the last decade, with marked improvements in spatial resolution, there has been a dramatic increase in the incidence of small renal masses (defined as renal cortical neoplasms measuring less than 4 cm in size). Although differentiating malignant from benign renal masses is problematic for lesions measuring more than 4 cm as well, it is particularly a problem for these small renal masses because anywhere between 15% and 30% of such masses are ultimately found to be benign (oncocytomas, lipid poor AMLs, adenomas, etc.). Unfortunately, multiple studies have found no reliable means, whether in terms of tumor morphology, histogram analysis, or enhancement characteristics, to differentiate benign from malignant small renal masses (provided there is no evidence of intratumoral macroscopic fat) [45–49]. While many centers still treat such small renal masses with partial nephrectomy or ablation, active surveillance with MDCT has become an accepted practice, particularly in patients who are elderly with significant comorbidities or limited life expectancy.

Infiltrative Renal Masses: Lymphoma and Transitional Cell Carcinoma

In the vast majority of cases, RCCs and the other solid renal masses described appear as well circumscribed, well marginated renal

(a) (b)

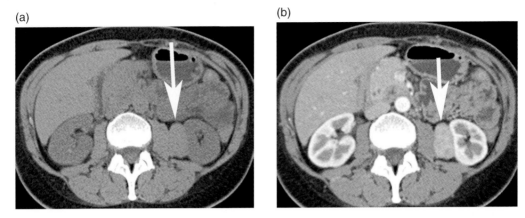

Figure 4.17 Axial noncontrast (a) and postcontrast (b) MDCT images demonstrates a intrinsically hyperdense (precontrast Hounsfield attenuation of greater than 35) mass (*arrows*) arising from the left kidney, found to represent a lipid-poor angiomyolipoma.

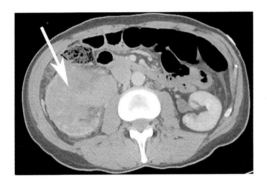

Figure 4.18 Axial contrast enhanced MDCT demonstrates a large aggressive infiltrating mass in the right kidney. Although this was thought to be a transitional cell carcinoma based on the imaging appearance, it was an aggressive variant of renal cell carcinoma.

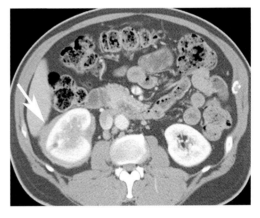

Figure 4.19 Axial postcontrast MDCT demonstrates a rind of soft tissue (*arrow*) in the right perinephric space, in keeping with lymphoma.

masses with clearly defined boundaries and margins. When confronted with an infiltrative renal mass, however, this is much less likely to be a RCC, but rather, is more likely to represent either a TCC extending beyond the renal collecting system into the renal parenchyma or renal lymphoma. It should be noted, however, that on rare occasions, particularly with more aggressive variants of RCC, a RCC could have an infiltrative appearance (Figure 4.18). Renal lymphoma can present as a solitary infiltrating hypovascular mass, multiple unilateral or bilateral poorly marginated renal masses, a perinephric soft-tissue mass encasing the kidney without an appreciable intraparenchymal component, or as a large extranodal mass secondarily involving the kidney (Figure 4.19). Although the distinction between TCC and lymphoma may not always be obvious, renal lymphoma virtually always represents secondary renal lymphoma, and there will typically be evidence of extrarenal nodal disease elsewhere [50].

Conclusion

Although other radiologic modalities such as magnetic resonance imaging (MRI) and positron emission tomography (PET) can now make significant contributions toward the imaging and staging of urologic malignancies, MDCT remains the first-line imaging modality for the identification, characterization, and diagnosis of urologic malignancies, regardless of whether they arise from the renal parenchyma or from the urothelium in the intrarenal collecting system, ureters, or bladder. However, accurate diagnosis and characterization is highly dependent on protocol design. Even in the hands of the best radiologist, an unequivocal malignancy can easily be missed if there are errors in study acquisition and technique.

References

1 Johnson PT, Horton KM, Fishman EK. Optimizing detectability of renal pathology with MDCT: Protocols, pearls, and pitfalls. AJR Am J Roentgenol. 2010;194:1001–12.

2 Chow LC, Kwan SW, Olcott EW, Sommer G. Split-bolus MDCT urography with synchronous nephrographic and excretory phase enhancement. AJR Am J Roentgenol. 2007;189:314–22.

3 Maheshwari E, O'Malley ME, Ghai S, Staunton M, Massey C. Split-bolus MDCT urography: Upper tract opacification and performance for upper tract tumors in patients with hematuria. AJR Am J Roentgenol. 2010;194:453–8.

4 Dillman JR, Caoili EM, Cohan RH, Ellis, JH, Francis IR, Nan Bm *et al.* Comparison of urinary tract distension and opacification using single-bolus 3-Phase vs split-bolus 2-phase multidetector row CT urography. J Comput Assist Tomogr. 2010;31:750–7.

5 Kekelidze M, Dwarkasing R, Dijkshoorn M, Sikorska K, Verhagen P, Krestin G. Kidney and urinary tract imaging: Triple-bolus multidetector CT urography as a one-stop shop. Protocol design, opacification, and image quality analysis. Radiology. 2010;255:508–16.

6 Caoili E, Inampudi P, Cohan R, Ellis J. Optimizatuion of multi-detector row CT urography: Effect of compression, saline administration, and prolongation of acquisition delay. Radiology. 2005;235:116–23.

7 Silverman SG, Akbar SA, Mortele KJ, Tuncali K, Bhagwat JG, Seifter JL. Multi-detector row CT urography of normal urinary collecting system: Furosemide versus saline as adjunct to contrast medium. Radiology. 2006;240:749–55.

8 Kawamoto S, Horton KM, Fishman EK. Opacification of the collecting system and ureters on excretory-phase CT using oral water as contrast medium. AJR Am J Roentgenol. 2006;86:136–40.

9 Raman SP, Horton KM, Fishman EK. Transitional cell carcinoma of the upper urinary tract: Pptimizing image interpretation with 3D reconstructions. Abdom Imaging. 2012;37:1129–40.

10 Fishman E, Ney D, Heath D, Corl F, Horton K, Johnson P. Volume rendering versus maximum intensity projection in CT angiography: What works best, when, and why. Radiographics. 2006;26:905–22.

11 Raman SP, Horton KM, Fishman EK. MDCT evaluation of ureteral tumors: Advantages of 3D reconstruction and volume visualization. AJR Am J Roentgenol. 2013;201:1239–47.

12 O'Connor OJ, McSweeney SE, Maher MM. Imaging of hematuria. Radiol Clin North Am. 2008;46:113–32, vii.

13 Vikram R, Sandler CM, Ng CS. Imaging and staging of transitional cell carcinoma: part 2, upper urinary tract. AJR Am J Roentgenol. 2009;192:1488–93.

14 Wang J, Wang H, Tang G, Hou Z, Wang G. Transitional cell carcinoma of upper urinary tract vs. benign lesions: distinctive MSCT features. Abdom Imaging. 2009;34:94–106.

15 Xu AD, Ng CS, Kamat A, Grossman HB, Dinney C, Sandler CM. Significance of

upper urinary tract urothelial thickening and filling defect seen on MDCT urography in patients with a history of urothelial neoplasms. AJR Am J Roentgenol. 2010;195:959–65.

16 Browne R, Meehan C, Colville J, Power R, Torreggiani W. Transitional cell carcinoma of the upper urinary tract: Spectrum of imaging findings. Radiographics. 2005;25:1609–27.

17 Anderson EM, Murphy R, Rennie AT, Cowan NC/Multidetector computed tomography urography (MDCTU) for diagnosing urothelial malignancy. Clin Radiol. 2007;62:324–32.

18 Atasoy C, Yagci C, Fitoz S, Sancak, Akyar G, Akyar S. Cross-sectional imaging in ureter tumors: Findings and staging accuracy of various modalities. J Clin Imag. 2001;25:197–202.

19 Turney BW, Willatt JM, Nixon D, Crew JP, Cowan NC. Computed tomography urography for diagnosing bladder cancer. BJU Int. 2006;98:345–8.

20 Sadow CA, Silverman SG, O'Leary MP, Signorovitch JE. Bladder cancer detection with CT urography in an Academic Medical Center. Radiology; 2008;249:195–202.

21 Shinagare AB, Sadow CA, Silverman SG. Surveillance of patients with bladder cancer following cystectomy: Yield of CT urography. Abdom Imaging. 2013;38:1415–21.

22 Gufler H, Schulze CG, Wagner S. Incidental findings in computed tomographic angiography for planning percutaneous aortic valve replacement: Advanced age, increased cancer prevalence? Acta Radiol. 2013;55:420–6.

23 Dighe MK, Bhargava P, Wright J. Urinary bladder masses: techniques, imaging spectrum, and staging. J Comput Assist Tomogr; 2011;35:411–24.

24 Shinagare AB, Sadow CA, Sahni VA, Silverman SG. Urinary bladder: normal appearance and mimics of malignancy at CT urography. Cancer Imag. 2011;11:100–8.

25 Kim JK, Park SY, Ahn HJ, Kim CS, Cho KS. Bladder cancer: Analysis of multi-detector row helical CT enhancement pattern and accuracy in tumor detection and perivesical staging. Radiology. 2004;231:725–31.

26 Xie Q, Zhang J, Wu PH, Jiang XQ, Chen SL, Wang QL, et al. Bladder transitional cell carcinoma: correlation of contrast enhancement on computed tomography with histological grade and tumour angiogenesis. Clin Radiol. 2005;60:215–23.

27 Bird VG, Kanagarajah P, Morillo G, Caruso DJ, Ayyathurai R, Levelillee R, et al. Differentiation of oncocytoma and renal cell carcinoma in small renal masses (<4cm): The role of 4-phase computerized tomography. World J Urol. 2011;29:787–92.

28 Kim J, Kim T, Ahn H, Kim C, Kim K, Cho K. Differentiation of subtypes of renal cell carcinoma on helical CT scans. AJR Am J Roentgenol. 2002;178:1499–1506.

29 Kim JH, Bae JH, Lee KW, Kim ME, Park SJ, Park JY. Predicting the histology of small renal masses using preoperative dynamic contrast-enhanced magnetic resonance imaging. Urology. 2012;80:872–6.

30 Shebel H, Elsayes K, Sheir KZ, Abou El Atta HM, El-Sherbiny AF, Ellis JH, et al. Quantitative enhancement washout analysis of solid cortical renal masses using multidetector computed tomography. J Comput Assist Tomogr. 2011;35:337–42.

31 Herts B, Coll D, Novick A, Obuchowski N, Linnell G, Wirth SL, et al. Enhancement characteristics of papillary renal neoplasms revealed on triphasic helical CT of the kidneys. AJR Am J Roentgenol. 2002;178:367–72.

32 Raman SP, Johnson PT, Allaf ME, Netto G, Fishman EK. Chromophobe renal cell carcinoma: multiphase MDCT enhancement patterns and morphologic features. AJR Am J Roentgenol. 2013;201:1268–76.

33 Choi S, Kim H, Ahn S, Park Y, Choi H. Differentiating radiological features of rapid- and slow-growing renal cell

carcinoma using multidetector computed tomography. J Comput Assist Tomogr. 2013;36:313–8.

34 Choi SK, Jeon SH, Chang SG. Characterization of small renal masses less than 4 cm with quadriphasic multidetector helical computed tomography: Differentiation of benign and malignant lesions. Korean J Urol. 2012;53:159–64.

35 Jinzaki M, Tanimoto A, Mukai M, Ikeda E, Kobayashi S, Yuasa Y, *et al.* Double-phase helical CT of small renal parenchymal neoplasms: Correlation with pathologic findings and tumor angiogenesis. J Comput Assist Tomogr. 2000;24:835–42.

36 Sheir KZ, El-Azab M, Mosbah A, El-Baz M, Shaaban AA. Differentiation of renal cell carcinoma subtypes by multislice computerized tomography. J Urol. 2005;174:451–5.

37 Zhang C, Li X, Hao H, Yu W, He Z, Zhou L. The correlation between size of renal cell carcinoma and its histopathological characteristics: a single center study of 1867 renal cell carcinoma cases. BJU Int. 2012;110:E481–5.

38 Zhang J, Lefkowitz R, Ishill N, Wang NM, Moskowitz CS, Russo P, *et al.* Solid renal cortical tumors: Differentiation with CT. Radiology. 2007;244:494–504.

39 Woo S, Cho JY, Kim SH, Kim SY. Comparison of segmental enhancement inversion on biphasic MDCT between small renal oncocytomas and chromophobe renal cell carcinomas. AJR Am J Roentgenol. 2013;201:598–604.

40 Young JR, Margolis D, Sauk S, Pantuck AJ, Sayre J, Raman SS. Clear cell renal cell carcinoma: discrimination from other renal cell carcinoma subtypes and oncocytoma at multiphasic multidetector CT. Radiology. 2013;267:444–53.

41 McGahan JP, Lamba R, Fisher J, Starshak P, Ramsamooj R, Fitgerald E, *et al.* Is segmental enhancement inversion on enhanced biphasic MDCT a reliable sign for the noninvasive diagnosis of renal oncocytomas? AJR Am J Roentgenol. 2011;197:W674–9.

42 Schieda N, McInnes MD, Cao L. Diagnostic accuracy of segmental enhancement inversion for diagnosis of renal oncocytoma at biphasic contrast enhanced CT: Systematic review. Eur Radiol. 2014;24:1421–9

43 O'Malley ME, Tran P, Hanbidge A, Rogalla P. Small renal oncocytomas: Is segmental enhancement inversion a characteristic finding at biphasic MDCT? AJR Am J Roentgenol. 2012;199:1312–5.

44 Yang CW, Shen SH, Chang YH, Chung HJ, Wang JH, Lin AT, *et al.* Are there useful CT features to differentiate renal cell carcinoma from lipid-poor renal angiomyolipoma? AJR Am J Roentgenol. 2013;201:1017–28.

45 Nishikawa M, Miyake H, Kitajima K, Takahashi S, Sugimura K, Fujisawa M. Preoperative differentiation between benign and malignant renal masses smaller than 4 cm treated with partial nephrectomy. Int J Clin Oncol. 2015;20:150–5.

46 Sahni VA, Silverman SG. Imaging management of incidentally detected small renal masses. Semin Intervent Radiol. 2014;31:9–19.

47 Wagstaff PG, Zondervan PJ, de la Rosette JJ, Laguna MP. The role of imaging in the active surveillance of small renal masses. Curr Urol Rep. 2014;15:386.

48 Millet I, Doyon FC, Hoa D, Thuret R, Merigeaud S, Serre I, *et al.* Characterization of small solid renal lesions: Can benign and malignant tumors be differentiated with CT? AJR Am J Roentgenol. 2013;197:887–96.

49 Chaudhry HS, Davenport MS, Nieman CM, Ho LM, Neville AM. Histogram analysis of small solid renal masses: differentiating minimal fat angiomyolipoma from renal cell carcinoma. AJR Am J Roentgenol. 2012;198:377–83.

50 Ganeshan D, Iyer R, Devine C, Bhosale P, Paulson E. Imaging of primary and secondary renal lymphoma. AJR Am J Roentgenol. 2013;201:W712–9.

5

MRI and Metabolic Imaging

Louise Dickinson, MRCS, PhD,[1] Francesco Fraioli, MD, FRCR,[2]
Athar Haroon, MBBS, FRCR,[3] and Clare Allen, MBBS, FRCR[1]

[1] *Department of Radiology, University College Hospital, London, UK*
[2] *Institute of Nuclear Medicine, University College Hospital, London, UK*
[3] *Department of Radiology, St Bartholomew's Hospital, London, UK*

Magnetic Resonance Imaging

Magnetic resonance imaging (MRI) uses information obtained from the movement and rotation of hydrogen atom protons within a strong magnet, following the application of radiofrequency fields. Following the reversal of the radiofrequency field, the protons return to a state of equilibrium at varying rates in different tissues. These characteristics are differentially exploited by the different MR parameters to depict contrast between soft tissues (including between benign and malignant tissue). Major advantages of MRI include excellent spatial resolution, multiplanar imaging, and the lack of radiation.

MRI Sequences

T1- and T2-Weighted

Traditionally, MRI has included T1- and T2-weighted sequences, which provide anatomical information for disease staging purposes. T1-weighted images differentiate fat from water and are interpreted for the presence of postbiopsy hemorrhage and metastatic disease within the pelvic bones and lymph nodes. T2-weighted images are used to assess anatomy, for localization and extent of visible cancer lesions (Figure 5.1).

Other MR sequences are now available that provide functional information on different tissues and which can be used to distinguish cancer lesions from normal tissue. The addition of any one or more of these sequences to standard T1- and T2-weighting is termed *multiparametric* MR imaging. Different sequence combinations are now in use to evaluate a variety of urological malignancies. Both diffusion-weighted and dynamic contrast-enhanced sequences assess physiological behavior, whereas MR spectroscopy assesses metabolic factors.

Diffusion-Weighted MRI

Diffusion-weighted (DW) imaging interprets the "diffusivity" or Brownian motion of water within tissue. Water movement is reduced where cells are tightly packed, such as within cancer tissue. This water movement restriction is represented by reduced signal intensity on DW imaging. This can be represented quantifiably by the apparent diffusion coefficient (ADC), which is a measure of average molecular motion.

Management of Urologic Cancer: Focal Therapy and Tissue Preservation, First Edition.
Edited by Mark P. Schoenberg and Kara L. Watts.
© 2017 John Wiley & Sons Ltd. Published 2017 by John Wiley & Sons Ltd.

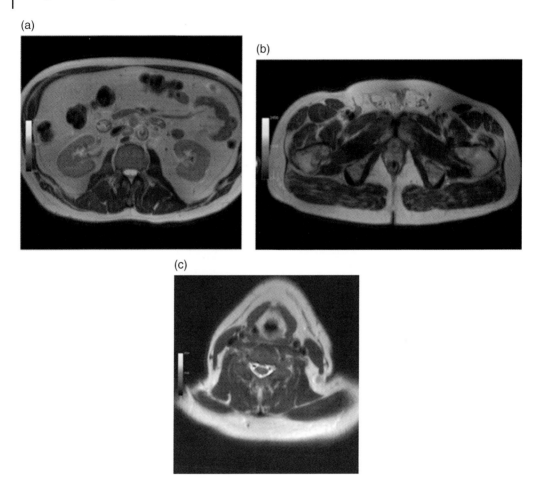

Figure 5.1 T2+ b1000 diffusion weighted (fused) whole-body magnetic resonance images showing (a) para-aortic lymphadenopathy, (b) femoral head and pelvic and (c) left cervical metastases in a man with advanced prostate cancer.

Dynamic Contrast-Enhanced MRI

Contrast-enhanced MRI uses the addition of a contrast agent, usually Gadolinium, to depict the vascular nature of cancer lesions shown as high signal on T1-weighted images. Dynamic contrast-enhanced (DCE) imaging captures the change in signal intensity over time following contrast agent intravenous administration, as the contrast distributes between the vasculature and the tissue. There is rapid uptake by the cancer tissue because of increased angiogenesis, micro-vasculature, and tissue permeability, and also rapid wash-out.

MR Spectroscopy

^{1}H-MR spectroscopy (MRS) depicts the concentrations of different metabolites in tissues. Spectroscopy itself observes the chemical changes in cancer cells, which tend to precede visually apparent anatomical changes. Once combined with MRI, which provides additional anatomical information, MRS theoretically provides an excellent tool for the early evaluation of cancers [1]. The spectra of metabolites within cells are visually inspected and can be depicted as a color map using computer-aided diagnosis (CAD) software. More recently, the use of metabolomics has

been introduced for MRS interpretation, in which a statistical method is applied instead of visual inspection [1]. This is thought to offer a more reliable and robust method, but it is not yet considered standard in MRS interpretation. MRS is currently considered a research tool and has not been fully integrated into clinical diagnostics.

Clinical Applications of MRI for Prostate Cancer

Introduction

Cancer lesions usually demonstrate low-signal intensity on T2-weighted images and are most easily visualized against the high-signal background of the peripheral zone. Identification of tumors within the transition zone is more challenging because of the heterogeneous T2-weighted signal in this area; however, malignant lesions tend to demonstrate homogenous signal and a lenticular shape on T2-weighted imaging. When these features are identified, sensitivity rates of 75–80% and specificity rates of 78–87%, respectively, can be obtained for cancer detection on T1- and T2-weighted MRI, against a reference standard of radical prostatectomy [2].

With any combination of additional functional sequences (DW, DCE, and MRS), multiparametric MRI (mpMRI), the accuracy for detecting lesions increases. In particular, recent data supports the ability of mpMRI with DW imaging to identify lesions of different Gleason grade and risk classification [3], and to predict aggressiveness [4]. The addition of DCE MRI to standard T1- and T2-weighted imaging has been shown to identify lesions of greater than 0.5 mL with sensitivity of 86% and specificity of 94%, respectively [5]. The value of MRS has been more equivocal with the ACRIN study demonstrating no clear benefit of its use for identifying prostate cancer lesions in the peripheral zone, over standard T2-weighting alone [6]. However, in another study, the addition of either MRS or DCE sequences to DW imaging increased the area-under-the-curve values for identifying tumors more than 1 mL from 0.65––0.71 to 0.94, with no additional benefit of adding a third sequence [7].

Most clinical centers currently use one or two additional sequences to T1- and T2-weighting, with scanning and interpretation time burden being a limitation with each additional sequence. The use of an endorectal coil, in addition to a pelvic-phased array coil, differs between centers dependent on the local imaging protocol. One of the controversies in mpMRI is the lack of consistency in its conduct and reporting. This was originally addressed by a European consensus group, with proposals for unification, including the use of five-point Likert-type scoring system for the interpretation of MR imaging results [8]. The consensus statements were followed up with the publication of European guidelines [9], in which the "PIRADs" scoring scale was proposed—so-called in recognition of its similarity to the BIRADs scoring system for breast imaging. Hopefully these combined consensus and guideline outputs, together with recent research studies aiming to validate the proposals, will result in more conformity in MR imaging and allow easier comparisons between research studies. Additionally, work on CAD systems is underway to help with the reporting and scoring of mpMRI to help reduce error.

mpMRI in Men with Suspected Prostate Cancer

Until fairly recently, the use of MRI in prostate cancer imaging has been limited to assessing tumor burden and staging disease, following a histological diagnosis, to aid management planning. Within this standard pathway, men receive a standard pelvic MRI around 3–6 weeks following a diagnostic transrectal ultrasound (TRUS) biopsy. There are many limitations to this pathway, however. Firstly, the TRUS biopsy is performed "blind" to tumor location and may miss or undercall disease burden. Secondly, postbiopsy hemorrhagic artifact results in accuracies in interpreting disease burden. In the last 5 years, there has been a shift toward performing mpMRI pre-biopsy, in at-risk men (raised PSA or abnormal digital rectal examination) to reduce these limitations [10], and this practice is now becoming standard of care in many centers.

Those with suspicious lesions on prebiopsy mpMRI can then undergo limited, targeted biopsies (either transperineal or transrectal) delivered to the area of concern. This targeted biopsy strategy appears to diminish the risk of understaging that currently occurs in up to 30% of men undergoing diagnostic TRUS biopsy [11]. Indeed, there is growing evidence to support equivalent or better risk stratification with image targeting, compared to sampling biopsies. A recent systematic review reported equivalence in the detection of clinically significant cancer with image-targeted biopsies against conventional TRUS-guided biopsy, with a smaller number of cores required (3.8 versus 12 cores) [12].

Another valuable attribute of mpMRI for prostate cancer is that the likelihood of a positive scan correlates closely with tumor burden. mpMRI has demonstrated poor sensitivity for low-grade, low-volume disease, in the range of approximately 30% for lesions <0.5 mL, increasing to more than 80% for detecting lesions >0.5 mL in one series.(5) Evidence is starting to accumulate that mpMRI is sensitive to tumor grade as well as tumor volume [3,13], resulting in a high negative predictive value (approximately 95%) for ruling out clinically significant disease [14]. Therefore, mpMRI may provide accurate information on the location and burden of clinically significant cancer lesions, while systematically overlooking clinically insignificant disease.

mpMRI for Planning Focal Treatment for Prostate Cancer

To date, most focal therapy studies have relied primarily on standard diagnostic sampling TRUS biopsy to detect and lateralize prostate cancer, without imaging correlation. However, there is significant potential for missing clinically significant lesions using TRUS biopsy alone, and it is likely that much of the variation in oncological outcomes from focal therapy can be attributed to differences in preoperative disease localization, rather than to the therapy itself. The adoption of mpMRI before focal therapy may improve accuracy of lesion identification and risk assessment for treatment planning.

Theoretically, the tighter the margin for focal treatment, the lower the rate of side effects. However, the potential trade-off of a more focal treatment is the risk of undertreatment and diminished oncological control. This risk could be minimized if highly accurate information were available on tumor locality, size, and peripheral (microscopic) extent. Although mpMRI is showing promise in the first two criteria, there is not currently sufficient research data on the accuracy of mpMRI for delineating peripheral cancer lesion margins. As a result, when planning focal therapy, a generous treatment margin is required to ensure adequate coverage.

Intraoperative mpMRI for Guiding Prostate Cancer Focal Therapy

Image guidance during treatment may reduce margin errors through direct visual assessment of the lesion. However, the majority of modalities adopted for focal therapy, such as cryotherapy and high-intensity focused ultrasound (HIFU), use an ultrasound platform for delivery of treatment without the provision for accurate lesion detection. This limitation has led most clinicians performing focal therapy to treat based on anatomical areas, such as the hemi- or quadrant gland, with avoidance of undertreatment at the margins. As prostate cancer detection by mpMRI has been found to correlate with grade and size, it could be hypothesised that margin errors might be reduced when treating MR-visible lesions, if imaging was appropriately incorporated into treatment planning and delivery.

There is a growing number of commercially available devices that coregister MR and ultrasound images to guide targeted prostate biopsies or to deliver focal treatment using an ultrasound platform. However, most devices are limited in accuracy because they do not perform "deformable" registration, with allowances for changes in prostate size and shape according to the position of the patient and the presence, or otherwise, or a rectal probe or endorectal coil. Early studies of deformable MR-ultrasound registration platforms in phantom models [15,16] demonstrated encouraging accuracy rates. Further, a deformable image registration technique that had demonstrated accuracy of 2.4 mm in phantom studies [17] was recently adopted with a prospective clinical study of focal therapy for localized prostate cancer. Although accuracy of the technique could not be assessed, coregistration of MR and ultrasound images within the operating theater was shown to be efficient and safe, with visual depiction of the lesion on the HIFU device during the ablation procedure [18].

MRI in the Follow-Up of Prostate Cancer Focal Therapy

MRI would appear an attractive, noninvasive means of follow-up after focal treatment, compared to serial biopsies, which carry a, not insignificant, procedure-related morbidity risk. Biochemical parameters (e.g., serum prostate-specific antigen [PSA]) may also be inaccurate in detecting residual or recurrent disease because of the presence of untreated prostate tissue. mpMRI has demonstrated reasonable accuracy in identifying residual disease after whole-gland HIFU for localized prostate cancer, when compared to postoperative biopsy [19]. Good correlation between ablated volumes and early postoperative MRI findings has been shown against radical prostatectomy specimens in small Phase I studies of focal laser ablation [20] and transperineal radiofrequency interstitial ablation [21].

However, longer-term oncological outcomes have not yet been formally assessed against an appropriate histological reference standard in men undergoing prostate focal treatment. Data is awaited in this area, before MRI can be recommended as a reliable follow-up tool. Additionally, consideration needs to be given to the cost implications of integrating long-term imaging in focal treatment protocols and the appropriate interval timescales for capturing new or residual disease.

Clinical Applications of MRI for Renal Cancer

Most renal lesions are evaluated using ultrasound and computed tomography (CT) and are often an incidental finding on imaging for alternative pathology. The majority of lesions can be classified as benign or malignant using ultrasound and CT, but MRI is considered a useful tool for equivocal lesions and also for posttreatment follow-up. Indeed, MRI has demonstrated more definitive diagnostic information of indeterminate lesions on ultrasound than contrast-enhanced CT but with likely cost implications [22].

Similar diagnostic techniques are adopted as for prostate cancer detection. Anatomical imaging using T1- and T2-weighted multiplanar scans followed by functional sequences using DW and contrast enhancement. Renal MRI is challenging because of respiratory motion, and various strategies need to be used to reduce artifact from this, including breath hold sequences and respiratory gating. MRI (without contrast enhancement) can be used in cases of renal failure in place of contrast-enhanced CT.

Correlation of ADC values between benign and malignant lesions has been reported in several recent studies. In one study of 26 renal lesions, renal tumors had significantly lower ADCs compared with benign cysts, and solid-enhancing tumors had significantly lower ADCs compared with nonenhancing necrotic or cystic regions [23]. A similar correlation was demonstrated by Kim *et al.* in comparing ADC values between renal cell carcinomas (RCCs) and benign cysts [24]. Furthermore, ADC values differed between solid and cystic components of complex cysts. Overall, however, DW imaging demonstrated equivalent performance to contrast-enhanced T1-weighted imaging across all lesion types. Although many studies are showing promise in the ability of DW imaging to differentiate benign from malignant renal lesions, and even to differentiate between tumor types, there is currently too much overlap of ADC values across the spectra of lesions to definitively recommend its routine use at present [25].

Ho *et al.* demonstrated promising diagnostic ability of contrast-enhanced MRI to distinguish malignant renal lesions from benign cysts [26]. However, a more contemporary series did not reproduce this encouraging result, with no differentiation in enhancement patterns shown between benign and malignant lesions on dynamic contrast-enhanced MRI [27]. However, there was moderate diagnostic differentiation between tumor subtypes in this study (i.e., papillary versus nonpapillary RCCs).

Despite some promising research findings, the performance characteristics of MRI are generally inferior to CT, particularly with the new generation of CT equipment. As such, CT remains the superior imaging test in the depiction of renal vascular anatomy, capsular margins, and renal sinus invasion for planning treatment management. Nephron-sparing surgery and ablation still rely on CT planning and assessment. Further, the majority of focal ablations are carried out using CT guidance and are operatively assessed using CT. However, MRI may be useful for long-term follow-up post ablation to reduce radiation burden.

Clinical Applications of MRI for Bladder Cancer

MRI has been shown to be accurate in the evaluation of bladder tumors in assessing local invasion and for staging and has the advantage over CT of excellent soft-tissue resolution and multiplanar ability. However, in both cases, imaging is conventionally performed following histopathological confirmation of cancer, from bladder biopsy or resection. Subsequently, the place of imaging within the bladder cancer pathway remains to be determined, particularly because resection causes local disturbance and inflammatory response, which limits imaging interpretation. MRI may, however, have a role in problem solving to assess large tumors before surgery including the presence of bladder neck, ureteric, urethral, cervical, and vaginal invasion. Additionally, MRI may be useful for assessing postneoadjuvant chemotherapy tumor response.

On T1-weighted images, the urine demonstrates low-signal intensity, with intermediate signal intensity of the bladder wall, and high-signal intensity of the surrounding fat. On T2-weighted images, the urine has high-signal intensity and the bladder wall has low-signal intensity. The T2-images are primarily used to assess involvement of the detrusor muscle and surrounding structures. Short tau inversion recovery (STIR) sequences can be applied to suppress perivesical fat, resulting in more distinct signal characteristics of tumors compared to the surrounding normal tissue. Further, MRI is superior to CT for determining muscle invasion and extravesicle disease, for local staging before radical treatment planning.

As with prostate cancer, use of a multiparametric approach appears to allow correlation with cancer aggressiveness. Increased cellular density of bladder tumors leads to increased signal intensity on diffusion-weighted images and a reduced ADC value. In one recent study evaluating diffusion-weighted MRI in 43 patients, ADC values inversely correlated with the grade of the disease [28]. Additionally, ADC values differed significantly between muscle invading tumors and those without muscle involvement. The area under the receiver operating characteristics (ROC) curve values were 0.884 for the prediction of muscle invasion and 0.906 for the prediction of high-grade disease, according to ADC values. As a result, DW imaging has been proposed as an excellent imaging parameter in identifying suitable candidates for organ-sparing treatment [29].

The addition of dynamic contrast enhancement to T2-weighting MRI has been shown to result in improved interobserver agreement and improved localization of small cancers, against a cystectomy histopathology specimen reference standard [30]. Additionally, bladder-cancer aggressiveness was significantly negatively correlated with a semi-quantitative assessment of DCE (wash-in and wash-out rates), as well as negatively correlating with ADC value on diffusion weighting in the same series, with marginally higher accuracy of the diffusion-weighting parameter over DCE [31].

New Advances in MRI

Whole-Body MRI

Research data is starting to emerge on the use of whole-body MRI with diffusion weighting to evaluate metastatic disease,

predominantly in cases of high-risk prostate cancer. It may be advantageous in offering a single-imaging technique as an alternative to bone scintigraphy and local staging CT and with potentially higher sensitivity and specificity rates. In particular, it has been proposed as a promising imaging tool in the follow-up of treatment, with a successful response usually depicted by a decrease in signal intensity, accompanied by an increase in ADC values [32].

In a study by Lecouvet *et al.* comparing the accuracy of whole-body MRI, CT and bone scintigraphy in the detection of metastases in men with high-risk prostate cancer, whole-body MRI outperformed bone scintigraphy (higher sensitivity rates) in the assessment of bone metastases but reached equivalence with CT in the detection of enlarged lymph nodes (Figure 5.2) [33]. However, the accompanying editorial to this study questioned whether the increased sensitivity of whole-body MRI in identifying bone metastases would confer clinical benefit in this group of patients and also raised attention on the issues associated with incidental findings from whole-body imaging. Further research data and cost-effectiveness analyses are awaited

(a)

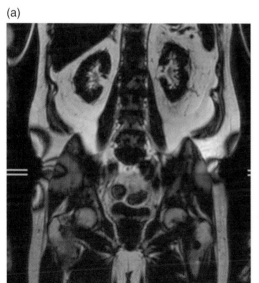

(b)

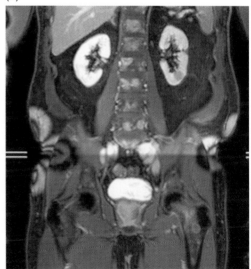

Figure 5.2 Coronal whole-body magnetic resonance images, (a) pre-contrast and (b) post-contrast. Multiple vertebral and bilateral femoral metastases from advanced prostate cancer.

before the potential role of whole-body MRI, including within the focal therapy pathway, can be determined.

Hyperpolarized 13-C MRI

Hyperpolarized 13-C MRI is a novel form of metabolic, MR spectroscopic, imaging. Although MRS provides information on metabolites in tissue, this is usually representative of a static snapshot of cellular activity. Hyperpolarized produces a far higher signal, not only from the intracellular 13-C labeled substrates but also their metabolic products. As a result, this type of MRI provides more dynamic information on the flux of 13-C labeled substrates. Overall, images with far higher signal-to-noise ratios and sensitivity rates are produced compared to standard MRS [34]. Indeed, dynamic nuclear polarization of 13C-labeled substrates has demonstrated increased enhancement in signal by 10,000-fold compared to conventional MRI [34]. Another potential advantage of hyperpolarized 13-C MRI is that it is purported to be a rapid technique, with evaluation of metabolite distributions within seconds, in vivo [35].

To date, in vitro studies have shown potential of this technique in earlier detection of primary cancer and earlier detection of tumor response to treatment [36]. The technique has also been investigated for a range of nononcological applications, such as early detection of renal tubular acidosis [37]. An early in vitro study of hyperpolarized 13-C MRI on unprocessed histological prostate specimens demonstrated good differentiation of cellular metabolite activity between cancer tissue and benign prostatic hyperplasia, such as differences in triacylglycerols, citrate, and acidic mucins [38].

The first-in-man clinical study was performed in 31 men with biopsy-proven prostate cancer, whom were injected with hyperpolarized 13-C-pyruvate [35]. Although the primary objectives of the study were to demonstrate safety of the technique, with no major adverse events reported, the authors also reported elevated 13-C-lactate/13-C-pyruvate in areas of biopsy-proven cancer tissue. They concluded that this novel metabolic technique has potential as a noninvasive tool for prostate cancer diagnosis and as a posttreatment monitoring tool.

Metabolic Imaging

Introduction

Beyond MRS, metabolic-imaging techniques include bone scintigraphy, single-photon emission computed tomography (SPECT), and positron emission tomography–computed tomography (PET–CT) (Figure 5.3). These are most commonly used in the evaluation of metastatic disease to plan management or assess response to treatment. In the context of focal therapy, metabolic imaging may be conducted to ensure localization of disease (primary or recurrent) before treatment. Additionally, these imaging techniques potentially offer significant advances in understanding the behavior of urological malignancies, including which lesions may be amenable to a more targeted treatment approach.

Bone Scan

Distant staging for bone metastases, particularly in prostate cancer, is usually assessed as standard using bone scintigraphy (bone scan) with 99mTc-phosphonates. Intravenously injected diphosphonates bond to hydroxyapatite crystals on the surface of bone, depicting osteoblastic activity (Figure 5.4). Although bone scintigraphy demonstrates reasonable sensitivity, it has low specificity for bone metastases, also demonstrating increased tracer activity with fractures and degenerative change. However, it remains part of the standard imaging armamentarium for staging in urological malignancies and in the follow-up of disease in association with biochemical parameters.

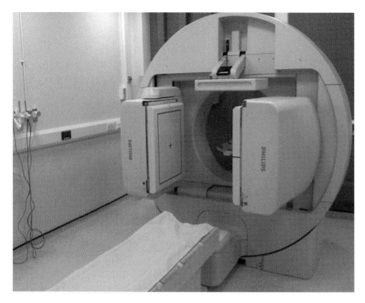

Figure 5.3 Single-photon emission computed tomography (SPECT) scanner is a nuclear medicine tomographic imaging technique using gamma rays.

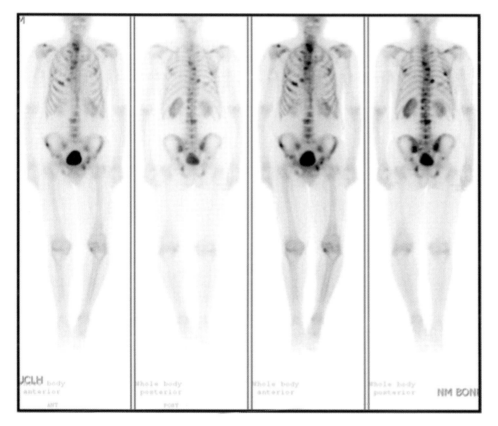

Figure 5.4 Anterior and posterior whole-body planar images demonstrating multiple foci of intense increased tracer uptake in the axial skeleton including ribs and pelvic bones in keeping with widespread osteoblastic bone metastastases.

PET–CT

PET is an imaging modality that provides a quantitative assessment of metabolic and functional tissue activity. The images are formed by detection of the activity of different positron emitting radiotracers, using multiple crystals fitted within 180-degree ring detectors. The detected emissions are converted into light signals, followed by electrical signal displayed on the monitor. The PET images are fused with CT images, usually performed within the same gantry, to provide a more accurate anatomical reference of tracer activity.

There are a growing number of radiotracers within PET imaging of urological cancers, which exploit different metabolic pathways within cancer tissue. However, a number of these demonstrate low specificity, with increased uptake within other disease processes, such as inflammation or infection. Newer radiotracers are emerging with improved specificity to individual tumor types.

Radiotracers Used in Urological Malignancies

Most radionuclides used in PET imaging are isotopes with short half-lives, ranging from approximately 2 minutes (oxygen-15) to 110 minutes (fluorine). They are bound to naturally occurring metabolites (e.g., glucose), or to receptor-specific molecules.

18F-flourodeoxyglucose (18F-FDG) is an established tracer in PET imaging. Its relatively long half-life (approximately 120 minutes) allows production off site, avoiding the requirement for a departmental cyclotron. FDG is a glucose analogue, with replacement of an oxygen molecule with 18-fluorine, which is actively transported into cells via structurally related transport proteins (GLUT). Both glucose and FDG are phosphorylated by hexokinase once intracellular. FDG then differs from glucose following phosphorylation (FDG-6-Phosphate) by remaining intracellular rather than continuing along the glycolysis pathway. The increased number of glucose transporters (GLUT) in cancer tissue, together with its high metabolic and glucose demand rates, results in increased uptake and retention of FDG compared to normal tissue. FDG is primarily excreted via the kidneys, resulting in high tracer activity in the collecting systems. This renders FDG a poor tracer for the detection of some urological malignancies. However, it has demonstrated good accuracy in the detection of metastatic disease and local lymph node involvement.

Choline and acetate derivatives, labeled with 11C or 18F, are incorporated within lipid metabolic pathways. Choline is an integral part of the phospholipid membrane. Tracers 11C-choline and 18F-fluorocholine are taken up by choline transporters of cancer cells and undergo intracellular phosphorylation by choline kinase. The half-life of the two isotopes is 20 minutes and 110 minutes, respectively. This has important logistic implications, with 11C-choline requiring an on-site cyclotron. However, the disadvantage of 18F-fluorocholine is that is has a higher urinary excretion than 11C-choline.

Acetate metabolites, usually labeled with 11C, are converted to acetyl-CoA by acetyl-CoA synthesase, and the substrate is then used to either synthesize cholesterol and fatty acids for incorporation within the cell membrane (anabolic pathway) or it is oxidized by the tricarboxylic acid cycle into CO_2 and H_2O (catabolic pathway). As tumor cells overexpress fatty acid synthesase, the majority of the tracer is incorporated into intracellular cell membranes via the anabolic pathway, which is promoted to allow tumor cell growth and metastasis. A major advantage of the acetate derivatives for urological imaging is that they are not excreted in the urinary tract, making them useful tracers for the primary detection of urological tumors.

The tracers 99mTc-labeled diphosphonate (MDP) and 18F-NaF are markers of bone turnover, used in the assessment of metastatic bone imaging, principally for prostate cancer. Unbound 99mTc-MDP tracer is taken up by bone, whereas 18F-NaF is transported unbound to plasma proteins via the bloodstream.

There are several newer tracers under investigation, which exploit other biochemical pathways. For example, 11C-methinonine and anti-FABC (1-amino-3-18F-fluorocyclobutane-1-carboxylic acid) are both amino acid analogues, which target the amino acid transport and protein synthesis pathways. Androgen-receptor binding activity is characterized by agents such as 18F-DHT (18F-fluoro-5α-dihydrotestosterone). Finally, there is an increasing body of work applying radiolabeled monoclonal antibodies to the challenge of imaging urologic cancers. These antibodies target specific antigens on cancer cells, such as Capromab pendetide labelled with 111-Indium to demonstrate prostate-specific membrane antigen (PSMA), which is overexpressed in prostate cancer.

Clinical Applications of PET–CT for Prostate Cancer

FDG

18F-FDG-PET is thought to have a limited role in the primary evaluation of localized prostate cancer [39]. This is firstly as a result of masking of pelvic pathology secondary to urinary excretion of the tracer with accumulation in the bladder. Secondly, it has poor specificity for prostate cancer, with increased uptake also seen in benign prostatic hypertrophy and prostatitis. Finally, only some prostate cancers demonstrate FDG avidity. Sensitivity and specificity levels in the primary diagnostic setting for localized prostate cancer are reported at around 50% and 75%, respectively.

Tumor grade may correlate with FDG–PET avidity (Figure 5.5). Improved accuracy was shown in tumors of higher grade (Gleason 7 or higher) in one study, with a sensitivity of 80% and a positive predictive value of 87% [40], compared to overall rates of 52% and 43%, respectively, across all tumor grades. Conversely, only a weak correlation was found between FDG–PET alone, and prostatectomy Gleason grade, in a recent

study by another group [41]. Incidental detection of prostate cancer can also occur when FDG–PET is used to investigate other malignancies, even amongst men with normal PSA values [42]. FDG–PET does not, therefore, appear to be a reliable method in the primary evaluation of localized prostate cancer. FDG–PET also has a limited role in the staging of prostate cancer, with higher accuracy rates seen with alternative radiotracers.

Choline

Because of the described limitations of 18F-FDG for prostate cancer, 11C-choline and 18F-FCH are now the more commonly used tracers. 11C-choline gained approval as a radiotracer in PET imaging for suspected recurrent prostate cancer in 2012. Two recent meta-analyses have been performed by the same study group on the accuracy of 18F-choline and 11C-choline PET-CT for both staging and restaging (for biochemical failure after local treatment) of prostate cancer. The meta-analysis of choline PET for detection of lymph node involvement in newly diagnosed intermediate to high-risk prostate cancer showed a pooled sensitivity of only 49.2% but with a higher pooled specificity of 95% (Figure 5.6) [43]. Low sensitivity rates were thought secondary to poor detection of small lymph node metastases (less than 0.4 cm). In the setting of recurrent disease, however, choline PET–CT demonstrated overall sensitivity of 92.6%, for detecting any site of recurrent disease (within the prostatic bed and lymph node and bone involvement) [44]. Overall, the highest accuracy rates in the recurrent setting were demonstrated in detecting lymph node metastases.

A further recent systematic review of PET imaging with choline tracers for prostate cancer staging and restaging, there appeared to be "high diagnostic evidence" toward its use for restaging purposes, as supported by other recent evidence, but no clear indication for primary staging purposes [45]. However,

(a)

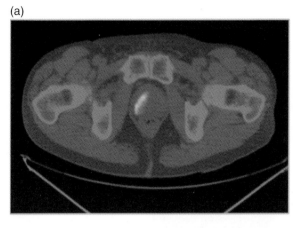

(b)

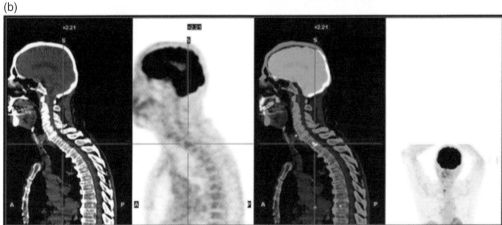

Figure 5.5 (a) 18F FDG axial fused positron emission tomography–computed tomography (PET–CT) demonstrating intense increased tracer uptake within the prostate extending from 9-o'clock to 12-o'clock position in keeping with a metabolically active lesion (biopsy-proven prostate cancer). (b) From left to right: Sagittal low dose CT, PET, 18F FDG PET–CT and maximum intensity projection (MIP) images demonstrating metabolically active focus in the thoracic vertebra in keeping with bone metastases.

the authors concluded that there is currently insufficient evidence to make recommendations on routine clinical use of choline PET–CT for prostate cancer at this stage.

Acetate

An early study of 11C-acetate demonstrated higher sensitivity than 18F-FDG PET in the detection of primary prostate cancers and high lymph node and bone metastasis avidity, albeit in a small study group (*n*=18), with a high proportion of advanced disease [46]. However, the study demonstrated no correlation between 11C-acetate accumulation and parameters of risk, including Gleason score, clinical stage, and serum PSA value. Similarly, when 11C-acetate PET–CT was compared to MRS for the primary detection of localized prostate cancer against TRUS-guided biopsy, neither test showed a correlation with tumor aggressiveness [47].

As with choline tracers, 11C-acetate PET has demonstrated higher accuracy in the recurrent setting for prostate cancer. A recent study showed good and comparable accuracy rates of 18F-FCH and 11C-acetate PET-CT in detecting recurrent disease in

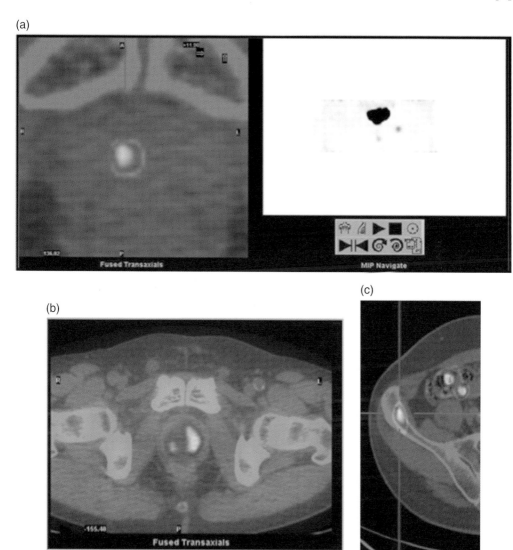

Figure 5.6 (a) 18F choline positron emission tomography–computed tomography (PET–CT) axial images showing focal area of increased choline uptake in the prostate and metabolically active left inguinal nodal metastases. (b) 18F choline PET–CT axial reformats demonstrating focal uptake in the right lobe and diffuse uptake in the left lobe of the prostate gland. In addition there is a choline-avid bone metastases (c) in the right iliac bone.

men who had undergone previous radical treatment (radical prostatectomy, radiotherapy, or radical prostatectomy with salvage radiotherapy), but with a low PSA (</=5ng/ml) [48].

18F-FACBC

Anti-18F-FACBC has also been evaluated in the primary and recurrent settings for prostate cancer, having demonstrated excellent in vitro uptake in prostate cancer cell lines and in prostate cancers implanted within nude rats [49]. A small clinical study was performed in a mixed cohort of men with newly diagnosed prostate carcinoma (*n*=9) or suspected recurrent disease (*n*=6) and both localized and metastatic disease, and it showed good visual analysis correlation of Anti-18F-FABC PET uptake with the presence or absence of focal disease [50]. Recurrent disease was correctly identified both within the prostatic bed and extraprostatic tissue, albeit among a cohort of only four men with proven recurrence. The study did demonstrate a significantly higher tracer uptake in malignant versus benign lymph nodes, within both staging and restaging cases, with intense uptake persisting up to 65 minutes.

18F-FDHT

Dihydrotestosterone (DHT) is the primary ligand of the androgen receptor, which is usually overexpressed in prostate cancer. The tracer 16β-18F-fluoro-5α-dihydrotestosterone (18F-FDHT) has been developed for selective androgen receptor binding. Early clinical studies demonstrated that the tracer was able to localize cancer lesions in progressive disease of clinically metastatic prostate cancer [51].

Radiolabeled Antibodies to PSMA

PSMA, also known as glutamate carboxypeptidase II (GCPII), is a transmembrane protein with high specificity and expression for prostate cancer cells, as well as the neovasculature of new lesions. It could serve as an effective and specific prostate cancer target. Various antibodies are under early evaluation for both diagnostic and therapeutic purposes [52].

A retrospective comparison of 68Ga-labelled-PSMA and 18F-fluoromethylcholine PET–CT showed superiority of the 68Ga-PSMA tracer in detecting biochemically recurrent prostate cancer [53]; however, PSMA antibody PET–CT performed less well in a recent prospective study in 93 patients with recurrent prostate cancer [54]. All patients received PET–CT with both tracers anti-18F-FACBC PET–CT and (111)In-capromab pendetide (ProstaScint®). The imaging outcomes were agreed by consensus, and histological

verification of index lesions was achieved in 96.1%. Anti-18F-FACBC achieved an accuracy rate of 90.2% for disease within the prostate or prostatic bed, compared to 67.2% with (111)In-capromab pendetide. Consensus was only reached in 70 of 93 patients with regard to the presence of extraprostatic disease with 72.9% and 50.0% accuracy for anti-3-(18)F-FACBC and (111)In-capromab pendetide, respectively. Anti-3-(18)F-FACBC was better than (111)In-capromab pendetide at identifying positive prostate bed recurrences and extraprostatic involvement.

A recent systematic review of current PET tracers for prostate cancer concluded that PSMA antibodies may prove valuable in the detection of extraprostatic disease and metastases, but the data are too limited at present to draw final conclusions [55].

Renal Cancer

FDG

RCC overexpresses glucose transporter proteins (GLUTs). In addition, cytoplasmic accumulation of glycogen is a prominent feature of many RCCs [56]. Accordingly, FDG-PET can be used for evaluation of RCCs. However, as already stated, a major limitation is that the tracer also accumulates in the renal parenchyma and undergoes urinary excretion, with subsequent poor detection of primary renal lesions. Furthermore, large renal tumors often have a central focus of necrosis, with absent FDG uptake. There is varied uptake of FDG tracer by oncocytomas, and therefore this imaging technique has not proven useful in preoperatively distinguishing these benign lesions from clear-cell renal tumors [57].

In a prospective study of 29 patients undergoing FDG PET–CT imaging before surgical resection of suspicious renal lesions, 77% were correctly identified with RCC [58]. False-positive results included the presence of other renal lesions (e.g., angiomyolipoma and phaeochromocytoma). Other, more recent studies of FDG-PET for detection of primary RCC have demonstrated suboptimal accuracy rates compared to conventional imaging, such as abdominal CT. In particular, sensitivity rates are reported at approximately 50–60%, compared to 90% for CT [59]. However, there may be a correlation between standardized uptake values (SUVs) and clear-cell tumor size and Fuhrman grade [60]. Further, SUV has been reported as correlative with survival outcome in patients with suspected locally advanced or metastatic disease [61].

As with prostate cancer, FDG-PET performs a little better in the identification of metastatic disease of renal cancers. Although a study comparing CT with FDG-PET in patients with suspected renal cancers showed poor sensitivity (47%) of FDG-PET for identifying the primary renal masses, it did better with identifying metastases [62]. Overall, the accuracy rates for identifying distant metastases on FDG-PET and CT were 97% and 83%, respectively. However, only a small subset of the cohort studied ($n=53$) was identified as having distant metastases (32%).

Acetate

Despite the lack of urinary excretion offering a potential advantage as a tracer in renal imaging, inconsistent results have limited its use. Comparative uptake was observed in tumors compared to surrounding normal parenchyma in one study [63], other than oncocytomas, which had the highest uptake. However, another group has reported excellent uptake by renal tumors compared to normal parenchyma, even in the presence of renal impairment [64].

Radiolabeled Antibodies

G250 is a monoclonal antibody that binds specifically to clear-cell renal cancers cells. A Phase I study of iodine-124 labeled antibody chimeric G250 (124I-cG250) PET has demonstrated differential tracer uptake between clear-cell renal tumors and more indolent papillary tumors, with extremely promising early results (sensitivity 94%, specificity 100%, negative predictive value 90%, positive predictive value 100%). A Phase III multicenter study is currently underway evaluating Iodine-124 labeled G250 in the identification of clear-cell versus nonclear-cell tumors in preoperative patients (clinicaltrials.gov NCT00606632).

Clinical Applications of PET–CT for Bladder Cancer

FDG

PET–CT does not have an established role in the primary evaluation of bladder tumors. One systematic review identified only two studies evaluating the FDG-PET in the detection of primary bladder lesions, preventing analysis of its diagnostic accuracy [65]. The paucity of data is likely the result of the, already discussed, inherent problems of urinary excretion of the tracer (Figure 5.7). To combat these limitations, several techniques have been employed, including voiding, catheterization with bladder irrigation, and increased diuresis with intravenous furosemide [66]. Although irrigation has can lead to a high false-positive rate for detection of recurrent or residual bladder tumors, forced diureses with furosemide has allowed good visualization of intravesical lesions, with improved sensitivity rates of FDG-PET [67].

On systematic review of FDG-PET for staging or restaging bladder cancer, a pooled sensitivity of 82% and pooled specificity of 89% were reported [65]. The meta-analysis was limited by the inclusion of only six studies. Lower sensitivity rates have been reported in individual studies in the diagnosis of metastatic disease [68].

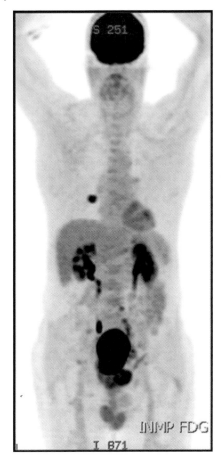

Figure 5.7 18F FDG positron emission tomography–computed tomography (PET–CT) maximum intensity projection (MIP) images demonstrating a metabolically active mass in the left hemi-pelvis, which was invading the left bladder wall and prostate. There is dilatation of the pelvicalyceal system bilaterally and a metabolically active deposit in the right lung which was a metastatic lesion.

Choline

Avid choline uptake has been shown in bladder tumors before cystectomy, with very little tracer found in the urine [69]. In a study of 25 patients with transurethrally resected tumors, 11C-choline PET correctly identified residual disease in 96%, compared to 84% using contrast-enhanced CT, using

subsequent cystectomy specimen as the reference standard [70]. PET was reported as superior to CT for identifying lymph node involvement, albeit with limited sensitivity in both cases (50% versus 62%, respectively). Additionally, there were no cases of false-positive lymph node involvement with PET versus a 22% rate with CT.

Novel Advances in PET Imaging: PET–MRI

Although PET–CT imaging has undergone significant advances within oncological imaging, it has several limitations. These include the requirement for separate sequential imaging of the PET and CT components, followed by coregistration. This can result in imprecision because of motion between scans, such as from respiration. Furthermore, CT is limited in its soft-tissue contrast and uses a significant radiation dose.

PET–MRI is a new technique that avoids these limitations (Figure 5.8). PET and MRI data can be acquired simultaneously with certain gantry systems. However, others are also available that use sequential techniques. Additionally, different MR sequences (DW, DCE, and MRS) can be applied to provide further functional information, which is not possible with PET–CT. PET–MRI could prove particularly useful in the context of focal therapy, combining the functional sequences that have shown promise in the detection and localization of index lesions, combined with additional metabolic information provided by PET, which may further inform on suitable lesions for targeted treatment (Figures 5.9 and 5.10).

Although PET–MRI has only limited availability so far, research and clinical outcomes of this new technique are keenly awaited. Furthermore, cost-effectiveness analyses will be required as part of an overall assessment and comparison with PET–CT imaging.

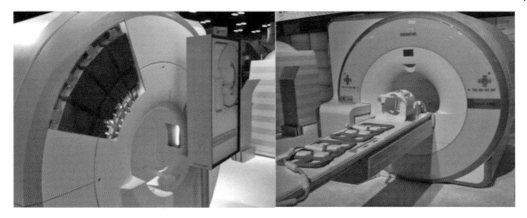

Figure 5.8 The new-generation positron emission tomography–magnetic resonance imaging (PET–MRI) scanners have intrinsic ability to acquire PET and MRI images at the same time (simultaneous PET MRI).

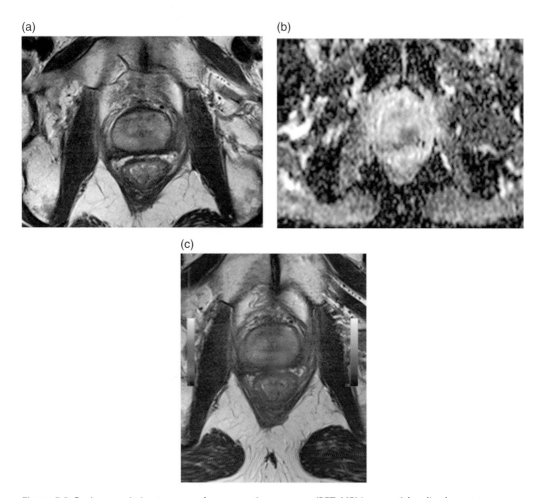

Figure 5.9 Positron emission tomography–magnetic resonance (PET–MR) images. A localized prostate cancer lesion within the left peripheral zone on (a) T2-weighted, (b) diffusion-weighted, and (c) PET–MRI images.

(a)

(b)

(c)

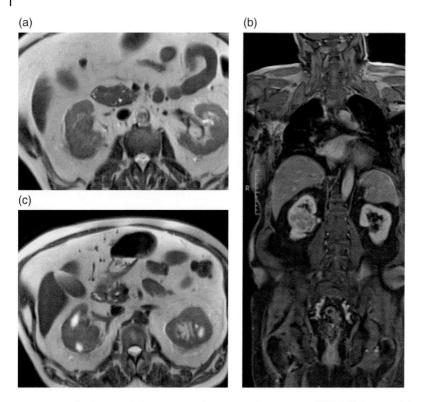

Figure 5.10 Positron emission tomography–magnetic resonance (PET–MR) images. A large right-sided central renal malignant mass, which was well visualized on (a) axial and (b) coronal MR images, but with only poor FDG PET tracer uptake as demonstrated on (c) PET–MRI. Excreted activity from the kidneys is a limiting factor in detection of renal lesions.

Summary

Metabolic imaging with PET–CT has improved our knowledge of the behavior of tumors and proven a valuable imaging tool for disease detection to plan appropriate management. Within urological malignancies, it has offered most value in the detection of metastatic disease and recurrent disease. Limitations in diagnostic PET–CT imaging have mostly stemmed from the urinary excretion of the majority of tracers. Exciting recent advances include the use of radiolabeled antibodies, which may prove highly specific to certain tumor cells and may lead to advances in targeted therapies in the future. Additionally, PET–MRI offers potential opportunities for obtaining functional information together with excellent soft-tissue resolution. These advances may prove particularly valuable for informing the location, burden, and metabolic behavior of cancer lesions in the context of targeted, focal treatments.

References

1 Bezabeh T, Ijare OB, Nikulin AE, Somorjai RL, Smith IC. MRS-based metabolomics in cancer research. Magn Reson Insights. 2014;7:1–14.

2 Akin O, Sala E, Moskowitz CS, Kuroiwa K, Ishill NM, Pucar D, *et al.* Transition zone prostate cancers: Features, detection,

localization, and staging at endorectal MR imaging. Radiology. 2006 Jun;239(3):784–92.

3 Vargas HA, Akin O, Franiel T, Mazaheri Y, Zheng J, Moskowitz C, *et al.* Diffusion-weighted endorectal MR imaging at 3 T for prostate cancer: Tumor detection and assessment of aggressiveness. Radiology. 2011 Jun;259(3):775–84.

4 Verma S, Rajesh A, Morales H, Lemen L, Bills G, Delworth M, *et al.* Assessment of aggressiveness of prostate cancer: Correlation of apparent diffusion coefficient with histologic grade after radical prostatectomy. AJR Am J Roentgenol. 2011 Feb;196(2):374–81.

5 Puech P, Potiron E, Lemaitre L, Leroy X, Haber GP, Crouzet S, *et al.* Dynamic contrast-enhanced-magnetic resonance imaging evaluation of intraprostatic prostate cancer: Correlation with radical prostatectomy specimens. Urology. 2009 Nov; 74(5):1094–9.

6 Weinreb JC, Blume JD, Coakley FV, Wheeler TM, Cormack JB, Sotto CK, *et al.* Prostate cancer: Sextant localization at MR imaging and MR spectroscopic imaging before prostatectomy—results of ACRIN prospective multi-institutional clinicopathologic study. Radiology. 2009 Apr;251(1):122–33.

7 Riches SF, Payne GS, Morgan VA, Sandhu S, Fisher C, Germuska M, *et al.* MRI in the detection of prostate cancer: Combined apparent diffusion coefficient, metabolite ratio, and vascular parameters. AJR Am J Roentgenol. 2009 Dec;193(6):1583–91.

8 Dickinson L, Ahmed HU, Allen C, Barentsz JO, Carey B, Futterer JJ, *et al.* Magnetic resonance imaging for the detection, localisation, and characterisation of prostate cancer: Recommendations from a european consensus meeting. Eur Urol. 2011 Apr;59(4):477–94.

9 Barentsz JO, Richenberg J, Clements R, Choyke P, Verma S, Villeirs G, *et al.* ESUR prostate MR guidelines 2012. Eur Radiol. 2012 Apr;22(4):746–57.

10 Sciarra A, Barentsz J, Bjartell A, Eastham J, Hricak H, Panebianco V, Witjes JA. Advances in magnetic resonance imaging: How they are changing the management of prostate cancer. Eur Urol. 2011 Jun; 59(6):962–77.

11 Berglund RK, Masterson TA, Vora KC, Eggener SE, Eastham JA, Guillonneau BD. Pathological upgrading and up staging with immediate repeat biopsy in patients eligible for active surveillance. J Urol. 2008 Nov;180(5):1964–7; discussion 1967–8.

12 Moore CM, Robertson NL, Arsanious N, Middleton T, Villers A, Klotz L, *et al.* Image-guided prostate biopsy using magnetic resonance imaging-derived targets: A systematic review. Eur Urol. 2013 Jan;63(1):125–40.

13 Shimizu T, Nishie A, Ro T, Tajima T, Yamaguchi A, Kono S, Honda H. Prostate cancer detection: The value of performing an MRI before a biopsy. Acta Radiol. 2009 Nov; 50(9):1080–8.

14 Villers A, Puech P, Mouton D, Leroy X, Ballereau C, Lemaitre L. Dynamic contrast enhanced, pelvic phased array magnetic resonance imaging of localized prostate cancer for predicting tumor volume: Correlation with radical prostatectomy findings. J Urol. 2006 Dec; 176(6 Pt 1):2432–7.

15 Makni N, Puech P, Colin P, Azzouzi A, Mordon S, Betrouni N. Elastic image registration for guiding focal laser ablation of prostate cancer: Preliminary results. Comput Methods Programs Biomed. 2012 Oct; 108(1):213–23.

16 Makni N, Toumi I, Puech P, Issa M, Colot O, Mordon S, Betrouni N. A non rigid registration and deformation algorithm for ultrasound & MR images to guide prostate cancer therapies. Conf Proc IEEE Eng Med Biol Soc. 2010;2010:3711–4.

17 Hu Y, Ahmed HU, Taylor Z, Allen C, Emberton M, Hawkes D, Barratt D. MR to ultrasound registration for image-guided prostate interventions. Med Image Anal. 2012 Apr;16(3):687–703.

18 Dickinson L, Hu Y, Ahmed HU, Allen C, Kirkham AP, Emberton M, Barratt D. Image-directed, tissue-preserving focal

therapy of prostate cancer: A feasibility study of a novel deformable magnetic resonance-ultrasound (MR-US) registration system. BJU Int. 2013, Sep; 112(5):594–601.

19 Punwani S, Emberton M, Walkden M, Sohaib A, Freeman A, Ahmed H, *et al.* Prostatic cancer surveillance following whole-gland high-intensity focused ultrasound: Comparison of MRI and prostate-specific antigen for detection of residual or recurrent disease. Br J Radiol. 2012 Jun;85(1014):720–8.

20 Lindner U, Lawrentschuk N, Weersink RA, Davidson SR, Raz O, Hlasny E, *et al.* Focal laser ablation for prostate cancer followed by radical prostatectomy: Validation of focal therapy and imaging accuracy. Eur Urol. 2010 Jun;57(6):1111–4.

21 Djavan B, Zlotta AR, Susani M, Heinz G, Shariat S, Silverman DE, *et al.* Transperineal radiofrequency interstitial tumor ablation of the prostate: Correlation of magnetic resonance imaging with histopathologic examination. Urology. 1997 Dec;50(6):986–92; discussion 992–3.

22 Margolis NE, Shaver CM, Rosenkrantz AB. Indeterminate liver and renal lesions: Comparison of computed tomography and magnetic resonance imaging in providing a definitive diagnosis and impact on recommendations for additional imaging. J Comput Assist Tomogr. 2013;37(6):882–6.

23 Zhang J, Tehrani YM, Wang L, Ishill NM, Schwartz LH, Hricak H. Renal masses: Characterization with diffusion-weighted MR imaging—a preliminary experience. Radiology. 2008 May;247(2):458–64.

24 Kim S, Jain M, Harris AB, Lee VS, Babb JS, Sigmund EE, *et al.* T1 hyperintense renal lesions: Characterization with diffusion-weighted MR imaging versus contrast-enhanced MR imaging. Radiology. 2009 Jun;251(3):796–807.

25 Nikken JJ, Krestin GP. MRI of the kidney-state of the art. Eur Radiol. 2007 Nov; 17(11):2780–93.

26 Ho VB, Allen SF, Hood MN, Choyke PL. Renal masses: Quantitative assessment of enhancement with dynamic MR imaging. Radiology. 2002 Sep;224(3):695–700.

27 Sevcenco S, Ponhold L, Javor D, Kuehhas FE, Mauermann J, Miernik A, *et al.* Three-Tesla dynamic contrast-enhanced MRI: A critical assessment of its use for differentiation of renal lesion subtypes. World J Urol. 2014 Feb;32(1):215–20.

28 Sevcenco S, Ponhold L, Heinz-Peer G, Fajkovic H, Haitel A, Susani M, *et al.* Prospective evaluation of diffusion-weighted MRI of the bladder as a biomarker for prediction of bladder cancer aggressiveness. Urol Oncol. 2014 Nov; 32(8):1166–71.

29 Yoshida S, Koga F, Kobayashi S, Tanaka H, Satoh S, Fujii Y, Kihara K. Diffusion-weighted magnetic resonance imaging in management of bladder cancer, particularly with multimodal bladder-sparing strategy. World J Radiol. 2014 Jun 28; 6(6):344–54.

30 Nguyen HT, Pohar KS, Jia G, Shah ZK, Mortazavi A, Zynger DL, *et al.* Improving bladder cancer imaging using 3-T functional dynamic contrast-enhanced magnetic resonance imaging. Invest Radiol. 2014 Jun;49(6):390–5.

31 Zhou G, Chen X, Zhang J, Zhu J, Zong G, Wang Z. Contrast-enhanced dynamic and diffusion-weighted MR imaging at 3.0T to assess aggressiveness of bladder cancer. Eur J Radiol. 2014 Nov;83(11):2013–8.

32 Padhani AR, Makris A, Gall P, Collins DJ, Tunariu N, de Bono JS. Therapy monitoring of skeletal metastases with whole-body diffusion MRI. J Magn Reson Imaging. 2014 May;39(5):1049–78.

33 Lecouvet FE, El Mouedden J, Collette L, Coche E, Danse E, Jamar F, *et al.* Can whole-body magnetic resonance imaging with diffusion-weighted imaging replace tc 99m bone scanning and computed tomography for single-step detection of metastases in patients with high-risk prostate cancer? Eur Urol. 2012 Jul; 62(1):68–75.

34 Day SE, Kettunen MI, Gallagher FA, Hu DE, Lerche M, Wolber J, *et al.* Detecting tumor

response to treatment using hyperpolarized 13C magnetic resonance imaging and spectroscopy. Nat Med. 2007 Nov; 13(11):1382–7.

35 Nelson SJ, Kurhanewicz J, Vigneron DB, Larson PE, Harzstark AL, Ferrone M, *et al.* Metabolic imaging of patients with prostate cancer using hyperpolarized $[1^{-13}C]$ pyruvate. Sci Transl Med. 2013 Aug 14; 5(198):198ra108.

36 Brindle KM, Bohndiek SE, Gallagher FA, Kettunen MI. Tumor imaging using hyperpolarized 13C magnetic resonance spectroscopy. Magn Reson Med. 2011, Aug; 66(2):505–19.

37 Clatworthy MR, Kettunen MI, Hu DE, Mathews RJ, Witney TH, Kennedy BW, *et al.* Magnetic resonance imaging with hyperpolarized [1,4-(13)C2]fumarate allows detection of early renal acute tubular necrosis. Proc Natl Acad Sci USA. 2012 Aug 14;109(33):13374–9.

38 Halliday KR, Fenoglio-Preiser C, Sillerud LO. Differentiation of human tumors from nonmalignant tissue by natural-abundance 13C NMR spectroscopy. Magn Reson Med. 1988 Aug;7(4):384–411.

39 Takahashi N, Inoue T, Lee J, Yamaguchi T, Shizukuishi K. The roles of PET and PET/CT in the diagnosis and management of prostate cancer. Oncology. 2007;72(3–4):226–33.

40 Minamimoto R, Uemura H, Sano F, Terao H, Nagashima Y, Yamanaka S, *et al.* The potential of FDG-PET/CT for detecting prostate cancer in patients with an elevated serum PSA level. Ann Nucl Med. 2011 Jan;25(1):21–7.

41 Chang JH, Lim Joon D, Lee ST, Hiew CY, Esler S, Gong SJ, *et al.* Diffusion-weighted MRI, 11c-choline PET and 18f-fluorodeoxyglucose PET for predicting the gleason score in prostate carcinoma. Eur Radiol. 2014 Mar;24(3):715–22.

42 Bartoletti R, Meliani E, Bongini A, Magno C, Cai T. Fluorodeoxyglucose positron emission tomography may aid the diagnosis of aggressive primary prostate cancer: A case series study. Oncol Lett. 2014 Feb;7(2):381–6.

43 Evangelista L, Guttilla A, Zattoni F, Muzzio PC, Zattoni F. Utility of choline positron emission tomography/computed tomography for lymph node involvement identification in intermediate- to high-risk prostate cancer: A systematic literature review and meta-analysis. Eur Urol. 2013 Jun;63(6):1040–8.

44 Evangelista L, Zattoni F, Guttilla A, Saladini G, Zattoni F, Colletti PM, Rubello D. Choline PET or PET/CT and biochemical relapse of prostate cancer: A systematic review and meta-analysis. Clin Nucl Med. 2013 May; 38(5):305–14.

45 Umbehr MH, Müntener M, Hany T, Sulser T, Bachmann LM. The role of 11c-choline and 18f-fluorocholine positron emission tomography (PET) and PET/CT in prostate cancer: A systematic review and meta-analysis. Eur Urol. 2013 Jul; 64(1):106–17.

46 Oyama N, Akino H, Kanamaru H, Suzuki Y, Muramoto S, Yonekura Y, *et al.* 11C-acetate PET imaging of prostate cancer. J Nucl Med. 2002 Feb;43(2):181–6.

47 Jambor I, Borra R, Kemppainen J, Lepomäki V, Parkkola R, Dean K, *et al.* Functional imaging of localized prostate cancer aggressiveness using 11c-acetate PET/CT and 1H-MR spectroscopy. J Nucl Med. 2010 Nov;51(11):1676–83.

48 Buchegger F, Garibotto V, Zilli T, Allainmat L, Jorcano S, Vees H, *et al.* First imaging results of an intraindividual comparison of (11)c-acetate and (18)f-fluorocholine PET/CT in patients with prostate cancer at early biochemical first or second relapse after prostatectomy or radiotherapy. Eur J Nucl Med Mol Imaging. 2014 Jan;41(1):68–78.

49 Oka S, Hattori R, Kurosaki F, Toyama M, Williams LA, Yu W, *et al.* A preliminary study of anti-1-amino-3-18f-fluorocyclobutyl-1-carboxylic acid for the detection of prostate cancer. J Nucl Med. 2007 Jan;48(1):46–55.

50 Schuster DM, Votaw JR, Nieh PT, Yu W, Nye JA, Master V, *et al.* Initial experience with the radiotracer anti-1-amino-3-18f-fluorocyclobutane-1-carboxylic acid with

PET/CT in prostate carcinoma. J Nucl Med. 2007 Jan;48(1):56–63.

51 Larson SM, Morris M, Gunther I, Beattie B, Humm JL, Akhurst TA, *et al.* Tumor localization of 16beta-18f-fluoro-5alpha-dihydrotestosterone versus 18F-FDG in patients with progressive, metastatic prostate cancer. J Nucl Med. 2004 Mar; 45(3):366–73.

52 Tykvart J, Navrátil V, Sedlák F, Corey E, Colombatti M, Fracasso G, *et al.* Comparative analysis of monoclonal antibodies against prostate-specific membrane antigen (PSMA). Prostate. 2014 Dec;74(16):1674–90.

53 Afshar-Oromieh A, Zechmann CM, Malcher A, Eder M, Eisenhut M, Linhart HG, *et al.* Comparison of PET imaging with a (68)ga-labelled PSMA ligand and (18)f-choline-based PET/CT for the diagnosis of recurrent prostate cancer. Eur J Nucl Med Mol Imaging. 2014 Jan; 41(1):11–20.

54 Schuster DM, Nieh PT, Jani AB, Amzat R, Bowman FD, Halkar RK, *et al.* Anti-3-[(18)F] FACBC positron emission tomography-computerized tomography and (111)in-capromab pendetide single photon emission computerized tomography-computerized tomography for recurrent prostate carcinoma: Results of a prospective clinical trial. J Urol. 2014 May;191(5):1446–53.

55 Yu CY, Desai B, Ji L, Groshen S, Jadvar H. Comparative performance of PET tracers in biochemical recurrence of prostate cancer: A critical analysis of literature. Am J Nucl Med Mol Imaging. 2014;4(6):580–601.

56 Ozcan A, Shen SS, Zhai QJ, Truong LD. Expression of GLUT1 in primary renal tumors: Morphologic and biologic implications. Am J Clin Pathol. 2007 Aug; 128(2):245–54.

57 Kochhar R, Brown RK, Wong CO, Dunnick NR, Frey KA, Manoharan P. Role of FDG PET/CT in imaging of renal lesions. J Med Imaging Radiat Oncol. 2010 Aug;54(4):347–57.

58 Bachor R, Kotzerke J, Gottfried HW, Brändle E, Reske SN, Hautmann R. [Positron emission tomography in diagnosis of renal cell carcinoma]. Urologe A. 1996, Mar; 35(2):146–50.

59 Kang DE, White RL, Zuger JH, Sasser HC, Teigland CM. Clinical use of fluorodeoxyglucose F 18 positron emission tomography for detection of renal cell carcinoma. J Urol. 2004 May; 171(5):1806–9.

60 Polat EC, Otunctemur A, Ozbek E, Besiroglu H, Dursun M, Ozer K, Horsanali MO. Standardized uptake values highly correlate with tumor size and fuhrman grade in patients with clear cell renal cell carcinoma. Asian Pac J Cancer Prev. 2014;15(18):7821–4.

61 Ferda J, Ferdova E, Hora M, Hes O, Finek J, Topolcan O, Kreuzberg B. 18F-FDG-PET/CT in potentially advanced renal cell carcinoma: A role in treatment decisions and prognosis estimation. Anticancer Res. 2013 Jun;33(6):2665–72.

62 Aide N, Cappele O, Bottet P, Bensadoun H, Regeasse A, Comoz F, *et al.* Efficiency of [(18)F]FDG PET in characterising renal cancer and detecting distant metastases: A comparison with CT. Eur J Nucl Med Mol Imaging. 2003 Sep; 30(9):1236–45.

63 Kotzerke J, Linné C, Meinhardt M, Steinbach J, Wirth M, Baretton G, *et al.* [1-(11)C]acetate uptake is not increased in renal cell carcinoma. Eur J Nucl Med Mol Imaging. 2007 Jun;34(6):884–8.

64 Shreve P, Chiao PC, Humes HD, Schwaiger M, Gross MD. Carbon-11-acetate PET imaging in renal disease. J Nucl Med. 1995 Sep;36(9):1595–601.

65 Lu YY, Chen JH, Liang JA, Wang HY, Lin CC, Lin WY, Kao CH. Clinical value of FDG PET or PET/CT in urinary bladder cancer: A systemic review and meta-analysis. Eur J Radiol. 2012 Sep; 81(9):2411–6.

66 Vesselle HJ, Miraldi FD. FDG PET of the retroperitoneum: Normal anatomy, variants, pathologic conditions, and

strategies to avoid diagnostic pitfalls. Radiographics. 1998;18(4):805–23; discussion 823–4.

67 Harkirat S, Anand S, Jacob M. Forced diuresis and dual-phase f-fluorodeoxyglucose-pet/CT scan for restaging of urinary bladder cancers. Indian J Radiol Imaging. 2010 Feb; 20(1):13–9.

68 Drieskens O, Oyen R, Van Poppel H, Vankan Y, Flamen P, Mortelmans L. FDG-PET for preoperative staging of bladder cancer. Eur J Nucl Med Mol Imaging. 2005 Dec;32(12):1412–7.

69 de Jong IJ, Pruim J, Elsinga PH, Jongen MM, Mensink HJ, Vaalburg W. Visualisation of bladder cancer using (11)c-choline PET: First clinical experience. Eur J Nucl Med Mol Imaging. 2002 Oct; 29(10):1283–8.

70 Picchio M, Treiber U, Beer AJ, Metz S, Bössner P, van Randenborgh H, *et al.* Value of 11c-choline PET and contrast-enhanced CT for staging of bladder cancer: Correlation with histopathologic findings. J Nucl Med. 2006 Jun; 47(6):938–44.

6

Biopsy Strategies in the Analysis of Urologic Neoplasia

Nabeel A. Shakir, MD,[1] Soroush Rais-Bahrami, MD,[2] and Peter A. Pinto, MD[3]

[1] Department of Urology, University of Texas Southwestern Medical Center, Dallas, TX, USA
[2] Departments of Radiology and Urology, University of Alabama at Birmingham, Birmingham, AL, USA
[3] Urologic Oncology Branch, National Cancer Institute, National Institutes of Health, Bethesda, MD, USA

Kidney

The scope and goals of renal mass biopsy have evolved from solely characterizing candidates for nonsurgical intervention to the present paradigm of also identifying patients who may benefit from early and focal therapy. Broadly, biopsy may be a consideration in four scenarios, the first three of which will be expanded on throughout this chapter.

- Evaluation and follow-up of a small renal mass, as defined herein.
- Before focal ablative therapy or during follow-up thereafter.
- In the setting of known metastatic primary renal malignancy.
- The traditional indications for renal biopsy: clinical suspicion for a hematalogic-based malignancy (e.g., lymphoma), renal abscess, or metastases to the kidney, all of which are primarily managed nonsurgically.

Background

The explosion in the number of imaging studies performed in the past two decades has redefined the epidemiological statistics for renal malignancy. Small renal masses (SRMs), those less than 4 cm in diameter, now represent 48–66% of new renal cancers [1].

An increasing proportion of SRMs are found in the elderly, and 20–30% of these lesions may be benign [2–4]. Given the aging population and taking into account medical comorbidities, including poor renal reserve and limited life expectancy, it is important to determine which patients will benefit from definitive surgical treatment (i.e., total or partial nephrectomy) compared with those patients who will benefit from alternative management strategies.

Unfortunately, conventional imaging techniques perform poorly in definitively differentiating benign from malignant renal masses [5,6]. Less than 20% of benign tumors are correctly identified on computed tomography (CT), and diagnostic accuracy decreases with decreasing mass diameter [7,8]. Additionally, monitoring for disease progression for patients with known renal malignancy on active surveillance may not be possible with imaging alone. Serial CT or ultrasound do not always correlate with the natural history of SRMs, and initial lesion size does not consistently predict the rate of growth [9]. To stratify treatment strategies for patients by the potential aggressiveness of their disease, biopsy is increasingly seen as an integral component of active surveillance for renal cancer [10].

The Evolution and Performance of Renal Biopsy

Historically, percutaneous renal biopsy was limited by low-tissue yield, inaccuracy in diagnosis, minimal change in management, and poor concordance with histologic subtype and aggressiveness. However, since 2001 the diagnostic accuracy of renal mass biopsy has been reported as high as 86–98% [11]. Overall, biopsy yield (for all modalities) ranges from 78% to 100% with increasing operator experience, with sensitivities and specificities of 86–100% and 100%, respectively, in multiple large studies [12]. This performance appears to be unique to the management of SRMs, and a greater risk for biopsy failure has been reported for each 1-cm increase in tumor diameter beyond a 4-cm threshold [13,14]. Furthermore, biopsy of the SRM alters clinical management in nearly 50% of patients [15].

Technical considerations include needle gauge, core-versus-aspiration biopsy technique, and image guidance. Core-needle biopsy demonstrates advantages over fine-needle aspiration (FNA) in terms of sensitivity; specifically, prediction of nuclear grade by FNA is particularly compromised (28% vs. 76%) [16,17]. Two passes with a core needle are sufficient to obtain a reliable sample in 97% of cases [18], and use of a biopsy sheath standardizes the depth of penetration to obtain consistent samples that may be more important than number of cores [19]. Needles that 18 gauge or larger demonstrate the greatest accuracy in terms of correlation with final surgical pathology [20].

Potential complications of either FNA or core-needle biopsy include bleeding, perirenal hematoma, pneumothorax, arteriovenous fistula, or tract seeding. However, the incidence of these is quite low [21]. The incidence of tract seeding in particular has been quoted as 0.01% and has been successfully managed with percutaneous ablation [22]. It may be prevented by the use of a coaxial guide or cannula, which also improves patients comfort and allows for better visualization on image

Table 6.1 Technique for Renal Mass Biopsy [23].

- The patient should be in a prone, semiprone, or lateral decubitus position.
- FNA should be done before core biopsy to reduce the number of clots in the specimen.
- The cannula with stylet is inserted into the target.
- Negative pressure is applied while passes are made with the needle.
- If the initial return is blood only, repeat the procedure using a capillary technique.

FNA, fine-needle aspiration.

guidance [23]. Recommended techniques for renal mass biopsy are summarized in Table 6.1.

Biopsy in the Settings of Diagnosis, Focal Therapy, or Metastatic Disease

Diagnostic Biopsy

The diagnostic yield is reportedly equivalent whether ultrasound or CT guidance is used [14]. Better spatial resolution and avoidance of necrotic areas is possible with CT-guided biopsy, but it is more expensive, does not yet allow for in-gantry needle visualization, and exposes the patient to ionizing radiation. On the other hand, ultrasound allows for real-time needle guidance and is portable and less costly, but it is highly operator-dependent [21]. CT guidance is recommended over ultrasound in the face of high accuracy with comparatively low false-negative rates.

Focal Therapy

Because the majority of new renal cancers are diagnosed in the elderly and frail population, focal therapies such as cryoablation or radiofrequency ablation (RFA) are attractive treatment options to consider. Histologically proven treatment success is high for cryoablation [24]. With regard to RFA, pretreatment biopsy has a diagnostic yield of >94%; 46% of post-RFA positive biopsy demonstrated no enhancement on CT or magnetic resonance imaging (MRI). This is supported in a small analysis of patients undergoing RFA for renal cell carcinoma (RCC); at 1-year follow-up biopsy, all histology demonstrated tumor eradication with only coagulative necrosis and inflammatory cells visible. These patients had stable imaging by contrast CT [25].

In light of all of this, all patients should be considered for core-needle biopsy of the lesion before ablation to exclude benign processes. Post ablation, all patients should undergo follow-up with CT or MRI; three to four imaging studies in the first year. Any persistently nonshrinking, enhancing tumor should be rebiopsied. In cases where central contrast enhancement is present, biopsy should be performed at 6 months; for peripheral contrast enhancement, at 12 months [26]. It is important to note that these suggestions have not been consistently or definitively agreed on.

Metastatic Disease

The role of biopsy in metastatic renal carcinoma remains to be elucidated. A study of patients undergoing cytoreductive nephrectomy who received preoperative biopsy of both the primary mass and the metastatic sites demonstrates some limitations. Although biopsy and pathologic specimens were in accordance in 96% of clear-cell RCC, they were in agreement in only 73% cases of non-clear-cell RCC. Furthermore, biopsy was exceedingly poor at identifying sarcomatoid de-differentiation (a poor prognostic factor and a relative contraindication to cytoreductive nephrectomy in most series) [27,28]. Furthermore, Fuhrman grade was concordant only for 38% of patients [29]. To overcome these limitations, the authors recommend biopsy from multiple sites within the primary tumor to obtain a better representation of the tumor being evaluated.

Current Challenges

Although the accuracy of renal mass biopsy has improved, its performance in assessing Fuhrman nuclear grade remains poor, regardless of the modality used. Because Fuhrman grade is an important prognostic indicator for clear-cell RCC and should ideally

be determined by biopsy, various refinements of technique and guidance have been reported, with accuracies ranging from 43% to 76% [23,30,31]. Nevertheless, when evaluating solely on the basis of low- versus high-grade tumors, biopsy correctly identified grade in 93% of cases [32].

Core-needle biopsy may outperform FNA in terms of nuclear grading; however, it is less informative for cystic lesions, with higher rates of biopsy failure and false-negative results [13,33,34]. As such, when evaluating cystic lesions, core biopsy may be more useful in Bosniak IV cysts where solid components are present or should be used in combination with FNA [35]. Using this strategy, 39% of Bosniak III and 70% of Bosniak IIF/III patients avoided potentially unnecessary surgery after biopsy [36,37].

The delineation of histologic subtype apart from clear-cell RCC has historically been poor with any biopsy modality; particularly, differentiation between oncocytic neoplasms: benign oncocytoma compared with chromophobe RCC [31]. However, with refinement in technique, the detection of chromophobe RCC has improved [18,32]. Previously, the incidence of hybrid malignant tumors coexisting with benign processes such as oncocytoma was thought to be as high as 20%, meaning that a biopsy result of oncocytoma may not have been adequate to rule out malignancy and that tumor heterogeneity may contribute to inaccurate biopsy results [38,39]. A more recent study demonstrated that only 2.7% of patients with solitary sporadic benign renal masses harbored malignant pathology—all low-grade chromophobe RCC in the setting of oncocytoma—and that no patient had regional or metastatic progression at 44 months of follow-up [40]. Therefore, biopsy may be more meaningful in this setting than previously thought. Nevertheless, benign biopsy findings in patients with multifocal tumors and known genetic syndromes, (i.e. Birt-Hogg-Dubé) should be scrutinized more carefully. In the setting of multiple synchronous renal tumors, it cannot be assumed that the histology of one is representative of all, and therefore special consideration of this factor must be made, particularly if biopsy of multiple lesions is undertaken, potentially increasing the risk of complications [21].

Nondiagnostic biopsy (most commonly inflammatory or necrotic tissue) may represent approximately 5% of renal biopsy results [11]. Repeat biopsy is one approach to this problem and appears to perform similarly to initial biopsy and results in similar long-term outcomes in terms of recurrence or metastasis [23,41]. There is relatively little data available on whether tumor location plays a role in the accuracy of biopsy; however, longitudinal (upper/mid/lower pole) location may predict a diagnostic biopsy [14]. Finally, although diagnostic performance is greatest for SRMs, biopsy failure for technical reasons such as erroneous targeting, difficult visualization, or blood contamination is also more common in smaller tumors [42].

Laparoscopic Biopsy

In the setting of failed percutaneous renal biopsy, solitary kidney or risk of complications as a result of cysts or anomalous anatomy, or where obesity inhibits the utility of ultrasound- or CT-guided biopsy, laparoscopic renal biopsy may be preferred. A two-trocar technique is adequate to obtain tissue suitable for diagnosis in 96% of cases with a 13.5% complication rate, primarily hemorrhage [43].

Future Directions

Imaging modalities are improving and show promise in their applications. Real-time fluoroscopic guidance of the biopsy needle may be ideal for lesions that are inaccessible by CT or ultrasound guidance [44]. Three-dimensional volumetric data from a C-arm can be fused with real-time fluoroscopy for stereotactic biopsy with a mean radiation dose-area product value of 44.0 Gy cm^2 and no major complications. However, the procedures necessitated a steep trajectory angle, which is challenging to achieve with fluoroscopy [45].

Advanced immunohistochemistry panels, molecular profiling, and genomic analysis are maturing and may help select patients for individualized targeted therapy; the samples from core biopsies are suitable for use in genomic analyses and for predicting clinical outcomes [46]. The addition of radiation therapy–polymerase chain reaction (RT–PCR) in the analysis of biopsy specimens increased overall diagnostic accuracy from 83% to 95% and the negative predictive value for clear-cell RCC to nearly 100% [47]. In addition, the use of interphase fluorescence in situ hybridization (FISH) specifically led to greater diagnostic fidelity [48]. However, the prognostic role of these new tools has only begun to be evaluated. One recent study demonstrated a significant association between disease-free survival as well as cancer-specific survival in patients evaluated with an immunohistochemistry (IHC) panel of six cell-cycle and proliferative markers [49]. The number of abnormal markers was found to correlate with disease aggressiveness, which may further support the routine use of renal biopsy for risk stratification.

Table 6.2 presents the recommendations of the American Urological Association (AUA) and the European Association of Urology (EAU) on the indications for renal mass biopsy.

Penile

Introduction

Accurate assessment of the grade and depth of invasion of penile squamous cell carcinoma (SCC) is vital because it is recognized that a significant proportion of patients with intermediate- and high-grade disease progress to nodal involvement. Biopsy should be considered for all penile lesions that appear suspicious and do not resolve with a course of antibiotics [50].

There are several strategies for this initial biopsy: incisional, tissue core, FNA, and brush or excisional biopsy. Superficial biopsies,

Table 6.2 Recommendations on the Use of Percutaneous Renal Biopsy

Guideline	AUA Recommendation	EAU Recommendation
Evaluation of a cT1 renal mass	Core biopsy with or without FNA especially if there is suspicion for lymphoma, abscess, or metastasis	Biopsy always required before ablative and systemic therapy. **Grade: A**
Before ablation	Core biopsy with or without FNA **Grade: C**	
In patients undergoing active surveillance	Consider biopsy **Grade: C**	Recommend biopsy to stratify follow-up **Grade: B**
Treatment failure	Biopsy after considering observation, repeat treatment, or surgical intervention	—
Biopsy technique	—	Obtain needle cores with a coaxial technique **Grade: B**

AUA, American Urological Association; EAU, European Association or Urology.

however, are grossly inadequate for determining depth of invasion and fail to identify the correct grade of tumor in approximately 30% of cases [51]. As such, incisional or excisional biopsies are acceptable, but in terms of determining treatment decisions and prognostic value, excisional biopsies are preferred.

Assessing Nodal Involvement at Time of Diagnosis

Assessment of inguinal and regional nodal involvement is a crucial issue to address after the diagnosis of penile or distal urethral SCC has been made. A careful physical examination should be performed to assess for palpable nodes because these may be biopsied via FNA [52]. Inguinal ultrasound can reveal abnormal nodes and is useful as a modality of image guidance for FNA [53].

However, 20% of patients with nonpalpable nodes but who have high-risk tumor features—stage T2 or greater, lymphovascular invasion, or higher grade—have presence of clinically occult nodal metastases [54]. Patients suspected of having micrometastatic disease who undergo prophylactic lymphadenectomy have greatly improved 5-year survival as compared to controls (83% vs. 36%, respectively), but this procedure carries

with it potential morbidity. Addressing the diagnostic dilemma posed by this group of patients spurred the development of dynamic sentinel lymph node biopsy (DSNB.)

Initially, sentinel node dissection was performed for penile cancer using lymphoscintigraphy alone, but this suffered from a high false-negative rate (20%) and recurrences [54]. The modification by Catalona reduced the rate of morbidity from 50% to 22%. In 1994, the Netherlands Cancer Institute used lymphoscintigraphy with intradermal peritumoral Tc-99 nanocolloid the day before surgery, followed by dynamic imaging with a portable gamma camera and static imaging to locate sentinel nodes. With the addition of ultrasound with FNA in 2001, the false-negative rate decreased to 4.8% and the morbidity to 5.7%.

Since the introduction of DSNB, the technique has been refined further. DSNB alone, before the use of ultrasound or FNA in conjunction, yielded a sensitivity of 80% with a false-negative rate of 22% [55]. Studies evaluating patients undergoing DSNB before and after the modification of the technique found improved 5 year disease-specific survival (91% vs. 82%) with the addition of ultrasound and FNA [56] and dramatic improvements in the false-negative rate (4.8% from 19.2%) and

Table 6.3 Summary of Key Steps in Dynamic Sentinel Node Biopsy.

- Day before surgery: peritumoral radiotracer injection (intradermal) followed by dynamic and static image acquisition using lymphoscintigraphy and SPECT–CT
- Day of surgery: blue dye injection
- Intraoperatively: inguinal exploration with a portable gamma probe plus blue dye visualization for precise anatomic localization
- Care must be taken with handling of specimens before tissue processing.

SPECT–CT, single-photon emission computed tomography–computed tomography.

rate of complications nearly halved (5.7% from 10.2%) [57]. Poor prognostic factors included greater number of positive nodes, extranodal extension, and pelvic lymph node involvement.

The technique itself may only be feasible in high-volume referral centers. Close collaboration between urologists and uropathologists is necessary [58]. However, the learning curve itself is short. Table 6.3 presents a summary of key steps in DSNB.

Patients with biopsy-proven positive nodes should undergo complete inguinal lymphadenectomy [52]. Only patients with high-risk features (as previously defined) and no apparent nodal disease should undergo DSNB [58]. For patients with intermediate-risk penile SCC (G2T1), the risk of lymph node metastasis was 9%. This is too low to justify prophylactic lymphadenectomy but may perhaps provide an argument for advocating DSNB in this patient population [59]. Furthermore, patients with intermediate-grade disease who have delayed DSNB (so called postresection DSNB) have recurrence and survival rates similar to those for DSNB performed at the time of primary resection [60].

Nodal Involvement after Primary Resection

After primary resection, 29.3% of patients with penile SCC had local, regional, or distant recurrences, with the majority (63%) being local. Of the recurrences, 92% occurred within 5 years of treatment, with 5-year survival being 92% for local recurrence and 33% for regional recurrence [61]. In patients who received primary resection and DSNB, ultrasound-guided FNA was used to diagnose recurrence in 80% of nonpalpable nodes, with a sensitivity and specificity of 87% and 99.9%, respectively [62].

The role of postresection DSNB is not well-defined. In a small study of patients with recurrence after undergoing DSNB and primary resection, the sentinel node could be identified in 79% of groins and was involved in 33% of cases [63].

A decision flowchart summarizing recommendations for DSNB is presented in Table 6.4.

Table 6.4 EAU Recommendations for the Role of Biopsy in Managing Penile Cancer.

Context	Recommendation	Grade
Initial evaluation	Cytological and histological diagnosis plus physical examination of both groins	C
After diagnosis:		
Palpable nodes	Ultrasound-guided FNA; however, core-needle, or open biopsy may be performed	—
Nonpalpable nodes	DSNB is indicated for >T1G2 tumors; otherwise, consider surveillance	**B**
Negative nodal biopsy	Repeat biopsy is indicated	**B**

DSNB, dynamic sentinel node biopsy; EAU, European Association of Urology; FNA, fine-needle aspiration.

Prostate

Background

Prostate cancer is unique among urologic neoplasia in that until recently, it was not possible to accurately or reliably identify suspicious intraprostatic lesions under image guidance. Consequently, the most widespread modality in use today is systematic regional needle biopsy of the gland. Widespread use of prostate-specific antigen (PSA) as a screening tool for these essentially random biopsies has shifted the demographics of prostate cancer significantly. Of the estimated quarter-million men in the United States who will be newly diagnosed with prostate cancer in 2014, the majority will present with localized disease and nearly half with low-grade cancer [64]. The fact that most patients with localized disease may die of causes other than prostate cancer has spurred the adoption of active surveillance (AS), in which repeat biopsy is a confirmatory strategy [65].

Broadly speaking, prostate biopsy is a consideration in four classes of patients.

- Men with elevated PSA level or suspicious digital rectal examination (DRE); however, to establish a diagnosis though the definitions of "elevated PSA" remains controversial. The National Comprehensive Cancer Network (NCCN) recommends biopsy at a threshold of PSA >2.6 ng/mL with a caveat against doing so if life expectancy is less than 10 years, whereas the AUA does not recommend a specific threshold [66,67].
- Men whose PSA is rising or remains elevated after an initial negative biopsy or who have suspicious findings on the initial biopsy. "Suspicious findings" include atypical small acinar proliferation (ASAP) and multifocal prostatic intraepithelial neoplasia (PIN) because their presence may portend prostatic adenocarcinoma [68,69]. Isolated PIN does not necessitate repeat biopsy [70].
- Men with clinically localized disease who are candidates for ablative therapy or AS to monitor for disease progression.
- Rarely, in men who have received definitive therapy to monitor for disease persistence or recurrence.

Before any prostate biopsy strategy, one should take into account the patient's age, medical comorbidities, functional status, and potential consequences of undergoing therapy if needed. Screening algorithms using risk assessments may reduce unnecessary biopsies [71]. Verification of an initially high PSA level after several weeks under standardized conditions before biopsy is considered standard of care [72]. Although optimal dosing and schedules vary, administration of antibiotics (commonly quinolones) before biopsy is recommended [73]. Patient comfort should be a priority and ultrasound-guided peri-prostatic block has been shown to be superior to intrarectal anesthetic in terms of pain control [74].

The Refinement of Needle-Guided Biopsy

Before the introduction of transrectal ultrasound (TRUS), biopsy of the prostate was accomplished via the operator performing DRE to locate suspicious nodules and then using a transrectal needle approach to approximately target the lesion. However, this technique suffered from poor accuracy and was highly operator-dependent. TRUS-guided needle biopsy quickly became the most widely used approach in a baseline prostate biopsy. Substantial data is now available regarding its performance, but questions remain about the ideal number of cores, the detection of clinically insignificant cancer, value in staging disease extent, and concordance with final surgical pathology when available.

Initially, a sextant template was used; in the parasagittal plane, biopsies are taken from the right and left sides of the prostate base, mid-gland, and apex. These sites are chosen arbitrarily by the operator [75]. However, multiple large studies have demonstrated an increase in cancer detection rate (CDR) with 4 to 6 additional cores for a total of 10 to 12 cores.

This extended 12-core approach is reported to increase the CDR by 12–33% as compared to the standard sextant biopsy [76,77]. Furthermore, laterally directed biopsies demonstrate a 31% greater detection rate than the standard sextant method [78]. However, rates of detecting cancer overall remain less than 40% for either the sextant or extended-template approach, with reported false-negative rates of 15–34% [79,80]. This poor negative predictive value implies that rebiopsy after an initial negative result would diagnose substantially more cancers, which has been borne out in prospective studies [81].

Correlation between biopsy Gleason grade with that of final surgical pathology is greater with either a 10- or 12-core approach as compared to standard sextant biopsy [79,82]. Upgrading from biopsy to final pathology is also less likely with an extended biopsy template, but rates of upgrading remain 14–25% overall [83,84]. The detection of clinically insignificant cancer does not appear to be significantly increased with the extended sextant 12-core approach [85,86].

Determining the ideal locations of the additional cores beyond those in the standard template has been challenging. With regard to anterior lesions, which are commonly missed by biopsy, tumor frequency is greatest in the mid-gland followed by the apex; apical biopsies have demonstrated several advantages [87]. Biopsy directed toward the bilateral anterior horns and midline increased the CDR by 31% in one study; the majority of nonsextant positive cores originated from the anterior horns [88]. Furthermore, the positive predictive value for a positive apical biopsy core identifying tumor location on final pathology appears to be high [89].

Biopsy of the transitional zone (TZ) has proven elusive in terms of yield and performance. Although 15–25% of all prostate cancer is located anteriorly within the TZ, there is discordance with the CDR of TZ biopsy [90,91]. With regard to concordance with the final pathology specimen, cancer detected by TZ-directed cores either was not actually from the TZ or did not reflect a dominant lesion in 80% of cases [92]. As a consequence, upgrading because of TZ biopsy is quite rare [93]. Laterally directed biopsies of the base, mid-gland, and apex result in up to a 17% increase in the overall CDR and outperform the mid-lobar sextant approach [94,95]. Furthermore, laterally directed cores independently predict total tumor volume and final Gleason score [96].

There are conflicting data on the ability of transrectal biopsy to predict extracapsular extension (ECE) or surgical margin status. Of several multivariate analyses evaluating predictors of ECE, the common variables include positive basal cores and tumor length or percentage of core involvement. No such association was found for positive apical biopsy [97-99]. Men with more than three positive biopsy cores had a greater risk for a positive surgical margin, but the predictive value for an individual core was low [100].

Obtaining more than 12 cores as an initial biopsy strategy may be suited to carefully selected populations. The overall CDR of an 18-core biopsy does not appear to differ significantly from that of 12-core biopsy, and the increase in diagnostic yield is comparatively low [101,102]. However, the CDR in men with PSA <10 ng/mL was 51.6% for 18-core compared with 42.6% for 12-core biopsy. The 18-core biopsy cases detected more cancer than 12-core biopsy in men with prostate volume >65 mL [103,104]. In addition, the rate of insignificant cancer detection increases with the number of additional cores taken, reported as 22–33% [105,106]. Nevertheless, the false-negative rate between 24-core and 12-core biopsy in a population of men with previously negative biopsy was equivalent [107].

In summary, per AUA recommendations, the use of a 12-core systematic template incorporating apical and far-lateral sampling may maximize CDR and negative predictive value as an initial biopsy strategy [75]. The EAU issues a grade B recommendation for at least 8 cores [72]. Both organizations do not recommend biopsy of the TZ with more than 12 cores as an initial strategy. However, these may be a consideration with persistently negative biopsy and continued clinical suspicion.

Issues with TRUS-Guided Biopsy

Despite the refinements to technique and large volume of data acquired regarding its performance, TRUS-guided biopsy has several persistent flaws. First, the overall CDR with any number of randomly targeted cores remains less than 40%, and a significant proportion of these tumors are not clinically significant [95]. This performance is especially problematic considering that repeat biopsy is used routinely in monitoring men on AS. Second, up to one-third of men on AS are undergraded on their initial biopsy as compared to final surgical pathology [108]. Third, there is a large degree of variability in the volume of cancer detected by serial biopsy [109].

Additionally, anterior cancers are still missed by extended-template biopsy [110]. African American men more often have anterior lesions that are more often upgraded on surgical pathology versus biopsy, as compared with Caucasian men [111]. This was found in a cohort of men on AS and argues for improved sampling of the anterior gland as well as better risk stratification for African American men.

Finally, 3.5% of men undergoing TRUS-guided biopsy had infectious complications, of whom the majority required hospitalization; the odds of infection increases by 1.3 for each successive biopsy session [112]. Fluoroquinolone resistant and extended-spectrum beta-lactamase–producing organisms are increasingly common. The overall rates of hospitalization post biopsy are reported at 4% [113].

However, multiple studies have demonstrated no increased risk of lower urinary tract symptoms [114], worsening of sexual function [115,116], or predilection for biochemical recurrence [117] with multiple TRUS-directed biopsies.

Transperineal Biopsy

Transperineal prostate biopsy is one strategy that may be useful in men with previously negative biopsies and in monitoring candidates for AS. Specifically in a population of men with a negative TRUS-guided biopsy and rising PSA, template-guided transperineal biopsy detected 46.6% of cancers of which 86.7% were clinically significant by the Epstein criteria [118]. The most common location was in the anterior apex. Furthermore, good access to the anterior gland has been afforded by the transperineal approach [119].

Although biopsy progression on AS is often missed by standard TRUS-guided biopsy, template-guided transperineal biopsy reclassified 41–85% of men as having clinically significant disease on repeat biopsy as compared to 8–22% for TRUS-guided biopsy [120]. Whole-mount pathological simulations of 12-core, 14-core, and transperineal mapping biopsies demonstrate significantly poorer performance in detecting clinically significant disease with the transrectal approach [121]. A targeted biopsy approach using image guidance for templating may increase performance further. Fewer cores are needed overall (4 vs. 12) to diagnose nearly 50% more high-risk cancers with image-guided transperineal biopsy [122]. Overall, up to an additional 38% of cancer may be detected using a transperineal approach with a possible avoidance of the infectious complications of transrectal biopsy [123]. The major drawback of transperineal biopsy is a comparatively high rate of postprocedure urinary retention (10%).

MRI-Guided Biopsy

MRI-guided biopsy is a promising tool in the initial diagnosis and in the follow-up of men with prostate cancer. Improved resolution, the addition of an endorectal coil, and the refinement of multiple modalities including MR spectroscopy (MRS) dynamic contrast enhancement (DCE), and diffusion-weighted imaging (DWI) has resulted in the ability of multiparametric MRI (mpMRI) to not only detect lesions and stage disease but also potentially determine biologic aggressiveness of tumors with high sensitivity and specificity [124,125]. Furthermore, mpMRI can detect tumors in more occult locations, commonly missed by traditional random biopsy, including central and anterior gland lesions [126]. Three strategies exist for targeting lesions based on imaging information.

First, transrectal or transperineal biopsy performed directly in the MR bore can be used to target visualized lesions [127]. There are limited data on this method, which is laborious because it necessitates serial MRI scans to confirm needle placement, requires sedation and specialized equipment, limits the working space, and is costly. However, small studies of in-bore mpMRI biopsy have demonstrated improved CDR as compared to TRUS-guided biopsy [128].

The second strategy is one of "cognitive biopsy" and is based on the operator's review of MRI scans before a standard TRUS-guided biopsy in which suspicious areas are attempted to be targeted. This approach does appear to increase the CDR and concordance with final pathology as compared to ultrasound-only biopsy [129]. However, there is a lack of reproducibility and inherent subjectivity in the scheme, which largely hinges on operator experience.

A third approach is one of MRI-ultrasound targeted biopsy, which uses software to fuse a previously acquired mpMRI volumetric data set with ultrasound images acquired in real time. A comparatively greater amount of experimental data available for fusion biopsy as compared to either in-bore or cognitive biopsy. This modality can be performed in an outpatient setting with only local anesthetic. Presently several competing fusion biopsy platforms are on the market and have been reviewed comprehensively by Logan *et al.* [124].

MRI-ultrasound fusion biopsy has demonstrated several advantages over TRUS-guided random biopsy: the overall CDR is greater and more cancer per core is detected via fusion-guided as compared to 12-core biopsy [130–132]. Of men with an initial negative 12-core TRUS-guided biopsy, 34–37% were found to have cancer on fusion biopsy and 72% had high-grade disease. Twelve-core biopsy missed 54% of clinically significant cancers [133,134]. This was true regardless of the fusion platform used. Furthermore, in patients with a negative initial fusion biopsy who underwent rebiopsy, the follow-up CDR was lower than the initial rate, and 93% of cancers were low grade (≤3+4) [135].

Detection rates appear to be consistently greater for fusion-guided biopsy across prostate volume (71.1% for glands <40 mL) [136]. More clinically significant cancers (≥ Gleason 4+3) are detected by targeted versus TRUS-guided biopsy with fewer cores needed to establish a diagnosis; the majority of cancers missed by fusion biopsy appear to be clinically insignificant [137]. The software platform enables documentation of targets and needle tracks, avoiding undersampling and representing an attractive option for serial follow-up with rebiopsy of old lesions [138]. Lastly, any strategy of true focal therapy of the prostate (i.e., targeting localized lesions) must necessarily use image-guided biopsy in selecting patients [139].

Nevertheless, there are significant barriers to implementing MRI-guided biopsy in routine clinical practice. A primary hurdle is that the majority of the data evaluating fusion biopsy has been retrospective in nature. However, a prospective trial evaluating a hybrid transrectal-transperineal fusion system demonstrated a CDR of 82.6%, of which targeted cores detected significantly more cancer than systematic biopsy (30% vs. 8.2%), with a low false-negative rate of 3.2% [140].

In addition, the performance of fusion biopsy relative to that of transperineal template biopsy is not well studied. One meta-regression analysis pooled 46 studies, representing 4,657 patients in comparing transrectal, transperineal, and MRI-guided biopsy. MRI-guided biopsy was found to be superior to transrectal biopsy in terms of

CDR, but the differences with transperineal biopsy were unclear. A major limitation of this study was that cognitive and software-fusion biopsies were pooled [141].

Furthermore, a small proportion of clinically significant lesions are detected by TRUS-guided biopsy but not MRI/ultrasound fusion biopsy. This may represent several possibilities: software errors in needle registration or tracking, the inability of mpMRI to detect cancer foci below a set threshold, or nonimageable tumors [124]. As a consequence, 12-core extended biopsy is currently still recommended to be performed as standard of care alongside fusion biopsy, though data are emerging in investigating the role of targeted biopsies in isolation.

There is presently no consensus on grading of suspicious lesions on mpMRI, with several competing score systems in use. However, the PI-RADS metric is currently being refined and demonstrates promise in standardizing prostate MRI interpretation and reporting [142].

With regard to active surveillance protocols, the various current thresholds of eligibility are based on percentage of core involvement and number of cores that are not applicable to targeted biopsies; new standards will need to be developed and validated. There are as yet no prospective studies detailing the performance of MRI guidance in repeat or follow-up biopsy. However, a study of progression from very low-risk disease with median follow-up of 18 months demonstrated a negative predictive value of 84%, with sensitivity and specificity of 70% and 72%, respectively, of mpMRI findings for Gleason score progression. Furthermore, the natural history of small index lesions (≤5 mm) on mpMRI may represent benign findings in 87.5% of cases or low-grade cancer in the remainder [143].

Lastly, the start-up costs are relatively steep. However, one model demonstrated that with a sensitivity of MRI of ≥20%, cost effectiveness of fusion biopsy could be achieved over 10 years with an improvement in quality-adjusted life years as compared to a strategy of serial systematic TRUS-guided biopsy [144]. Additional efforts are underway to investigate the diagnostic value of a more time-efficient, screening prostate MRI with limited parameters, which would further minimize cost [145,146].

Alternative Prostate Biopsy Modalities

Several alternative biopsy strategies have been proposed but suffer from poor specificity or accuracy:

- Real-time transrectal elastography, using the principle that cancerous lesions will manifest in more dense tissue, has been evaluated prospectively in one trial. CDR were significantly greater with elastography as opposed to 12-core biopsy; however, overall sensitivity and specificity were 60.8% and 68.4%, respectively, as compared to 15% and 92.3%, respectively, for TRUS-guided biopsy.
- Contrast-enhanced TRUS-guided biopsy, using sulfur hexafluoride microbubbles as a contrast agent, has demonstrated variable results but does not outperform standard TRUS-guided biopsy [147,148].
- Transurethral resection of the prostate (TURP) is a poor modality for detecting prostate adenocarcinoma but may be used in men with obstructive symptoms [149].

Table 6.5 summarizes the details of the prostate biopsy modalities discussed.

Table 6.5 Take-Home Message: Prostate Biopsy.

- In the initial evaluation for suspected prostate cancer, obtain 12 cores using a transrectal ultrasound-guided extended sextant-template.
- Rebiopsy, saturation biopsy, or transperineal approach are options for persistently negative biopsy.
- Multiparametric prostate MRI and lesion-targeted biopsies may be more representative of whole-gland pathology than 12-core TRUS biopsy.

MRI, magnetic resonance imaging; TRUS, transrectal ultrasound.

Seminal Vesicle Biopsy

The role of seminal vesicle biopsy in the setting of prostate cancer is poorly defined. At PSA >15–20 ng/mL, the odds of seminal vesicle involvement are 20–25% [150]. However, it is not recommended to biopsy the seminal vesicles unless doing so will impact treatment (i.e., in the choice of radiotherapy compared with surgical management) [72]. An intriguing small study of MRI-ultrasound guided seminal vesicle biopsy triggered by suspicious MRI findings demonstrated seminal vesicle invasion in 65% of cases; further studies are necessary to determine if this modality may be useful in preoperative staging.

Testis

Background

The role of testicular biopsy remains controversial. For a suspected testicular mass, surgical exploration is recommended, with biopsy (enucleation) only if the diagnosis is unclear [151]. However, patients with known testicular cancer may harbor synchronous or metachronous disease in the contralateral testicle.

Assessment of the Contralateral Testicle

Testicular intraepithelial neoplasia (TIN) is the precursor lesion for all testicular germ cell tumors except for spermatocytic seminoma [152]. Approximately 70% of all TIN progresses to invasive cancer [153]. The prevalence of TIN in the contralateral testicle in men who are diagnosed with testicular cancer was previously estimated as high as 5%, with testicular atrophy and age 30 and younger being risk factors for progression [154,155]. However, a population study of nearly 30,000 cases of testicular cancer in the United States found that the 15-year cumulative risk for either synchronous or metachronous contralateral disease was 1.9%, and the

10-year overall survival after metachronous diagnosis was 93% and for synchronous disease, 85% [156].

Biopsy of the contralateral testicle may be beneficial in evaluating patients with confirmed cancer. In German studies, the sensitivity and overall accuracy of contralateral testicular random biopsy assessing for the presence of TIN were 91% and 99.5% respectively, with a false-negative rate of 0.5% [157]. Men with testicular volume <12 mL, a history of cryptorchidism, or age 30 years or younger were at elevated risk for contralateral TIN. The greatest risk factor was testicular atrophy (4.3-fold increase in risk) [158]. Furthermore, there is an increase in diagnostic yield of taking two random biopsies compared with one [159]. The risk of complications is low (2.8%), the majority of which (96%) were minor, including focal hematoma and edema, and which resolved within 1 week [160].

However, several concerns remain regarding testicular biopsy. More than 10% of the testicular volume should be tubules with TIN for a random biopsy to be positive [158]. Despite a false-negative rate of 0.5%, patients with testicular cancer who have a negative biopsy still require meticulous follow-up. Furthermore, Although TIN can be treated by irradiation, this results in irreversible infertility as well as impairment of the endocrine function of Leydig cells in 25% of men necessitating testosterone replacement [158]. The overall cure rate for secondary germ cell tumors is high, and it is questionable if biopsy improves disease-specific survival; in fact, patients undergoing platinum-based chemotherapy had significantly reduced risk of metachronous testicular cancer, especially in those undergoing more than four cycles [154,161].

Consequently, biopsy of the contralateral testicle is ideally to be restricted to two groups of patients:

- Men with testicular volume <12 mL, history of cryptorchidism, or poor spermatogenesis (Johnson score 1–3). Ultrasound findings of testicular microlithiasis may be a further indicator of TIN specifically in this population but not others [162,163].

- Men with extragonadal germ cell tumors, especially those with retroperitoneal tumors. Up to one-third of these patients may present with metachronous testicular cancer [164].

Nevertheless, the quandary of offering treatment remains the same in these groups. Dieckmann *et al.* reviewed the technique for biopsy comprehensively; however, it has not been widely adopted [165]. Unfortunately, minimally invasive alternatives to this technique such as FNA with immunostaining have performed poorly in terms of sensitivity and accuracy [166].

The EAU recommends biopsy to be offered to the high-risk group defined previously, with double biopsy preferred; biopsy is not necessary in patients older than 40 years of age [151].

Urothelium

Bladder

Introduction

The mainstay of diagnosis, as well as treatment, of the majority of bladder malignancies revolves around urethrocystoscopy and transurethral biopsy and resection. Several recent innovations have augmented this modality or demonstrated promise in increasing its accuracy, yield, or safety.

This section deals primarily with biopsy strategies for urothelial carcinoma and its precursor lesions. Bladder small cell carcinoma, sarcomas, and other malignancies are addressed separately.

The population of patients in whom biopsy is a consideration can be divided broadly into two subgroups:

- Patients suspected of harboring disease on the basis of clinical history of microscopic or gross hematuria, environmental risk factors, abnormal urine cytology or urinary molecular marker tests, or on the basis of concerning imaging findings, and

- Patients being monitored for disease recurrence after focal or definitive therapy.

Goals of Biopsy

Urothelial carcinoma spans noninvasive papillary carcinoma (Ta), carcinoma-in-situ (Tis), and stage T1 tumors, characterized as nonmuscle-invasive, as well as muscle-invasive bladder carcinoma (≥T2 tumors). Because treatment modalities vary significantly depending on the histologic diagnosis, knowledge of the extent of disease is critical. Recently, practice has shifted toward individualized risk assessments that must be tailored on the basis of accurate staging data.

It is recommended that patients with suspected bladder tumor undergo initial cystoscopy with transurethral resection as necessary [167]. Inspection of the entire urothelial lining of the bladder is essential. When abnormal areas of urothelium (velvet-like, erythematous) are seen, it is advised to take cold-cup biopsies or biopsies with a resection loop. All findings should be documented on a bladder map for future localization of tissue sampling.

Tumors visualized on cystoscopy should be resected en-bloc if 1 cm or smaller in diameter. Larger tumors should be removed in a piecemeal fashion, including the exophytic portion of the tumor, underlying bladder wall with muscle, and the edges of resection. The yield of biopsy of normal mucosa ("random mapping") is 2% or less in patients with solitary Ta or T1 tumors and is therefore discouraged [168].

If the tumor is located in the trigone or bladder neck, or if there are multiple tumors, the risk of ductal involvement appears to be elevated [169]. The incidence of carcinoma-in-situ in the prostatic urethra in these patients has been reported to be 11.7% [170]. Where abnormalities of the prostatic urethra can be seen, or there is suspicion for bladder CIS, or urine cytology is positive without evidence of a bladder tumor, prostatic urethral biopsies should be taken. Biopsies should be taken from abnormal-appearing areas and from the precollicular area (5- to 7-o'clock) using a resection loop. Where stromal invasion is not suspected, a cold-cup biopsy can be performed with forceps instead [171].

For patients with positive cytology and in whom no bladder tumor can be seen, random mapping biopsy is recommended in addition to an upper-tract workup (see Upper-Tract Urothelial Carcinoma section). Biopsies should be taken from the trigone, bladder dome, and walls. In addition, the prostatic urethra should be biopsied as described previously.

Critically Examining TUR

The rate of recurrence for initial transrectal resection (TUR) is alarmingly high (50–70% in some series) [172]. This has been attributed to incomplete TUR, tumor cell implantation, or aggressive tumor biology. Understaging of the tumor is also quite common. Disease progression also occurs at a high rate in patients with initially nonmuscle-invasive bladder cancer, with high-grade lesions, multiple tumors, lesion size greater than 3.0 cm, concomitant CIS, and presence of tumor at the first cystoscopy after TUR, constituting accepted risk factors for progression [173].

Residual tumor was found in the location of the initial resection on repeat transurethral resection of bladder (TURB) and high rates of upstaging are reported [174,175]. Furthermore, repeat TUR can identify patients at risk of progression [176]. Clinical management was changed in a third of patients who underwent repeat TURB because of upstaging [177]. Therefore, a second-look TUR should be considered standard of care for patients with high-grade T1 disease because of its prognostic and therapeutic benefit. The role of repeat TUR in patients with high-grade Ta disease remains a topic of scholarly debate. Patients with low- and intermediate-risk bladder cancer can be considered for repeat TUR based on an individual assessment of risk [174].

Improving on or replacing the TUR technique has been suggested. TUR violates the oncologic principle of tissue integrity for large tumors. Several modifications (e.g., en-bloc resection using a knife electrode, resectoscope cutting loop modifications, and use of bipolar cautery) have been proposed [172]. The use of a modified polypectomy snare may allow for improved biopsy of the tumor base and preserved tumor integrity; however, it was practical only for pedunculated tumors and those small enough to be removed transurethrally [178]. Although in principle these new modalities should reduce recurrence (if caused by tumor implantation), no data exists to validate their use.

Mapping Biopsy

Systematic mapping of normal-appearing bladder mucosa is performed after initial TURB because CIS is especially important to detect; its presence in biopsies can herald upstaging as compared to patients with normal mucosa in biopsies [179]. The incidence of positive random biopsies is significantly greater in patients with high-grade disease. In a large series of patients with nonmuscle-invasive bladder cancer, 12.4% of 1033 patients were found to have abnormal random biopsies, which altered therapy in 7% of cases [180].

Mapping biopsy may be performed with cold-cup forceps or a resection loop. Abnormal-appearing mucosa should be biopsied as well; however, there are few data on the rates of positive biopsy in patients undergoing initial TUR. The sensitivity of random mapping bladder biopsy for the detection of CIS was reported as 51% in one study; therefore, negative results should be interpreted with caution [181].

Vesical diverticula may warrant investigation through mapping biopsy because their presence may portend a greater risk of developing urothelial carcinoma; patients with positive diverticular biopsy had a significantly higher percentage of high-grade and invasive disease [182].

Novel Diagnostic and Biopsy Aids in Urothelial Carcinoma

Photodynamic diagnosis (PDD) has demonstrated promise in terms of improved diagnostic accuracy and yield as compared to traditional white-light cystoscopy (WLC). The data are most convincing for hexylaminolevulinate (HAL)-PDD (as opposed to the older 5-aminolevulinic acid) as a photosensitive marker. With regard to biopsy of abnormal-appearing mucosa in patients with known bladder tumor, HAL-PDD detects CIS more frequently than WLC [183]. Furthermore, the improved detection of bladder tumors may lead to a reduction in recurrence at 9–12 months independently of the level of risk and across patients with Ta, T1, CIS, and primary or recurrent cancer as compared to WLC [184]. Figure 6.1 illustrates these recommendations.

(a)

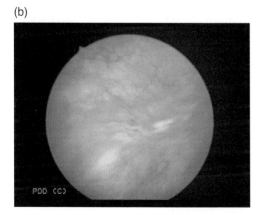

(b)

Figure 6.1 Bladder biopsy in the patient with hematuria. Biopsies may be obtained using cold-cup forceps versus a resection loop. All biopsy findings should be documented on a bladder map. "Abnormal urothelium" includes velvet-like areas or erythema versus sessile/flat tumor. PDD, photodynamic diagnosis.

The rates and types of adverse events are similar between PDD and WLC. However, the technique is costly and requires specialized equipment, has a higher false-positive rate, and long-term outcomes are lacking. In addition, there are no data regarding detection of high-risk cancer or correlation of disease progression with PDD [185].

Narrow-band imaging (NBI) is another optical modality that has shown a benefit in the identification of bladder mucosal lesions. NBI also improves the detection rates for CIS, Ta, and overall nonmuscle-invasive bladder cancer as compared to WLC [186]. The rate of repeat TUR overall and primary site residual tumor rates as well as the 1-year recurrence rates were significantly decreased with the use of NBI [187]. As with PDD, the false-positive rate for NBI is greater than that for WLC mostly as a result of inflammation. There are limited data on recurrence following NBI-assisted TUR or biopsy (Table 6.6).

Confocal laser endomicroscopy (CLE) is an intriguing technique in its infancy. Clear visual differences between normal mucosa, low-grade disease, and high-grade disease could be visualized in a small study of patients with biopsy-confirmed bladder cancer. This could portend "optical biopsy," which could augment tissue sampling techniques [190]. Follow-up studies have demonstrated the possibility of cataloguing tumor growth patterns to assess malignant potential [191]. Furthermore, the learning curve of CLE appears to be low, and interobserver agreement (between urologists and pathologists) appears to be greater than that of traditional WLC [192]. However, apart from cost and training, the performance of this test remain to be determined.

Follow-Up Biopsy

The role of biopsy in patients who have received definitive therapy (i.e., TURB) is to assess for disease recurrence and progression. After TUR in both nonmuscle- and muscle-invasive disease, second-look cystoscopy is necessary at least at 3 months and scheduled per individual risk thereafter.

Table 6.6 Diagnostic Aids in Diagnosing Urothelial Carcinoma.

Technique	Advantages	Disadvantages	Recommendation
Photodynamic diagnosis using ALA or HAL	More sensitive for detection of malignant tumors, particularly for CIS [188]	Recurrence rate for ALA-guided TURB has not been shown to be lower than that of white light [189]; poor specificity	Use in patients suspected of harboring high-grade disease (positive cytology or history)
Narrow-band imaging	Improved cancer detection [186]	No large studies	—

ALA, delta-aminolevulinic acid; CIS, carcinoma in situ; HAL, hexylaminolevulinate; TURB, transurethral resection of bladder.

Table 6.7 Recommendations for Follow-Up Biopsy in Nonmuscle- and Muscle-Invasive Bladder Cancer.

Context	Recommendation	Grade
Nonmuscle invasive	*Regular cystoscopy; stratify risk*	**A**
Low risk	**Cystoscopy** at 3 months, then 9 months, then yearly for 5 years	**C**
High risk	**Cystoscopy plus cytology** at 3 months, repeated every 3 months for 2 years, then every 6 months for 5 years, then yearly.	**C**
Suspicious findings on cystoscopy	*Biopsy*	**B**
Positive cytology without visible tumor	*Random biopsies vs. biopsies with PDD **and** biopsy of the prostatic urethra with upper-tract workup*	**B**
Muscle-invasive	*Full assessment of upper urinary tracts*	
Imaging	Excretory-phase CT urography is preferred to MR urography	**C**
Biopsy	Ureteroscopic-guided biopsy where upper-tract involvement is suspected	**C**

CT, computed tomography; MR, magnetic resonance; PDD, photodynamic diagnosis.

Patients with muscle-invasive, node-positive disease should be observed most stringently. Bladder biopsies should be performed when cystoscopy shows suspicious findings or cytology is positive [193]. If only cytology is positive, random mapping should be performed. Biopsy may be omitted in patients with normal cystoscopy and normal urine cytology even if erythematous findings are present [194]. These guidelines are summarized in Table 6.7.

Follow-up biopsy after initial bacillus Calmette-Guérin (BCG) treatment is more complex. In one study of random-mapping biopsy performed after initial BCG treatment, 32% of patients had positive biopsy, with a combination of negative cytology and normal cystoscopy associated with negative biopsy in 94% of cases [195]. Predictors time to recurrence, progression, and disease-related mortality in patients with grade 3 T1 disease treated with TUR and an induction course of BCG were female and CIS in the prostatic urethra [170]. Therefore, routine TUR biopsies may not be necessary in patients receiving BCG treatment. However, it is important to perform biopsy of the prostatic urethra in patients with high-grade disease because of the prognostic implications.

Bladder Cancer Variants

Data are scant to support the performance of cystoscopic biopsy in the detection of small-cell bladder cancer or squamous differentiation.

A comparison of biopsy findings to final pathology specimens after cystectomy found poor sensitivity overall for predicting bladder cancer variants via bladder biopsy (20–54%) [196]. However, for small-cell bladder cancer specifically, the combined sensitivity of TURB and biopsy was 81%. These findings may be as a result of poor sampling as well as tumor heterogeneity.

Upper-Tract Urothelial Carcinoma

As described in the previous section, cases in which to assess for upper-tract carcinoma include:

- Patients with hematuria or positive urinary cytology and no bladder tumor visualized or sampled on cystoscopy (in addition to random mapping biopsy as previously described); and
- Muscle-invasive bladder carcinoma.

Diagnostic Strategies

Initial evaluation includes CT urography, MR urography, or ureteroscopy. CT urography with an excretory phase is used for diagnosis in preference to MR [197]. Biopsies obtained via flexible ureteroscopy have demonstrated value in staging and prognosis.

The advantages of ureteroscopic biopsy include accurate quantification of disease as well as opportunities for focal therapy. Ureteroscopic biopsy has consistently demonstrated good performance in the detection of urothelial carcinoma as well as determining specific grade of disease when compared to final pathologic specimens. Although staging is not presently as accurate, invasion of lamina propria in biopsy specimens can be determined [198]. This is true regardless of the biopsy volume [199].

The accuracy of ureteroscopic biopsy has been called into question with regard to conservative (endoscopic) management of upper-tract urothelial carcinoma. There is a high risk of recurrence and a grade-related risk of progression in endoscopically managed patients and up to 20% may proceed to radical nephroureterectomy [200]. Furthermore, repeat ureteroscopic biopsy (median interval, 6 weeks) in patients managed conservatively demonstrated upgrading in one-third of cases [201]. Therefore, a highly selected patient population (low-grade, 5-year disease-specific survival) may contain the ideal candidates for endoscopic treatment.

Biopsies are usually performed via a flexible ureteroscope using 3Fr cup forceps. However, biopsy yield may be greater and grading may be more accurate with the use of a wire basket as opposed to cup forceps [202]. Basket biopsy also provided larger specimens than forceps, and larger biopsy forceps may provide less distorted specimens than traditional forceps [203].

Combining urine cytology, the presence or absence of hydronephrosis, and ureteroscopic biopsy grade in a multivariate model yielded high-positive predictive values for muscle-invasive and nonorgan-confined upper-tract urothelial carcinoma (89% and 78%, respectively, if all three variables were abnormal), and a negative predictive value of 100% if all three were normal [204]. These combined modalities may identify patients at risk for advanced disease but need to be validated prospectively.

Primary Urethral Carcinoma

Because the majority of urethral carcinomas arise from the urothelium, and as with bladder urothelial carcinoma, the preferred modality for diagnosis is via urethrocystoscopy. As primary urethral carcinoma is quite rare, there are few recommendations with regard to follow-up.

Patients with larger lesions should undergo transurethral loop resection [205]. However, transurethral biopsy may not determine prostatic involvement or depth of invasion accurately, although negative predictive value was high [206]. The technique most commonly used is loop biopsy of the prostatic urethra at 5- and 7-o'clock positions from the bladder neck and distally around the verumontanum.

References

1 Cooperberg MR, Mallin K, Ritchey J, Villalta JD, Carroll PR, Kane CJ. Decreasing size at diagnosis of stage 1 renal cell carcinoma: analysis from the National Cancer Data Base, 1993 to 2004. J Urol. 2008;179(6):2131–5.

2 Remzi M, Ozsoy M, Klingler HC, Susani M, Waldert M, Seitz C, *et al.* Are small renal tumors harmless? Analysis of histopathological features according to tumors 4 cm or less in diameter. J Urol. 2006;176(3):896–9.

3 Frank I, Blute ML, Cheville JC, Lohse CM, Weaver AL, Zincke H. Solid renal tumors: An analysis of pathological features related to tumor size. J Urol. 2003;170(6 Pt 1): 2217–20.

4 Chow WH, Devesa SS, Warren JL, Fraumeni JF, Jr. Rising incidence of renal cell cancer in the United States. JAMA. 1999;281(17):1628–31.

5 Choudhary S, Rajesh A, Mayer NJ, Mulcahy KA, Haroon A. Renal oncocytoma: CT features cannot reliably distinguish oncocytoma from other renal neoplasms. Clin Radiol. 2009;64(5):517–22.

6 Rosenkrantz AB, Hindman N, Fitzgerald EF, Niver BE, Melamed J, Babb JS. MRI features of renal oncocytoma and chromophobe renal cell carcinoma. AJR Am J Roentgenol. 2010;195(6):W421–7.

7 Remzi M, Katzenbeisser D, Waldert M, Klingler HC, Susani M, Memarsadeghi M, *et al.* Renal tumour size measured radiologically before surgery is an unreliable variable for predicting histopathological features: Benign tumours are not necessarily small. BJU Int. 2007;99(5):1002–6.

8 Millet I, Doyon FC, Hoa D, Thuret R, Merigeaud S, Serre I, *et al.* Characterization of small solid renal lesions: can benign and malignant tumors be differentiated with CT? AJR Am J Roentgenol. 2011;197(4):887–96.

9 Chawla SN, Crispen PL, Hanlon AL, Greenberg RE, Chen DY, Uzzo RG. The natural history of observed enhancing renal masses: meta-analysis and review of the world literature. J Urol. 2006;175(2):425–31.

10 Raman JD. Percutaneous renal biopsy may aid management of small renal masses on active surveillance. Can J Urol. 2013;20(2):6742.

11 Lane BR, Samplaski MK, Herts BR, Zhou M, Novick AC, Campbell SC. Renal mass biopsy—a renaissance? J Urol. 2008;179(1):20–7.

12 Volpe A, Finelli A, Gill IS, Jewett MA, Martignoni G, Polascik TJ, *et al.* Rationale for percutaneous biopsy and histologic characterisation of renal tumours. Eur Urol. 2012;62(3):491–504.

13 Rybicki FJ, Shu KM, Cibas ES, Fielding JR, vanSonnenberg E, Silverman SG. Percutaneous biopsy of renal masses: sensitivity and negative predictive value stratified by clinical setting and size of masses. AJR Am J Roentgenol. 2003;180(5):1281–7.

14 Leveridge MJ, Finelli A, Kachura JR, Evans A, Chung H, Shiff DA, *et al.* Outcomes of small renal mass needle core biopsy, nondiagnostic percutaneous biopsy, and the role of repeat biopsy. Eur Urol. 2011;60(3):578–84.

15 Maturen KE, Nghiem HV, Caoili EM, Higgins EG, Wolf JS, Jr., Wood DP, Jr. Renal mass core biopsy: Accuracy and impact on clinical management. AJR Am J Roentgenol. 2007;188(2):563–70.

16 Schmidbauer J, Remzi M, Memarsadeghi M, Haitel A, Klingler HC, Katzenbeisser D, *et al.* Diagnostic accuracy of computed tomography-guided percutaneous biopsy of renal masses. Eur Urol. 2008;53(5): 1003–11.

17 Volpe A, Kachura JR, Geddie WR, Evans AJ, Gharajeh A, Saravanan A, *et al.* Techniques, safety and accuracy of sampling of renal tumors by fine needle aspiration and core biopsy. J Urol. 2007;178(2):379–86.

18 Neuzillet Y, Lechevallier E, Andre M, Daniel L, Coulange C. Accuracy and clinical role of fine needle percutaneous

biopsy with computerized tomography guidance of small (less than 4.0 cm) renal masses. J Urol. 2004;171(5):1802–5.

19 Rapp DE, Orvieto M, Sokoloff MH, Shalhav AL. Use of biopsy sheath to improve standardization of renal mass biopsy in tissue-blative procedures. J Endourol. 2004;18(5):453–4.

20 Breda A, Treat EG, Haft-Candell L, Leppert JT, Harper JD, Said J, *et al.* Comparison of accuracy of 14-, 18- and 20-G needles in ex-vivo renal mass biopsy: A prospective, blinded study. BJU international. 2010;105(7):940–5.

21 Phe V, Yates DR, Renard-Penna R, Cussenot O, Roupret M. Is there a contemporary role for percutaneous needle biopsy in the era of small renal masses? BJU Int. 2012;109(6):867–72.

22 Sainani NI, Tatli S, Anthony SG, Shyn PB, Tuncali K, Silverman SG. Successful percutaneous radiologic management of renal cell carcinoma tumor seeding caused by percutaneous biopsy performed before ablation. J Vasc Interv Radiol. 2013;24(9):1404–8.

23 Lebret T, Poulain JE, Molinie V, Herve JM, Denoux Y, Guth A, *et al.* Percutaneous core biopsy for renal masses: indications, accuracy and results. J Urol. 2007;178(4 Pt 1): 1184–8; discussion 8.

24 Weight CJ, Kaouk JH, Hegarty NJ, Remer EM, O'Malley CM, Lane BR, *et al.* Correlation of radiographic imaging and histopathology following cryoablation and radio frequency ablation for renal tumors. J Urol. 2008;179(4):1277–81; discussion 8–-3.

25 Raman JD, Stern JM, Zeltser I, Kabbani W, Cadeddu JA. Absence of viable renal carcinoma in biopsies performed more than 1 year following radio frequency ablation confirms reliability of axial imaging. J Urol. 2008;179(6):2142–5.

26 Klingler HC, Susani M. Focal therapy and imaging in prostate and kidney cancer: Renal biopsy protocols before and after focal therapy. J Endourol. 2010;24(5):701–5.

27 Golshayan AR, George S, Heng DY, Elson P, Wood LS, Mekhail TM, *et al.* Metastatic sarcomatoid renal cell carcinoma treated with vascular endothelial growth factor-targeted therapy. J Clin Oncol. 2009;27(2):235–41.

28 Shuch B, Bratslavsky G, Shih J, Vourganti S, Finley D, Castor B, *et al.* Impact of pathological tumour characteristics in patients with sarcomatoid renal cell carcinoma. BJU Int. 2012;109(11):1600–6.

29 Abel EJ, Carrasco A, Culp SH, Matin SF, Tamboli P, Tannir NM, *et al.* Limitations of preoperative biopsy in patients with metastatic renal cell carcinoma: Comparison to surgical pathology in 405 cases. BJU Int. 2012;110(11):1742–6.

30 Ficarra V, Martignoni G, Maffei N, Brunelli M, Novara G, Zanolla L, *et al.* Original and reviewed nuclear grading according to the Fuhrman system: A multivariate analysis of 388 patients with conventional renal cell carcinoma. Cancer. 2005;103(1):68–75.

31 Blumenfeld AJ, Guru K, Fuchs GJ, Kim HL. Percutaneous biopsy of renal cell carcinoma underestimates nuclear grade. Urology. 2010;76(3):610–3.

32 Millet I, Curros F, Serre I, Taourel P, Thuret R. Can renal biopsy accurately predict histological subtype and Fuhrman grade of renal cell carcinoma? J Urol. 2012;188(5):1690–4.

33 Park SY, Park BK, Kim CK, Kwon GY. Ultrasound-guided core biopsy of small renal masses: diagnostic rate and limitations. J Vasc Interv Radiol. 2013;24(1):90–6.

34 Wood BJ, Khan MA, McGovern F, Harisinghani M, Hahn PF, Mueller PR. Imaging guided biopsy of renal masses: Indications, accuracy and impact on clinical management. J Urol. 1999;161(5):1470–4.

35 Parks GE, Perkins LA, Zagoria RJ, Garvin AJ, Sirintrapun SJ, Geisinger KR. Benefits of a combined approach to sampling of renal neoplasms as demonstrated in a series of 351 cases. Am J Surg Pathol. 2011;35(6):827–35.

36 Lang EK, Macchia RJ, Gayle B, Richter F, Watson RA, Thomas R, *et al.* CT-guided biopsy of indeterminate renal cystic masses (Bosniak 3 and 2F): Accuracy and impact on clinical management. Eur Radiol. 2002;12(10):2518–24.

37 Harisinghani MG, Maher MM, Gervais DA, McGovern F, Hahn P, Jhaveri K, *et al.* Incidence of malignancy in complex cystic renal masses (Bosniak category III): Should imaging-guided biopsy precede surgery? AJR Am J Roentgenol. 2003;180(3):755–8.

38 Dechet CB, Bostwick DG, Blute ML, Bryant SC, Zincke H. Renal oncocytoma: Multifocality, bilateralism, metachronous tumor development and coexistent renal cell carcinoma. J Urol. 1999;162(1):40–2.

39 Waldert M, Klatte T, Haitel A, Ozsoy M, Schmidbauer J, Marberger M, *et al.* Hybrid renal cell carcinomas containing histopathologic features of chromophobe renal cell carcinomas and oncocytomas have excellent oncologic outcomes. Eur Urol. 2010;57(4):661–5.

40 Ginzburg S, Uzzo R, Al-Saleem T, Dulaimi E, Walton J, Corcoran A, *et al.* Coexisting hybrid malignancy in a solitary sporadic solid benign renal mass: Implications for treating patients following renal biopsy. J Urol. 2014;191(2):296–300.

41 Somani BK, Nabi G, Thorpe P, N'Dow J, Swami S, McClinton S, *et al.* Image-guided biopsy-diagnosed renal cell carcinoma: Critical appraisal of technique and long-term follow-up. European urology. 2007;51(5):1289–95; discussion 96–7.

42 Shannon BA, Cohen RJ, de Bruto H, Davies RJ. The value of preoperative needle core biopsy for diagnosing benign lesions among small, incidentally detected renal masses. J Urol. 2008;180(4):1257–61; discussion 61.

43 Louis R. Kavoussi, Michael J. Schwartz, Gill IS. Laparoscopic Surgery of the Kidney. In: Alan J. Wein, Louis R. Kavoussi, Andrew C. Novick, Alan W. Partin, Peters CA, editors. Campbell-Walsh Urology. 10th ed. Philadelphia: Saunders; 2011.

44 Kroeze SG, Huisman M, Verkooijen HM, van Diest PJ, Ruud Bosch JL, van den Bosch MA. Real-time 3D fluoroscopy-guided large core needle biopsy of renal masses: A critical early evaluation according to the IDEAL recommendations. Cardiovasc Interv Radiol. 2012;35(3):680–5.

45 Braak SJ, van Melick HH, Onaca MG, van Heesewijk JP, van Strijen MJ. 3D cone-beam CT guidance, a novel technique in renal biopsy—results in 41 patients with suspected renal masses. Eur Radiol. 2012;22(11):2547–52.

46 Yang XJ, Sugimura J, Schafernak KT, Tretiakova MS, Han M, Vogelzang NJ, *et al.* Classification of renal neoplasms based on molecular signatures. J Urol. 2006;175(6):2302–6.

47 Barocas DA, Rohan SM, Kao J, Gurevich RD, Del Pizzo JJ, Vaughan ED, Jr., *et al.* Diagnosis of renal tumors on needle biopsy specimens by histological and molecular analysis. J Urol. 2006;176(5):1957–62.

48 Chyhrai A, Sanjmyatav J, Gajda M, Reichelt O, Wunderlich H, Steiner T, *et al.* Multi-colour FISH on preoperative renal tumour biopsies to confirm the diagnosis of uncertain renal masses. World J Urol. 2010;28(3):269–74.

49 Gayed BA, Youssef RF, Bagrodia A, Kapur P, Darwish OM, Krabbe LM, *et al.* Prognostic role of cell cycle and proliferative biomarkers in patients with clear cell renal cell carcinoma. J Urol. 2013;190(5):1662–7.

50 Heyns CF, Mendoza-Valdes A, Pompeo AC. Diagnosis and staging of penile cancer. Urology. 2010;76(2 Suppl 1):S15–23.

51 Velazquez EF, Barreto JE, Rodriguez I, Piris A, Cubilla AL. Limitations in the interpretation of biopsies in patients with penile squamous cell carcinoma. Int J Surg Pathol. 2004;12(2):139–46.

52 Pizzocaro G, Algaba F, Horenblas S, Solsona E, Tana S, Van Der Poel H, *et al.* EAU penile cancer guidelines 2009. Eur Urol. 2010;57(6):1002–12.

53 Kroon BK, Horenblas S, Deurloo EE, Nieweg OE, Teertstra HJ. Ultrasonography-guided fine-needle aspiration cytology before sentinel node biopsy in patients with penile carcinoma. BJU Int. 2005;95(4):517–21.

54 Yeung LL, Brandes SB. Dynamic sentinel lymph node biopsy as the new paradigm for the management of penile cancer. Urol Oncol. 2013;31(5):693–6.

55 Tanis PJ, Lont AP, Meinhardt W, Olmos RA, Nieweg OE, Horenblas S. Dynamic sentinel node biopsy for penile cancer: Reliability of a staging technique. J Urol. 2002;168(1):76–80.

56 Djajadiningrat RS, Graafland NM, van Werkhoven E, Meinhardt W, Bex A, van der Poel HG, *et al.* Contemporary management of regional nodes in penile cancer-improvement of survival? J Urol. 2014;191(1):68–73.

57 Leijte JA, Kroon BK, Valdes Olmos RA, Nieweg OE, Horenblas S. Reliability and safety of current dynamic sentinel node biopsy for penile carcinoma. Eur Urol. 2007;52(1):170–7.

58 Nicolai N. Has dynamic sentinel node biopsy achieved its top performance in penile cancer? What clinicians still need to manage lymph nodes in early stage penile cancer. Eur Urol. 2013;63(4):664–6.

59 Hughes BE, Leijte JA, Kroon BK, Shabbir MA, Swallow TW, Heenan SD, *et al.* Lymph node metastasis in intermediate-risk penile squamous cell cancer: A two-centre experience. Eur Urol. 2010;57(4):688–92.

60 Graafland NM, Valdes Olmos RA, Meinhardt W, Bex A, van der Poel HG, van Boven HH, *et al.* Nodal staging in penile carcinoma by dynamic sentinel node biopsy after previous therapeutic primary tumour resection. Eur Urol. 2010;58(5):748–51.

61 Leijte JA, Kirrander P, Antonini N, Windahl T, Horenblas S. Recurrence patterns of squamous cell carcinoma of the penis: Recommendations for follow-up based on a two-centre analysis of 700 patients. Eur Urol. 2008;54(1):161–8.

62 Djajadiningrat RS, Teertstra HJ, van Werkhoven E, van Boven HH, Horenblas S. Ultrasound examination and fine needle aspiration cytology: Useful in followup of the regional nodes in penile cancer? J Urol. 2014;191(3):652–5.

63 Graafland NM, Leijte JA, Olmos RA, Van Boven HH, Nieweg OE, Horenblas S. Repeat dynamic sentinel node biopsy in locally recurrent penile carcinoma. BJU Int. 2010;105(8):1121–4.

64 Brawley OW. Trends in prostate cancer in the United States. J Natl Cancer Instit Monogr. 2012;2012(45):152–6.

65 Lu-Yao GL, Albertsen PC, Moore DF, Shih W, Lin Y, DiPaola RS, *et al.* Outcomes of localized prostate cancer following conservative management. JAMA. 2009;302(11):1202–9.

66 Kawachi MH, Bahnson RR, Barry M, Busby JE, Carroll PR, Carter HB, *et al.* NCCN clinical practice guidelines in oncology: Prostate cancer early detection. J Natl Compr Cancer Netw. 2010;8(2):240–62.

67 Carter HB, Albertsen PC, Barry MJ, Etzioni R, Freedland SJ, Greene KL, *et al.* Early detection of prostate cancer: AUA Guideline. J Urol. 2013;190(2):419–26.

68 Merrimen JL, Jones G, Walker D, Leung CS, Kapusta LR, Srigley JR. Multifocal high grade prostatic intraepithelial neoplasia is a significant risk factor for prostatic adenocarcinoma. J Urol. 2009;182(2):485–90; discussion 90.

69 Zhang M, Amberson JB, Epstein JI. Two sequential diagnoses of atypical foci suspicious for carcinoma on prostate biopsy: A follow-up study of 179 cases. Urology. 2013;82(4):861–4.

70 Moore CK, Karikehalli S, Nazeer T, Fisher HA, Kaufman RP, Jr., Mian BM. Prognostic significance of high grade prostatic intraepithelial neoplasia and atypical small acinar proliferation in the contemporary era. J Urol. 2005;173(1):70–2.

71 Roobol MJ, Steyerberg EW, Kranse R, Wolters T, van den Bergh RC, Bangma CH,

et al. A risk-based strategy improves prostate-specific antigen-driven detection of prostate cancer. Eur Urol. 2010;57(1):79–85.

72 Heidenreich A, Bastian PJ, Bellmunt J, Bolla M, Joniau S, van der Kwast T, *et al.* EAU guidelines on prostate cancer. Part 1: Screening, diagnosis, and local treatment with curative intent-update 2013. Eur Urol. 2014;65(1):124–37.

73 Aron M, Rajeev TP, Gupta NP. Antibiotic prophylaxis for transrectal needle biopsy of the prostate: a randomized controlled study. BJU Int. 2000;85(6):682–5.

74 von Knobloch R, Weber J, Varga Z, Feiber H, Heidenreich A, Hofmann R. Bilateral fine-needle administered local anaesthetic nerve block for pain control during TRUS-guided multi-core prostate biopsy: a prospective randomised trial. Eur Urol. 2002;41(5):508–14; discussion 14.

75 Bjurlin MA, Carter HB, Schellhammer P, Cookson MS, Gomella LG, Troyer D, *et al.* Optimization of initial prostate biopsy in clinical practice: Sampling, labeling and specimen processing. J Urol. 2013;189(6):2039–46.

76 Singh H, Canto EI, Shariat SF, Kadmon D, Miles BJ, Wheeler TM, *et al.* Improved detection of clinically significant, curable prostate cancer with systematic 12-core biopsy. J Urol. 2004;171(3):1089–92.

77 Presti JC, Jr., O'Dowd GJ, Miller MC, Mattu R, Veltri RW. Extended peripheral zone biopsy schemes increase cancer detection rates and minimize variance in prostate specific antigen and age related cancer rates: Results of a community multi-practice study. J Urol. 2003;169(1):125–9.

78 Eichler K, Hempel S, Wilby J, Myers L, Bachmann LM, Kleijnen J. Diagnostic value of systematic biopsy methods in the investigation of prostate cancer: A systematic review. J Urol. 2006;175(5):1605–12.

79 Elabbady AA, Khedr MM. Extended 12-core prostate biopsy increases both the detection of prostate cancer and the

accuracy of Gleason score. Eur Urol. 2006;49(1):49–53; discussion 53.

80 Roehrborn CG, Pickens GJ, Sanders JS. Diagnostic yield of repeated transrectal ultrasound-guided biopsies stratified by specific histopathologic diagnoses and prostate specific antigen levels. Urology. 1996;47(3):347–52.

81 Levine MA, Ittman M, Melamed J, Lepor H. Two consecutive sets of transrectal ultrasound guided sextant biopsies of the prostate for the detection of prostate cancer. The J Urol. 1998;159(2):471–5; discussion 5–6.

82 King CR, McNeal JE, Gill H, Presti JC, Jr. Extended prostate biopsy scheme improves reliability of Gleason grading: implications for radiotherapy patients. Int J Radiat Oncol Biol Phys. 2004;59(2):386–91.

83 Mian BM, Lehr DJ, Moore CK, Fisher HA, Kaufman RP, Jr., Ross JS, *et al.* Role of prostate biopsy schemes in accurate prediction of Gleason scores. Urology. 2006;67(2):379–83.

84 San Francisco IF, DeWolf WC, Rosen S, Upton M, Olumi AF. Extended prostate needle biopsy improves concordance of Gleason grading between prostate needle biopsy and radical prostatectomy. J Urol. 2003;169(1):136–40.

85 Meng MV, Elkin EP, DuChane J, Carroll PR. Impact of increased number of biopsies on the nature of prostate cancer identified. J Urol. 2006;176(1):63–8; discussion 69.

86 Siu W, Dunn RL, Shah RB, Wei JT. Use of extended pattern technique for initial prostate biopsy. J Urol. 2005;174(2):505–9.

87 Takashima R, Egawa S, Kuwao S, Baba S. Anterior distribution of Stage T1c nonpalpable tumors in radical prostatectomy specimens. Urology. 2002;59(5):692–7.

88 Babaian RJ, Toi A, Kamoi K, Troncoso P, Sweet J, Evans R, *et al.* A comparative analysis of sextant and an extended 11-core multisite directed biopsy strategy. J Urol. 2000;163(1):152–7.

89 Rogatsch H, Moser P, Volgger H, Horninger W, Bartsch G, Mikuz G, *et al.* Diagnostic effect of an improved preembedding method of prostate needle biopsy specimens. Hum Pathol. 2000;31(9):1102–7.

90 Epstein JI, Walsh PC, Sauvageot J, Carter HB. Use of repeat sextant and transition zone biopsies for assessing extent of prostate cancer. J Urol. 1997;158(5):1886–90.

91 Morote J, Lopez M, Encabo G, de Torres I. Value of routine transition zone biopsies in patients undergoing ultrasound-guided sextant biopsies for the first time. Eur Urol. 1999;35(4):294–7.

92 Haarer CF, Gopalan A, Tickoo SK, Scardino PT, Eastham JA, Reuter VE, *et al.* Prostatic transition zone directed needle biopsies uncommonly sample clinically relevant transition zone tumors. J Urol. 2009;182(4):1337–41.

93 Richard JL, Motamedinia P, McKiernan JM, DeCastro GJ, Benson MC. Routine transition zone biopsy during active surveillance for prostate cancer rarely provides unique evidence of disease progression. J Urol. 2012;188(6):2177–80.

94 Presti JC, Jr., Chang JJ, Bhargava V, Shinohara K. The optimal systematic prostate biopsy scheme should include 8 rather than 6 biopsies: results of a prospective clinical trial. J Urol. 2000;163(1):163–6; discussion 6–7.

95 Ravery V, Goldblatt L, Royer B, Blanc E, Toublanc M, Boccon-Gibod L. Extensive biopsy protocol improves the detection rate of prostate cancer. J Urol. 2000;164(2):393–6.

96 Singh H, Canto EI, Shariat SF, Kadmon D, Miles BJ, Wheeler TM, *et al.* Six additional systematic lateral cores enhance sextant biopsy prediction of pathological features at radical prostatectomy. J Urol. 2004;171(1):204–9.

97 Naya Y, Ochiai A, Troncoso P, Babaian RJ. A comparison of extended biopsy and sextant biopsy schemes for predicting the pathological stage of prostate cancer. J Urol. 2004;171(6 Pt 1):2203–8.

98 Badalament RA, Miller MC, Peller PA, Young DC, Bahn DK, Kochie P, *et al.* An algorithm for predicting nonorgan confined prostate cancer using the results obtained from sextant core biopsies with prostate specific antigen level. J Urol. 1996;156(4):1375–80.

99 Touma NJ, Chin JL, Bella T, Sener A, Izawa JI. Location of a positive biopsy as a predictor of surgical margin status and extraprostatic disease in radical prostatectomy. BJU Int. 2006;97(2):259–62.

100 Tigrani VS, Bhargava V, Shinohara K, Presti JC, Jr. Number of positive systematic sextant biopsies predicts surgical margin status at radical prostatectomy. Urology. 1999;54(4):689–93.

101 Scattoni V, Roscigno M, Raber M, Deho F, Maga T, Zanoni M, *et al.* Initial extended transrectal prostate biopsy--are more prostate cancers detected with 18 cores than with 12 cores? J Urol. 2008;179(4):1327–31; discussion 31.

102 de la Taille A, Antiphon P, Salomon L, Cherfan M, Porcher R, Hoznek A, *et al.* Prospective evaluation of a 21-sample needle biopsy procedure designed to improve the prostate cancer detection rate. Urology. 2003;61(6):1181–6.

103 Li YH, Elshafei A, Li J, Gong M, Susan L, Fareed K, *et al.* Transrectal saturation technique may improve cancer detection as an initial prostate biopsy strategy in men with prostate-specific antigen <10 ng/ml. Eur Urol. 2014;65(6):1178–83.

104 Rodriguez-Covarrubias F, Gonzalez-Ramirez A, Aguilar-Davidov B, Castillejos-Molina R, Sotomayor M, Feria-Bernal G. Extended sampling at first biopsy improves cancer detection rate: results of a prospective, randomized trial comparing 12 versus 18-core prostate biopsy. J Urol. 2011;185(6):2132–6.

105 Haas GP, Delongchamps NB, Jones RF, Chandan V, Serio AM, Vickers AJ, *et al.* Needle biopsies on autopsy prostates:

Sensitivity of cancer detection based on true prevalence. J Natl Cancer Instit. 2007;99(19):1484–9.

106 Zaytoun OM, Moussa AS, Gao T, Fareed K, Jones JS. Office based transrectal saturation biopsy improves prostate cancer detection compared to extended biopsy in the repeat biopsy population. J Urol. 2011;186(3):850–4.

107 Lane BR, Zippe CD, Abouassaly R, Schoenfield L, Magi-Galluzzi C, Jones JS. Saturation technique does not decrease cancer detection during followup after initial prostate biopsy. J Urol. 2008;179(5):1746–50; discussion 50.

108 Shapiro RH, Johnstone PA. Risk of Gleason grade inaccuracies in prostate cancer patients eligible for active surveillance. Urology. 2012;80(3):661–6.

109 Porten SP, Whitson JM, Cowan JE, Perez N, Shinohara K, Carroll PR. Changes in cancer volume in serial biopsies of men on active surveillance for early stage prostate cancer. J Urol. 2011;186(5):1825–9.

110 Miyake H, Sakai I, Harada K, Hara I, Eto H. Increased detection of clinically significant prostate cancer by additional sampling from the anterior lateral horns of the peripheral zone in combination with the standard sextant biopsy. Int J Urol. 2004;11(6):402–6.

111 Sundi D, Kryvenko ON, Carter HB, Ross AE, Epstein JI, Schaeffer EM. Pathological examination of radical prostatectomy specimens in men with very low risk disease at biopsy reveals distinct zonal distribution of cancer in black American men. J Urol. 2014;191(1):60–7.

112 Ehdaie B, Vertosick E, Spaliviero M, Giallo-Uvino A, Taur Y, Sullivan M, *et al.* The impact of repeat biopsies on infectious complications in men with prostate cancer on active surveillance. J Urol. 2014;191(3):660–4.

113 Loeb S, Carter HB, Berndt SI, Ricker W, Schaeffer EM. Is repeat prostate biopsy associated with a greater risk of

hospitalization? Data from SEER-Medicare. J Urol. 2013;189(3):867–70.

114 Glass AS, Hilton JF, Cowan JE, Washington SL, Carroll PR. serial prostate biopsy and risk of lower urinary tract symptoms: results from a large, single-institution active surveillance cohort. Urology. 2014;83(1):33–9.

115 Braun K, Ahallal Y, Sjoberg DD, Ghoneim T, Dominguez Esteban M, Mulhall J, *et al.* Effect of repeated prostate biopsies on erectile function in men on active surveillance for prostate cancer. J Urol. 2014;191(3):744–9.

116 Hilton JF, Blaschko SD, Whitson JM, Cowan JE, Carroll PR. The impact of serial prostate biopsies on sexual function in men on active surveillance for prostate cancer. J Urol. 2012;188(4):1252–8.

117 Kopp RP, Stroup SP, Schroeck FR, Freedland SJ, Millard F, Terris MK, *et al.* Are repeat prostate biopsies safe? A cohort analysis from the SEARCH database. J Urol. 2012;187(6):2056–60.

118 Bittner N, Merrick GS, Butler WM, Bennett A, Galbreath RW. Incidence and pathological features of prostate cancer detected on transperineal template guided mapping biopsy after negative transrectal ultrasound guided biopsy. J Urol. 2013;190(2):509–14.

119 Dimmen M, Vlatkovic L, Hole KH, Nesland JM, Brennhovd B, Axcrona K. Transperineal prostate biopsy detects significant cancer in patients with elevated prostate-specific antigen (PSA) levels and previous negative transrectal biopsies. BJU Int. 2012;110(2 Pt 2): E69–75.

120 Barzell WE, Melamed MR, Cathcart P, Moore CM, Ahmed HU, Emberton M. Identifying candidates for active surveillance: An evaluation of the repeat biopsy strategy for men with favorable risk prostate cancer. J Urol. 2012;188(3):762–7.

121 Lecornet E, Ahmed HU, Hu Y, Moore CM, Nevoux P, Barratt D, *et al.* The accuracy of different biopsy strategies for the

detection of clinically important prostate cancer: A computer simulation. J Urol. 2012;188(3):974–80.

122 Robertson NL, Hu Y, Ahmed HU, Freeman A, Barratt D, Emberton M. Prostate cancer risk inflation as a consequence of image-targeted biopsy of the prostate: A computer simulation study. Eur Urol. 2014;65(3):628–34.

123 Moran BJ, Braccioforte MH, Conterato DJ. Re-biopsy of the prostate using a stereotactic transperineal technique. J Urol. 2006;176(4 Pt 1):1376–81; discussion 81.

124 Logan JK, Rais-Bahrami S, Turkbey B, Gomella A, Amalou H, Choyke PL, *et al.* Current status of MRI and ultrasound fusion software platforms for guidance of prostate biopsies. BJU Int. 2014;114(5):641–52.

125 Sonn GA, Margolis DJ, Marks LS. Target detection: Magnetic resonance imaging-ultrasound fusion-guided prostate biopsy. Urol Oncol. 2014;32(6):903–11.

126 Komai Y, Numao N, Yoshida S, Matsuoka Y, Nakanishi Y, Ishii C, *et al.* High diagnostic ability of multiparametric magnetic resonance imaging to detect anterior prostate cancer missed by transrectal 12-core biopsy. J Urol. 2013;190(3):867–73.

127 Lichy MP, Anastasiadis AG, Aschoff P, Sotlar K, Eschmann SM, Pfannenberg C, *et al.* Morphologic, functional, and metabolic magnetic resonance imaging-guided prostate biopsy in a patient with prior negative transrectal ultrasound-guided biopsies and persistently elevated prostate-specific antigen levels. Urology. 2007;69(6):1208.e5–8.

128 Franiel T, Stephan C, Erbersdobler A, Dietz E, Maxeiner A, Hell N, *et al.* Areas suspicious for prostate cancer: MR-guided biopsy in patients with at least one transrectal US-guided biopsy with a negative finding—multiparametric MR imaging for detection and biopsy planning. Radiology. 2011;259(1):162–72.

129 Haffner J, Lemaitre L, Puech P, Haber GP, Leroy X, Jones JS, *et al.* Role of magnetic resonance imaging before initial biopsy: comparison of magnetic resonance imaging-targeted and systematic biopsy for significant prostate cancer detection. BJU Int. 2011;108(8 Pt 2):E171–8.

130 Pinto PA, Chung PH, Rastinehad AR, Baccala AA, Jr., Kruecker J, Benjamin CJ, *et al.* Magnetic resonance imaging/ultrasound fusion guided prostate biopsy improves cancer detection following transrectal ultrasound biopsy and correlates with multiparametric magnetic resonance imaging. J Urol. 2011;186(4):1281–5.

131 Rastinehad AR, Turkbey B, Salami SS, Yaskiv O, George AK, Fakhoury M, *et al.* Improving detection of clinically significant prostate cancer: MRI/TRUS fusion-guided prostate biopsy. J Urol. 2014;191(6):1749–54.

132 Rais-Bahrami S, Siddiqui MM, Turkbey B, Stamatakis L, Logan J, Hoang AN, *et al.* Utility of multiparametric magnetic resonance imaging suspicion levels for detecting prostate cancer. J Urol. 2013;190(5):1721–7.

133 Vourganti S, Rastinehad A, Yerram NK, Nix J, Volkin D, Hoang A, *et al.* Multiparametric magnetic resonance imaging and ultrasound fusion biopsy detect prostate cancer in patients with prior negative transrectal ultrasound biopsies. J Urol. 2012;188(6):2152–7.

134 Sonn GA, Chang E, Natarajan S, Margolis DJ, Macairan M, Lieu P, *et al.* Value of targeted prostate biopsy using magnetic resonance-ultrasound fusion in men with prior negative biopsy and elevated prostate-specific antigen. Eur Urol. 2014;65(4):809–15.

135 Hong CW, Walton-Diaz A, Rais-Bahrami S, Hoang AN, Turkbey B, Stamatakis L, *et al.* Imaging and pathology findings after an initial negative MRI-US fusion-guided and 12-core extended sextant prostate biopsy session. Diagnostic and interventional radiology. 2014;20(3):234–8.

136 Walton Diaz A, Hoang AN, Turkbey B, Hong CW, Truong H, Sterling T, *et al.* Can magnetic resonance-ultrasound fusion biopsy improve cancer detection in enlarged prostates? J Urol. 2013;190(6):2020–5.

137 Siddiqui MM, Rais-Bahrami S, Truong H, Stamatakis L, Vourganti S, Nix J, *et al.* Magnetic resonance imaging/ultrasound-fusion biopsy significantly upgrades prostate cancer versus systematic 12-core transrectal ultrasound biopsy. Eur Urol. 2013;64(5):713–9.

138 Turkbey B, Xu S, Kruecker J, Locklin J, Pang Y, Bernardo M, *et al.* Documenting the location of prostate biopsies with image fusion. BJU Int. 2011;107(1):53–7.

139 Metwalli AR, Pinto PA. Commentary on: "Focal cryosurgical ablation of the prostate: A single institute's perspective." BMC Urol. 2013;13(1):39.

140 Kuru TH, Roethke MC, Seidenader J, Simpfendorfer T, Boxler S, Alammar K, *et al.* Critical evaluation of magnetic resonance imaging targeted, transrectal ultrasound guided transperineal fusion biopsy for detection of prostate cancer. J Urol. 2013;190(4):1380–6.

141 Nelson AW, Harvey RC, Parker RA, Kastner C, Doble A, Gnanapragasam VJ. Repeat prostate biopsy strategies after initial negative biopsy: Meta-regression comparing cancer detection of transperineal, transrectal saturation and MRI guided biopsy. PloS One. 2013;8(2):e57480.

142 Westphalen AC, Rosenkrantz AB. prostate imaging reporting and data system (pi-rads): reflections on early experience with a standardized interpretation scheme for multiparametric prostate MRI. AJR Am J Roentgenol. 2014;202(1):121–3.

143 Rais-Bahrami S, Turkbey B, Rastinehad AR, Walton-Diaz A, Hoang AN, Siddiqui MM, *et al.* Natural history of small index lesions suspicious for prostate cancer on multiparametric MRI: recommendations for interval imaging follow-up. Diagn Interv Radiol. 2014;20(4):293–8.

144 de Rooij M, Crienen S, Witjes JA, Barentsz JO, Rovers MM, Grutters JP. Cost-effectiveness of magnetic resonance (MR) imaging and MR-guided targeted biopsy versus systematic transrectal ultrasound-guided biopsy in diagnosing prostate cancer: a modelling study from a health care perspective. Eur Urol. 2014; 66(3):430–6.

145 Rais-Bahrami S, Siddiqui MM, Vourganti S, Turkbey B, Rastinehad AR, Stamatakis L, *et al.* diagnostic value of biparametric MRI as an adjunct to PSA-based detection of prostate cancer in men without prior biopsies. BJU Int. 2015;115(3):381–3.

146 de Rooij M, Hamoen EH, Futterer JJ, Barentsz JO, Rovers MM. Accuracy of multiparametric MRI for prostate cancer detection: A meta-analysis. AJR Am J Roentgenol. 2014;202(2):343–51.

147 Cornelis F, Rigou G, Le Bras Y, Coutouly X, Hubrecht R, Yacoub M, *et al.* Real-time contrast-enhanced transrectal US-guided prostate biopsy: Diagnostic accuracy in men with previously negative biopsy results and positive MR imaging findings. Radiology. 2013;269(1):159–66.

148 Taverna G, Morandi G, Seveso M, Giusti G, Benetti A, Colombo P, *et al.* Colour Doppler and microbubble contrast agent ultrasonography do not improve cancer detection rate in transrectal systematic prostate biopsy sampling. BJU Int. 2011;108(11):1723–7.

149 Zigeuner R, Schips L, Lipsky K, Auprich M, Salfellner M, Rehak P, *et al.* Detection of prostate cancer by TURP or open surgery in patients with previously negative transrectal prostate biopsies. Urology. 2003;62(5):883–7.

150 Linzer DG, Stock RG, Stone NN, Ratnow R, Ianuzzi C, Unger P. Seminal vesicle biopsy: Accuracy and implications for staging of prostate cancer. Urology. 1996;48(5):757–61.

151 Albers P, Albrecht W, Algaba F, Bokemeyer C, Cohn-Cedermark G, Fizazi K, *et al.* EAU guidelines on testicular cancer: 2011 update. Eur Urol. 2011;60(2):304–19.

152 Rorth M, Rajpert-De Meyts E, Andersson L, Dieckmann KP, Fossa SD, Grigor KM, *et al.* Carcinoma in situ in the testis. Scand J Urol Nephrol Suppl. 2000(205):166–86.

153 von der Maase H, Rorth M, Walbom-Jorgensen S, Sorensen BL, Christophersen IS, Hald T, *et al.* Carcinoma in situ of contralateral testis in patients with testicular germ cell cancer: Study of 27 cases in 500 patients. Br Med J. 1986;293(6559):1398–401.

154 Winstanley AM, Mikuz G, Debruyne F, Schulman CC, Parkinson MC, European Association of Pathologists UDiF. Handling and reporting of biopsy and surgical specimens of testicular cancer. Eur Urol. 2004;45(5):564–73.

155 Dieckmann KP, Loy V. Prevalence of contralateral testicular intraepithelial neoplasia in patients with testicular germ cell neoplasms. J Clin Oncol. 1996;14(12):3126–32.

156 Fossa SD, Chen J, Schonfeld SJ, McGlynn KA, McMaster ML, Gail MH, *et al.* Risk of contralateral testicular cancer: a population-based study of 29,515 U.S. men. J Natl Cancer Instit. 2005;97(14):1056–66.

157 Dieckmann KP, Loy V. False-negative biopsies for the diagnosis of testicular intraepithelial neoplasia (TIN)–an update. Eur Urol. 2003;43(5):516–21.

158 Heidenreich A. Contralateral testicular biopsy in testis cancer: Current concepts and controversies. BJU Int. 2009;104(9 Pt B): 1346–50.

159 Dieckmann KP, Kulejewski M, Pichlmeier U, Loy V. Diagnosis of contralateral testicular intraepithelial neoplasia (TIN) in patients with testicular germ cell cancer: Systematic two-site biopsies are more sensitive than a single random biopsy. Eur Urol. 2007;51(1):175–83; discussion 83–5.

160 Dieckmann KP, Heinemann V, Frey U, Pichlmeier U, German Testicular Cancer Study G. How harmful is contralateral testicular biopsy?–an analysis of serial imaging studies and a prospective evaluation of surgical complications. Eur Urol. 2005;48(4):662–72.

161 Brabrand S, Fossa SD, Cvancarova M, Axcrona U, Lehne G. Probability of metachronous testicular cancer in patients with biopsy-proven intratubular germ cell neoplasia depends on first-time treatment of germ cell cancer. J Clin Oncol. 2012;30(32):4004–10.

162 de Gouveia Brazao CA, Pierik FH, Oosterhuis JW, Dohle GR, Looijenga LH, Weber RF. Bilateral testicular microlithiasis predicts the presence of the precursor of testicular germ cell tumors in subfertile men. J Urol. 2004;171(1):158–60.

163 Elzinga-Tinke JE, Sirre ME, Looijenga LH, van Casteren N, Wildhagen MF, Dohle GR. The predictive value of testicular ultrasound abnormalities for carcinoma in situ of the testis in men at risk for testicular cancer. Int J Androl. 2010;33(4):597–603.

164 Fossa SD, Aass N, Heilo A, Daugaard G, N ES, Stenwig AE, *et al.* Testicular carcinoma in situ in patients with extragonadal germ-cell tumours: The clinical role of pretreatment biopsy. Ann Oncol. 2003;14(9):1412–8.

165 Dieckmann KP, Kulejewski M, Heinemann V, Loy V. Testicular biopsy for early cancer detection—objectives, technique and controversies. Int J Androl. 2011;34(4 Pt 2):e7–13.

166 Tavolini IM, Bettella A, Boscolo Berto R, Bassi PF, Longo R, Menegazzo M, *et al.* Immunostaining for placental alkaline phosphatase on fine-needle aspiration specimens to detect noninvasive testicular cancer: A prospective evaluation in cryptorchid men. BJU Int. 2006;97(5):950–4.

167 Babjuk M, Burger M, Zigeuner R, Shariat SF, van Rhijn BW, Comperat E, *et al.* EAU guidelines on non-muscle-invasive urothelial carcinoma of the bladder: Update 2013. Eur Urol. 2013;64(4):639–53.

168 van der Meijden A, Oosterlinck W, Brausi M, Kurth KH, Sylvester R, de Balincourt C. Significance of bladder biopsies in Ta,T1 bladder tumors: A report from the EORTC Genito-Urinary Tract Cancer Cooperative Group. EORTC-GU Group Superficial Bladder Committee. Eur Urol. 1999;35(4):267–71.

169 Mungan MU, Canda AE, Tuzel E, Yorukoglu K, Kirkali Z. Risk factors for mucosal prostatic urethral involvement in superficial transitional cell carcinoma of the bladder. Eur Urol. 2005;48(5):760–3.

170 Palou J, Sylvester RJ, Faba OR, Parada R, Pena JA, Algaba F, *et al.* Female gender and carcinoma in situ in the prostatic urethra are prognostic factors for recurrence, progression, and disease-specific mortality in T1G3 bladder cancer patients treated with bacillus Calmette-Guerin. Eur Urol. 2012;62(1):118–25.

171 Huguet J, Crego M, Sabate S, Salvador J, Palou J, Villavicencio H. Cystectomy in patients with high risk superficial bladder tumors who fail intravesical BCG therapy: Pre-cystectomy prostate involvement as a prognostic factor. Eur Urol. 2005;48(1):53–9; discussion 9.

172 Kay T, Timothy O, x, Brien. Improving transurethral resection of bladder tumour: The gold standard for diagnosis and treatment of bladder tumours. Eur Urol.7(7):524–8.

173 Millan-Rodriguez F, Chechile-Toniolo G, Salvador-Bayarri J, Palou J, Vicente-Rodriguez J. Multivariate analysis of the prognostic factors of primary superficial bladder cancer. J Urol. 2000;163(1):73–8.

174 Vianello A, Costantini E, Del Zingaro M, Bini V, Herr HW, Porena M. Repeated white light transurethral resection of the bladder in nonmuscle-invasive urothelial bladder cancers: Systematic review and meta-analysis. J Endourol. 2011; 25(11):1703–12.

175 Schwaibold HE, Sivalingam S, May F, Hartung R. The value of a second transurethral resection for T1 bladder cancer. BJU Int. 2006;97(6):1199–201.

176 Herr HW, Donat SM. A re-staging transurethral resection predicts early progression of superficial bladder cancer. BJU Int. 2006;97(6):119–8.

177 Nieder AM, Brausi M, Lamm D, O'Donnell M, Tomita K, Woo H, *et al.* Management of stage T1 tumors of the bladder: International Consensus Panel. Urology. 2005;66(6 Suppl 1):108–25.

178 Maurice MJ, Vricella GJ, MacLennan G, Buehner P, Ponsky LE. Endoscopic snare resection of bladder tumors: Evaluation of an alternative technique for bladder tumor resection. J Endourol. 2012;26(6):614–7.

179 Sylvester RJ, van der Meijden A, Witjes JA, Jakse G, Nonomura N, Cheng C, *et al.* High-grade Ta urothelial carcinoma and carcinoma in situ of the bladder. Urology. 2005;66(6 Suppl 1):90–107.

180 May F, Treiber U, Hartung R, Schwaibold H. Significance of random bladder biopsies in superficial bladder cancer. Eur Urol. 2003;44(1):47–50.

181 Gudjonsson S, Blackberg M, Chebil G, Jahnson S, Olsson H, Bendahl PO, *et al.* The value of bladder mapping and prostatic urethra biopsies for detection of carcinoma in situ (CIS). BJU Int. 2012;110(2 Pt 2):E41–5.

182 Kong MX, Zhao X, Kheterpal E, Lee P, Taneja S, Lepor H, *et al.* Histopathologic and clinical features of vesical diverticula. Urology. 2013;82(1):142–7.

183 Fradet Y, Grossman HB, Gomella L, Lerner S, Cookson M, Albala D, *et al.* A comparison of hexaminolevulinate fluorescence cystoscopy and white light cystoscopy for the detection of carcinoma in situ in patients with bladder cancer: A phase III, multicenter study. J Urol. 2007;178(1):68–73; discussion

184 Burger M, Grossman HB, Droller M, Schmidbauer J, Hermann G, Dragoescu O, *et al.* Photodynamic diagnosis of non-muscle-invasive bladder cancer with hexaminolevulinate cystoscopy: a meta-analysis of detection and recurrence based on raw data. Eur Urol. 2013;64(5):846–54.

185 Liu JJ, Droller MJ, Liao JC. New optical imaging technologies for bladder cancer: considerations and perspectives. J Urol. 2012;188(2):361–8.

186 Cauberg EC, Kloen S, Visser M, de la Rosette JJ, Babjuk M, Soukup V, *et al.* Narrow band imaging cystoscopy improves the detection of non-muscle-invasive bladder cancer. Urology. 2010;76(3):658–63.

187 Geavlete B, Multescu R, Georgescu D, Stanescu F, Jecu M, Geavlete P. Narrow band imaging cystoscopy and bipolar plasma vaporization for large nonmuscle-invasive bladder tumors—results of a prospective, randomized comparison to the standard approach. Urology. 2012;79(4):846–51.

188 Kausch I, Sommerauer M, Montorsi F, Stenzl A, Jacqmin D, Jichlinski P, *et al.* Photodynamic diagnosis in non-muscle-invasive bladder cancer: a systematic review and cumulative analysis of prospective studies. Eur Urol. 2010;57(4):595–606.

189 Grossman HB, Stenzl A, Fradet Y, Mynderse LA, Kriegmair M, Witjes JA, *et al.* Long-term decrease in bladder cancer recurrence with hexaminolevulinate enabled fluorescence cystoscopy. J Urol. 2012;188(1):58–62.

190 Sonn GA, Jones SN, Tarin TV, Du CB, Mach KE, Jensen KC, *et al.* Optical biopsy of human bladder neoplasia with in vivo confocal laser endomicroscopy. J Urol. 2009;182(4):1299–305.

191 Wiesner C, Jager W, Salzer A, Biesterfeld S, Kiesslich R, Hampel C, *et al.* Confocal laser endomicroscopy for the diagnosis of urothelial bladder neoplasia: A technology of the future? BJU Int. 2011;107(3):399–403.

192 Chang TC, Liu JJ, Hsiao ST, Pan Y, Mach KE, Leppert JT, *et al.* Interobserver agreement of confocal laser endomicroscopy for bladder cancer. J Endourol. 2013;27(5):598–603.

193 Soukup V, Babjuk M, Bellmunt J, Dalbagni G, Giannarini G, Hakenberg OW, *et al.* Follow-up after surgical treatment of bladder cancer: A critical analysis of the literature. Eur Urol. 2012;62(2):290–302.

194 van der Aa MNM, Steyerberg EW, Bangma C, van Rhijn BWG, Zwarthoff EC, van der Kwast TH. Cystoscopy revisited as the gold standard for detecting bladder cancer recurrence: diagnostic review bias in the randomized, prospective CEFUB trial. J Urol. 2010;183(1):76–80.

195 Swietek N, Waldert M, Rom M, Schatzl G, Wiener HG, Susani M, *et al.* The value of transurethral bladder biopsy after intravesical bacillus Calmette-Guerin instillation therapy for nonmuscle invasive bladder cancer: A retrospective, single center study and cumulative analysis of the literature. J Urol. 2012;188(3):748–53.

196 Abd El-Latif A, Watts KE, Elson P, Fergany A, Hansel DE. The sensitivity of initial transurethral resection or biopsy of bladder tumor(s) for detecting bladder cancer variants on radical cystectomy. J Urol. 2013;189(4):1263–7.

197 Picozzi S, Ricci C, Gaeta M, Ratti D, Macchi A, Casellato S, *et al.* Upper urinary tract recurrence following radical cystectomy for bladder cancer: A meta-analysis on 13,185 patients. J Urol. 2012;188(6):2046–54.

198 Guarnizo E, Pavlovich CP, Seiba M, Carlson DL, Vaughan ED, Jr., Sosa RE. Ureteroscopic biopsy of upper tract urothelial carcinoma: Improved diagnostic accuracy and histopathological considerations using a multi-biopsy approach. J Urol. 2000;163(1):52–5.

199 Rojas CP, Castle SM, Llanos CA, Cortes JAS, Bird V, Rodriguez S, *et al.* Low biopsy volume in ureteroscopy does not affect tumor biopsy grading in upper tract urothelial carcinoma. Urol Oncol. 2013;31(8):1696–700.

200 Cutress ML, Stewart GD, Zakikhani P, Phipps S, Thomas BG, Tolley DA. Ureteroscopic and percutaneous management of upper tract urothelial carcinoma (UTUC): Systematic review. BJU Int. 2012;110(5):614–28.

201 Ishikawa S, Abe T, Shinohara N, Harabayashi T, Sazawa A, Maruyama S, *et al.* Impact of diagnostic ureteroscopy on intravesical recurrence and survival in patients with urothelial carcinoma of the upper urinary tract. J Urol. 2010;184(3):883–7.

202 Kleinmann N, Healy KA, Hubosky SG, Margel D, Bibbo M, Bagley D. Ureteroscopic biopsy of upper tract urothelial carcinoma: Comparison of basket and forceps. J Endourol. 2013;27(12):1450–4.

203 Wason SE, Seigne JD, Schned AR, Pais VM, Jr. Ureteroscopic biopsy of upper tract urothelial carcinoma using a novel ureteroscopic biopsy forceps. Can J Urol. 2012;19(6):6560–5.

204 Brien JC, Shariat SF, Herman MP, Ng CK, Scherr DS, Scoll B, *et al.* Preoperative hydronephrosis, ureteroscopic biopsy grade and urinary cytology can improve prediction of advanced upper tract urothelial carcinoma. J Urol. 2010;184(1):69–73.

205 Liedberg F, Chebil G, Mansson W. Urothelial carcinoma in the prostatic urethra and prostate: current controversies. Expert Rev Anticancer Ther. 2007;7(3):383–90.

206 Donat SM, Wei DC, McGuire MS, Herr HW. The efficacy of transurethral biopsy for predicting the long-term clinical impact of prostatic invasive bladder cancer. J Urol. 2001;165(5):1580–4.

7

Active Surveillance for Low-Risk Prostate Cancer

Laurence Klotz, MD, FRCSC

Division of Urology, Sunnybrook Health Sciences Center, University of Toronto, Toronto, Ontario, Canada

Introduction and Background

The history of surgery has been one of progressive movement toward less invasive, painful, and mutilating operations. The ultimate expression of this trend will be the management of disease without invasive procedures at all [1]. In prostate cancer, there has been a major shift toward tissue-conserving approaches, including active surveillance (AS) and focal therapy. Progress in AS will be reviewed in this chapter.

The advent of prostate-specific antigen (PSA) testing in the late 1980s resulted in a dramatic (threefold) increase in the annual age adjusted incidence of prostate cancer, followed by a gradual decrease. In conjunction with this increased incidence, there was a steady decrease in the average volume of cancer in newly diagnosed men. This was prototypical stage migration of cancer, occurring as a result of a new diagnostic test that detects cancer which was previously undiagnosed but highly prevalent. The new test resulted in the rapid diagnosis of hundreds of thousands of men who had harbored preclinical prostate cancer for many years. As the prevalent cases were identified and treated, the incidence of new cases drifted back toward baseline levels (although they never dropped down to baseline levels, reflecting the "true" incidence of the disease).

The U.S. Preventative Services Task Force (USPSTF) recommendation against PSA screening in 2012 largely reflected concerns about overdiagnosis and overtreatment of nonlife-threatening or nonclinically significant disease [2]. Previously, most men with prostate cancer were treated by either radical prostatectomy or high-dose radiation treatment. The recommendations of the USPSTF, enhanced by evidence regarding the indolent nature of low-grade disease and the very low cancer-specific mortality outcome achieved with conservative management, has resulted in a more widespread adoption of this approach, and an emerging consensus regarding the use of conservative management for patients with low- and selected intermediate-risk cancer.

Rationale

Prostate cancer develops with age in most men from all races and regions. In Caucasians and African Americans, the chance of harboring prostate cancer is approximately one's age as a percentage; in other words, as many as 30% of men in their 30s, 40% in their 40s, and 70 in their 70s, have some histologic prostate cancer [3]. Most of these are microfoci only

(<1 mm^3) and low grade. The high prevalence of microfocal prostate cancer has been confirmed in autopsy studies of Caucasians, Asians, and other racial groups going back more than 50 years. A recent autopsy study in Japanese and Russian men, two groups in whom PSA testing was uncommon, found that in those who died of other causes, 35% of both groups had prostate cancer. Surprisingly, 50% of the cancers in Japanese men aged 70 or older were Gleason score 7 or higher [4]. In Japanese men younger than age 60, the prevalence was lower than Caucasians, and there was no difference in men older than 60. This finding suggests that, particularly in men older than 70, microfocal Gleason $3+4$ might also represent "overdiagnosis" of clinically insignificant cancer.

Genetic Features of Low-Grade Prostate Cancer

Genetic analyses comparing Gleason 3 and 4 patterns, the two most common histologic patterns of prostate cancer, have found that their molecular hallmarks of cancer differ. The hallmarks of cancer, described by Hanahan and Weinberg, provide a context for comparing the degree to which these cancers are "malignant" [5]. The six original hallmarks of cancer include unlimited replicative potential, sustained angiogenesis, local tissue invasion, insensitivity to antigrowth signals, metastasis, and replicative self-sufficiency. The update in 2011 added two more: deregulating cellular energetics and evasion of immune destruction [6]. The genetic pathways responsible for these hallmarks of malignancy have been worked out in detail (Table 7.1). The assignment of Gleason pattern, particularly between 3 and 4, segregates prostate cancer between genetically normal and abnormal cells to a remarkable degree. There are many examples of this segregation. Genetic pathways mediating apoptosis resistance [7], angiogenesis [8], and the development of other pro-angiogenic factors [9], genes involved in regulating cellular metabolomics, and metastasis invasion processes, are overexpressed in Gleason 4 and normal in 3 [7–20]. Proliferation pathway associated genes, including Akt and HER2neu [10,11], are expressed normally in Gleason 3 and abnormally in Gleason 4 (see Table 7.1). Cell-cycle regulatory genes and

Table 7.1 Gleason 3 Lacks the Hallmarks of Cancer.

Characteristic of Cancer	Gleason 3	Gleason 4
Expression of pro-proliferation embryonic, neuronal, haematopoietic stem cell genes, EGF, EGFR [10]	Not present	Overexpressed
Akt pathway [10]	Not present	Aberrant
HER2/neu [11]	Not present	Amplified
Insensitivity to antigrowth signals such as cyclin D2 methylation, CKDN1β [12–14]	Expressed	Absent
Resistance to apoptosis: BCL2 [7]	Negative	Strong expression
Absence of senescence [17]	Normal	Increased
Sustained angiogenesis: VEGF [8]	Expression low	Increased
Other proangiogenic factors and microvessel density [9]	Normal	Increased
Tissue invasion and metastasis markers [10]	Normal	Overexpressed
PTEN [15,16]	Present (7% deleted)	Deleted
TMPRSS2-ERG translocation [18,19]	Present 45%	Present 50–60%
Clinical evidence of metastasis mortality [23,25]	Virtually absent	Present

proteins are present in Gleason 3 and absent in Gleason 4 [12–14]. Senescence is normal in Gleason 3, largely impaired in Gleason 4 [17]. Expression of invasion and metastasis associated genes are absent in pattern 3 but present in pattern 4 [20]. There are exceptions; for example, both Phosphatase and tensin homolog(pTEN) [15,16] and TMPRSS2-ERG [18–20], commonly upregulated and present respectively in most Gleason 4s, have been reported to be altered in a proportion of Gleason 3. Given the normal limits of histology at predicting genetic abnormalities, this is not surprising. However, these isolated genetic alterations do not appear to translate into an aggressive metastatic phenotype. At a genetic level, Gleason pattern 3 resembles normal prostate epithelium much more than it does cancer; Gleason pattern 4 has the features of cancer [21,22].

Metastatic Potential

Prostate cancers vary widely in their metastatic potential, from completely indolent to highly aggressive. Several large clinical series have reported a rate of metastasis for surgically confirmed Gleason 6 (where there is no possibility of occult higher-grade cancer lurking in the prostate) that is essentially zero. A natural limitation of the conservative (no treatment) management series is that because the diagnosis is based on needle biopsy, there is no way to exclude the possibility that the patients who progress to metastasis had occult higher-grade cancer at the time of diagnosis. About 25% of men initially diagnosed with Gleason 6 on biopsy have occult higher-grade cancer, and these appear to be responsible for most of the prostate cancer deaths reported in series of conservative management. These cases are wolves in sheeps' clothing, and their earlier identification is a major unmet need in the field.

One multicenter study of 24,000 men with long-term follow up after surgery included 12,000 with surgically confirmed Gleason 6 cancer [23]. The 20-year prostate cancer mortality was 0.2%. About 4,000 of these were treated at Memorial Sloan Kettering Cancer Center (MSKCC); of these, 1 died of prostate cancer; a pathological review of this patient revealed Gleason 4 + 3 disease [24]. A second study of 14,000 men with surgically confirmed Gleason 6 disease found only 22 with lymph node metastases; review of these cases showed that all had higher-grade cancer in the primary tumour. The rate of node-positive disease in the patients with no Gleason 4 or 5 disease in their prostates was therefore zero [25].

Occasional genetic mutations that confer an aggressive phenotype may be pre-histologic or may develop as a result of the accumulation of genetic alterations in normal cells or low-grade cancers. A recent genetic analysis of multiple metastatic sites from a patient who had extensive Gleason 4 + 3 pT3a N1 disease resected at age 47 and died 17 years later of metastatic castration-resistant prostate cancer (CRPC), reported that the metastatic lesions appeared to derive from a microfocus of Gleason pattern 3 disease, rather than, as expected, from the high-grade cancers elsewhere in the prostate [26]. A second case report from the same group described a patient on AS with 12 annual biopsies that were negative or showed Gleason 6 cancer only. Biopsies were discontinued for 5 years, until a repeat biopsy performed because of a rise in PSA showed Gleason 9 cancer, which had metastasized. Molecular characterization of the biopsies in this patient showed no homology at all between the previous low-grade cancer and the high-grade cancer [27]. These case reports are a challenge to the view that Gleason pattern 3 does not behave like a malignancy. It has been proposed that in the first patient, the low-grade cancer that shared genetic homology with the metastases, and was present in a sea of higher grade cancer, may have developed as a "re-differentiated clonal offspring of a higher grade cancer cell that had metastasized" [28]. Key points raised by these informative cases are that biology is complex, dynamic, and not 100%

predictable; these are single-case reports and should be viewed in that context; and it is possible that histological Gleason pattern 3, particularly when it coexists with higher-grade cancer, can harbor prehistological genetic alterations that confer a more-aggressive phenotype. This is the conceptual basis for genetically based predictive assays that disaggregate low-grade cancer into low- and higher-risk groups. Importantly, these cases should be balanced against the extensive clinical evidence supporting the absence of metastatic potential in the vast majority of cancers that are pure Gleason pattern 3.

Biomarkers

Two biomarkers have been approved by the U.S. Food and Drug Administration (FDA) based on their ability to predict progression in patients with low-grade prostate cancer: the Prolaris assay [29] (Myriad Genetics), which looks for abnormal expression of cell cycle related genes, and the Oncotype DX assay (Genome Health), which identifies a panel of genes linked to a more-aggressive phenotype [30]. The Decipher assay, a tissue-based 22-marker genomic classifier evaluating non-coding RNA sequences, has been demonstrated to accurately predict the risk of biochemical progression after radical prostatectomy [31]. The Mitomics assay, which identifies the presence of a functional mitochondrial DNA deletion associated with aggressive prostate cancer [32], is not yet FDA approved. These tests hold the promise of interrogating the microfocus of Gleason 6 found on biopsy for accurate information about the presence of higher-grade cancer elsewhere in the prostate or the future likelihood of progression to aggressive disease. That the biomarkers can achieve this confirms the inter-relationship of heterogeneous multifocal cancers.

Limitations of PSA Kinetics

PSA kinetics are currently used as a guide to identify patients at higher risk but not to drive the decision to treat. Until multiparametric MRI became available, men on AS with poor PSA kinetics (doubling time <3 years) were offered treatment. In the PRIAS multi-institutional AS registry, 20% of men being treated had intervention based on a PSA doubling time <3 years [33]. In a report of the five men dying of metastatic prostate cancer in the Toronto cohort, all had a PSA doubling time <2 years [34]. However, PSA kinetics has a crucial limitation: lack of specificity [35]. In a study of PSA kinetics in a large surveillance cohort, false-positive PSA triggers (doubling time <3 years, or PSA velocity >2 ng/year) occurred in 50% of stable untreated patients, none of whom went on to progress, require treatment, or die of prostate cancer [35]. Vickers, in an overview of all of the studies of more than 200 patients examining the predictive value of PSA kinetics in localized prostate cancer, concluded that kinetics had no independent predictive value beyond the absolute value of PSA [36].

Role of MRI

Systematic serial transrectal ultrasound (TRUS)-guided biopsies has been the primary tool for identification of the "wolf in sheep's clothing" in men with Gleason 6 cancer on surveillance. This technique has significant limitations. TRUS-guided biopsy undersamples the anterior prostate, apex, and antero-lateral horn. Thus, a confirmatory biopsy to target these areas in men on surveillance is essential. Because prostate cancer in most cases takes 10–20 years to reach the stage where clinical diagnosis is possible, the delay of 6–12 months in finding occult higher-grade cancer is unlikely to alter curability. MRI has an emerging role in the management of patients under AS. There are two potential benefits: reassurance that no higher risk disease is present in those with a negative MRI; and, in the patients harboring occult higher-grade disease, earlier identification of this cancer. With respect to the former benefit, the key metric is the negative predictive value (NPV). This has been reported to be

97% for a group of about 300 surveillance candidates at MSKCC [37]. This observation requires validation. An MRI lesion characterized as Prostate Imaging Reporting and Data System (PiRADS) score of 4 or 5/5 has a 90% positive predictive value for high-grade cancer. This abnormality is characterized by a hypodenselesion on T2-weighted image, with both restricted diffusion and enhanced contrast. These are significant and should lead at least to a targeted biopsy, if not definitive intervention. An equivocal lesion (PiRADS 3/5) should trigger a targeted biopsy. The diagnostic usefulness of MRI and targeted biopsy compared to systematic biopsy has recently been reported to be optimized in men with a PSA >5.2 [38].

Importantly, the favorable results of AS summarized herein have been achieved without incorporating MRI, which has been a recent development. It is thus, currently, an adjunct to surveillance and not a requirement. In centers where access to MRI is limited by either availability or resource restrictions, it should be used selectively. However, it is plausible that an MRI performed at diagnosis in all patients with newly diagnosed prostate cancer would enhance these excellent results further. This approach is currently the subject of prospective trials.

If the results of single-center cohorts are validated, the reliable performance of MRI as a diagnostic test would permit a level of confidence in a negative MRI that would allow it to replace the biopsy. This would decrease the number of men requiring biopsies (a major unmet need) and facilitate early identification of clinically significant disease. A limitation of multiparametric MRI is that the skill set for accurate interpretation is demanding and not yet widely prevalent.

A further area for research is to better understand how to integrate the results of genetic biomarker tests and MRI. For example, optimal management of the patient in whom results are discrepant (i.e., genetic test indicates high risk but MRI is negative) is currently unknown. False-positive and false-negative results undoubtedly occur with both diagnostic approaches, but how commonly this occurs is uncertain. Although they may meet the unmet need of better risk assignment, further validation of their performance is needed before they are widely adopted in the surveillance scenario.

Implications for Patient Management

The appreciation of the critical observation that Gleason pattern 3 has little or no metastatic phenotype has altered the approach to these patients. Gleason pattern 3, which can invade locally, does fulfill sufficient traditional pathological criteria to be called a *cancer*, despite its nonmetastasizing phenotype (analogous to basal cell carcinoma of the skin or gliomas). Both of these latter tumors are non-metastasizing, but are they called cancers because of their demonstrated ability to invade locally. However, it is not a lethal threat, in contrast to the implications of the cancer diagnosis for to lay people. Changing the terminology away from the emotionally loaded term *cancer* would significantly reassure the patient and derail the headlong rush into aggressive treatment. Terms like *pseudo-cancer, pseudo-disease, part of the aging process*, and *pre-cancer* are useful in counseling these men.

Young age does not exclude the option of conservative management. The benefits of avoiding treatment with respect to maintenance of erectile function and continence are greater in young men, and the risks of second malignancies as sequelae of radiation are also greater in men with a long life expectancy. Microfocal low-grade cancer is present in 30–40% of men in their 40s [3]. Diagnosing microfocal Gleason 6 cancer on a TRUS-guided biopsy does not mean that disease progression is inevitable. Many studies, however, have demonstrated that that men with high-volume Gleason pattern 3 have a higher risk of harboring higher-grade cancer. The volume threshold of Gleason 3 on biopsy at which point higher-grade cancer is more likely to be present is variable. A threshold of more than 8 mm of total cancer on systematic biopsy has recently been described [39]. Another approach to the question of the significance of higher volume Gleason 6 has been to use the European Randomized Study for Prostate Cancer (ERSPC) database to characterize the volume of cancer in those patients with clinically significant Gleason 6 disease. The threshold for clinically significant Gleason 6 disease was a cancer volume of >1.3 mL [40]. This is an important refinement of the traditional definition of >0.5 mL, defined by Stamey based on 149 cystoprostatectomy specimens from the pre-PSA era. The management of these patients is to exclude the presence of higher-grade cancer as rigorously as possible (based on MRI, targeted/template biopsies, and biomarkers). Such patients are unlikely to require treatment.

AS not only offers the prospect of reduced morbidity and improved quality of life, but should result in an improvement in survival. The logic is as follows. PSA screening has been discarded by policy makers such as the USPSTF because of concerns about overtreatment and a high number needed to treat (NNT) for each death avoided. Selective treatment employing AS would result in a decrease in the NNT for each death avoided. If widely adopted, AS would eventually result in a reappraisal of the benefits of PSA screening and a greater acceptance of its value by policy makers such as the USPSTF. The result will be "rehabilitation" of PSA screening, earlier identification of those with aggressive disease, lives saved, and an overall reduction in prostate cancer mortality (compared to no screening resulting from the perceived hazards of overtreatment).

Eligibility for Surveillance

Who Is a Candidate?

Low-risk disease based on biopsy is widely defined as Gleason 6 and PSA <10 ng/mL. (The 2005 reclassification of the Gleason scoring system resulted in Gleason 2–5 being eliminated from the needle biopsy grading. The National Comprehensive Cancer Network (NCCN) makes a distinction between very low-risk (fulfilling Epstein criteria of two or less cores positive, no more than 50% of any core involvement, and PSA density <0.15) and low-risk (Gleason 6, PSA <10). Technically patients with T stage > T2a are excluded; in fact, most eligible patients are T1c. This group includes around 45% of newly diagnosed patients in the United States and Canada, which is currently approximately 150,000 men per year The Epstein criteria were based on those biopsy criteria which predicted for the Stamey definition of clinically insignificant disease (<0.5 mL of Gleason 6 prostate cancer). As mentioned previously, this definition is too stringent and would exclude many patients with low-risk disease who would otherwise be excellent candidates. Based on the contemporary ERSPC definition of clinically insignificant disease as being a low-grade tumor volume >1.3 mL and because the number of cores taken at biopsy has increased (to more than 80 in patients having template biopsies), these criteria warrant redefinition. Informed by the genetic characterization of Gleason pattern 3 and the clinical experience with Gleason 6, we believe that all Gleason 6 cancer has a low risk of metastasis. The main significance of higher volume disease is as a predictor of occult higher-grade cancer. In the absence of higher-grade cancer, metastasis will not occur. Thus, these patients require close scrutiny to preclude as much as possible co-existent higher-grade disease, but do not necessarily require treatment in the absence of higher-grade cancer.

Most patients who are upgraded harbor occult higher-grade cancer at the time of diagnosis. Biological grade progression (Gleason 3 cells giving rise to Gleason 4 or 5 progeny) occurs over time, but it is uncommon. In the Toronto surveillance cohort, we observed that the likelihood of grade progression increased approximately 1% per year from the time of the original biopsy [41].

This is a likely estimate of the frequency of grade progression. The implication is that long-term follow up is required, although in most cases the Gleason grade remains stable.

Low prostate volume, and more specifically a high PSA density (PSA-to-prostate volume ratio), has been demonstrated in many studies to be a predictor for risk progression. A high PSA density in some surveillance candidates reflects PSA arising from a large occult cancer. Increased caution is warranted in these cases.

A few young men (50 years of age or younger) are found to have extensive Gleason 6 cancer on biopsy. In these patients, uncertainty exists about. the risk of true tumor progression over time, as well as the risk of harboring occult high-grade disease. These patients are clearly outliers, and it is reasonable to offer them treatment. Where exactly to draw the line in terms of age and cancer volume is a matter of clinical judgment.

Race is a relevant factor. African Americans on AS have a higher rate of risk reclassification and PSA failure when treated than Caucasians [42]. African American men who are surveillance candidates also have a higher rate of large anterior cancers than Caucasians [43]. Japanese men younger than age 60 have a lower rate of histological "autopsy" cancer than Caucasian men. Thus, the finding of low-grade prostate cancer in young Asian men may be less likely to represent overdiagnosis. However, African American and Asian patients diagnosed with low-grade prostate cancer includes many men who have little or no probability of a prostate cancer–related death during their remaining lives, and AS is still an appealing option for those who have been appropriately risk stratified.

Outcome of Surveillance

Cardiovascular disease is the most-common cause of death in men on AS. Death from prostate cancer is uncommon, although it occurs. In the most mature surveillance cohort [44,45], with a median follow up of 8 years, the cumulative hazard ratio (or relative risk) of death not related to prostate cancer was 10 times that for prostate cancer. To date, the published literature on surveillance includes 13 prospective studies, encompassing about 5,000 men [45–56]. Most of these studies have a follow up duration that is too short to identify an increased risk of prostate cancer mortality as a result of surveillance. For example, a pivotal Swedish study reported that the risk of prostate cancer mortality in patients managed by watchful waiting was low for many years, but tripled after 15 years of follow up [57,58]. ("Watchful waiting" meant no opportunity for selective delayed intervention, whereas about 30% of patients in most surveillance series have had radical treatment.) In the Toronto experience, 70 patients have been followed for 14 years or more; 1.5% have had late disease progression, but there is no evidence of a sharp increase in mortality in those with longer follow up [45]. A critical question in this field is what the long-term prostate cancer mortality will be beyond 15 years. It will be 5–7 years before the most mature cohorts have a median of 15 years of follow-up. Table 7.2 summarizes the results of the 13 prospective series. The key outcome measures include the proportion of patients treated, overall, and cause-specific survival. About one third of patients are treated; most series have few or no prostate cancer deaths. In the Toronto series, the actuarial prostate cancer mortality at 15 years is 5%. The rate of other cause mortality is 10 times greater than the prostate cancer mortality.

Modeling

The use of surveillance compared with surgery and radiation has been modeled by several groups. One propensity score analysis compared 452 men from the Toronto surveillance cohort to 6,485 men having radical prostatectomy, 2264 treated

Table 7.2 Outcomes of AS in Large Prospective Series.

Reference	n	Median Follow-Up (months)	Treated Overall (%); Treatment Free (%)	Overall and Disease-Specific Survival (%)	BCR postdeferred treatment (%)
Klotz *et al.* [45], University of Toronto	993	92	30; 72 at 5 years	79 and 97 at 10 years DSS 95% at 15 years	25% (6% overall)
Bul *et al.* [33], Multicenter, Europe	2500	47	32; 43 at 10 years	77 and 100 at 10 years	20%^
Dall'Era *et al.* [46], UCSF	328	43	24; 67 at 5 years	100 and 100 at 5 years	NR
Kakehi *et al.* [48] Multicenter, Japan	118	36	51; 49 at 3 years	NR	NR
Tosian J *et al.* [48], Johns Hopkins, United States	407	NR	36; NR	NR	NR: 50% 'incurable' based on RP pathology
Roemeling *et al.* [49], Rotterdam, Netherlands	273	41	29; 71 at 5 years	89 and 100 at 5 years	NR [31% of 13 RP positive margins]
Soloway *et al.* [50], Miami, United States	99	35	8; 85 at 5 years	NR	NR
Patel *et al.* [51], Memorial Sloan Kettering, United States	88	35	35; 58 at 5 years	NR	NR
Barayan GA [52], McGill, Canada	155	65	20%	NR	NR
Rubio-Briones [53], Spain	232	36	27%	93% and 99.5% at 5 years	
Godtman [54]	439		63%	81 and 99.8	14
Thomsen [55], Denmark	167	40	35%/60% at 5 years		
Selvadurai [56], United Kingdom	471	67	30	98 and 99.7	12

DSS, disease-specific survival.

with external beam, and 1680 with brachytherapy. There was no difference in prostate cancer mortality and an improved overall survival in the surveillance group (because of an increase in other-cause mortality in the patients who underwent radiation) [59]. A decision analysis of surveillance compared to initial treatment showed that surveillance had the highest quality-adjusted life expectancy (QALE), even if the relative risk of prostate cancer–specific death for initial treatment compared with AS was as low as 0.6 [60]. (In fact, it is 0.95 at 15 years in the Toronto series.)

Although surveillance has become more widely accepted over the last decade, the modification of the Gleason system in 2005 has, ironically, resulted in grade migration, a decrease in the number of newly diagnosed Gleason 6 compared to 7, and therefore a smaller proportion of patients with prostate cancer eligible for surveillance. There is an increasing recognition that patients with Gleason $3+4=7$, where the component of pattern 4 is small (<10%) have a similar natural history to those with Gleason $3+3$, perhaps reflecting the stage-migration phenomenon [61].

AS in Practice

Most clinicians use the following approach or a variation of it: Following the initial diagnosis of Gleason 6 prostate cancer on 10 or more core systematic biopsy, PSA is performed every 3–6 months. A confirmatory biopsy must be carried out within 6–12 months of the initial diagnostic biopsy on which cancer was identified. This confirmatory biopsy should target the areas that are typically under-sampled on the initial diagnostic biopsy. This includes the anterior prostate and the prostatic apex and base. If the confirmatory biopsy is either negative or confirms microfocal Gleason $3+3$ disease, subsequent biopsies are performed every 3–5 years until the patient reaches age 80 or has a life expectancy <5 years because of comorbidity. Multiparametric MRI should be performed on the patients whose PSA kinetics suggests more aggressive disease (usually defined as a PSA doubling time <3 years), whose biopsy shows substantial volume increase, or who is upgraded to Gleason $3+4$. and surveillance is still desired as a management option. Identification of an MRI target suspicious for high-grade disease should warrant a targeted biopsy, or if the lesion is large and unequivocal, intervention.

Over time, about one-third of patients will be reclassified as higher risk for progression and offered treatment. This will depend on the inclusion criteria used for eligibility for surveillance. An inclusive approach, offering surveillance to all patients with Gleason 6 and PSA <15, for example, will include more patients with occult high-grade disease than a narrower approach, restricting surveillance to those who meet Epstein criteria (two or less positive cores, <50% involvement of any

one core, and PSA density <0.15). However, the more stringent eligibility denies the benefits of AS to many men with indolent disease who do not fit the Epstein criteria and thus are discouraged from choosing AS.

Most cases that are upgraded on the confirmatory or initial subsequent biopsy are upgraded based on resampling (about 25% of patients). More than 85% are upgraded to Gleason $3+4$ [62]. We have developed a risk calculator (Figure 7.1), which incorporates the important clinical parameters associated with grade progression in a surveillance cohort [41]. Note that, based on simple clinical and pathological parameters, a patient's likelihood of upgrading can be stratified over a large range, from 10% to 70%.

Conclusions

AS is an appealing approach for patients with low-risk disease and an effective solution to the widely recognized problem of overtreatment. Widespread adoption of surveillance would result in a reduction in the number needed to treat for each death avoided without the risk of increasing disease mortality. A dispassionate reassessment of PSA screening based on these improved metrics should lead to a reconsideration of the value of prostate cancer screening by organizations such as the USPSTF. Ongoing improvements in diagnostic accuracy based on multiparametric MRI and genetic biomarkers should reduce the need for systematic biopsies, improve the early identification of occult higher-risk disease, and enhance the ability to detect patients destined to have grade progression over time. The minimum current standard is a confirmatory biopsy targeting the anterolateral horn and anterior prostate within 6–12 months. PSA should be performed every 6 months and subsequent biopsies every 3–5 years until patient is no longer a candidate for definitive therapy. MRI is indicated for men with a grade or volume increase or adverse PSA kinetics. Treatment should be offered for most patients with upgraded disease.

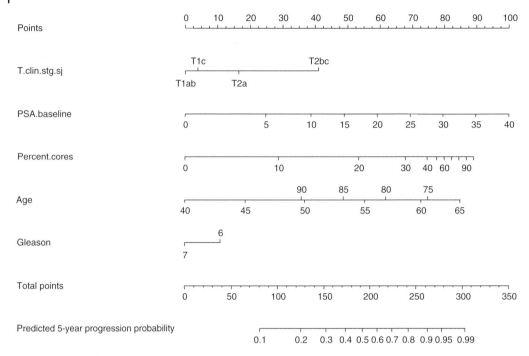

Figure 7.1 Risk of pathological upgrading or radical therapy 5 years after diagnosis in men on surveillance in the Sunnybrook cohort.

References

1 Gawende A. Two hundred years of surgery. N Engl J Med. 2012;366:1716–23.

2 http://ww.uspreventiveservicestaskforce.org/uspstf12/prostate/prostateart.htm

3 Sakr WA, Grignon DJ, Crissman JD, Heilbrun LK, Cassin BJ, Pontes JJ, *et al.* High grade prostatic intraepithelial neoplasia (HGPIN) and prostatic adenocarcinoma between the ages of 20–69: An autopsy study of 249 cases. In Vivo. 1994;May–Jun; 8(3):439–43.

4 Zlotta AR, Egawa S, Pushkar D, Govorov A, Kimura T, Kido M, *et al.* Prevalence of prostate cancer on autopsy: Cross-sectional study on unscreened Caucasian and Asian men. J Natl Cancer Inst. 2013;Jul 17;105(14):1050–8.

5 Hanahan D, Weinberg RA. The hallmarks of cancer. Cell. 2000;100:57–70

6 Hanahan D, Weinberg RA Hallmarks of cancer: The next generation. Cell. 2011; Mar 4;144(5):646–74.

7 Fleischmann A, Huland H, Mirlacher M, Wilczak W, Simon R, Erbersdobler A, *et al.* Prognostic relevance of Bcl-2 overexpression in surgically treated prostate cancer is not caused by increased copy number or translocation of the gene. Prostate.2012;72:991–97.

8 West AF, O'Donnell M, Charlton RG, Neal DE, Leung HY. Correlation of vascular endothelial growth factor expression with fibroblast growth factor-8 expression and clinico-pathologic parameters in human prostate cancer. Br J Cancer. 2001;85:576–83.

9 Erbersdobler A, Isbarn H, Dix K, Steiner I, Schlomm T, Mirlacher M, *et al.* Prognostic value of microvessel density in prostate cancer: a tissue microarray study. World J Urol. 2010; 28: 687–692.

10 Ross AE, Marchionni L, Vuica-Ross M, Cheadle C, Fan J, Berman DM, *et al.* Gene expression pathways of high grade localized prostate cancer. Prostate. 2011;71:1568–77.

11 Skacel M, Ormsby AH, Pettay JD, *et al.* Aneusomy of chromosomes 7, 8, and 17 and amplification of HER-2/neu and epidermal growth factor receptor in Gleason score 7 prostate carcinoma: A differential fluorescent in situ hybridization study of Gleason pattern 3 and 4 using tissue microarray. Hum Pathol. 2001;32:1392–97.

12 Padar A, Sathyanarayana UG, Suzuki M, Maruyama R, Hsieh JT, Frenkel EP, *et al.* Inactivation of cyclin D2 gene in prostate cancers by aberrant promoter methylation. Clin Cancer Res. 2003; 9:4730–34.

13 Susaki E, Nakayama KI. Multiple mechanisms for p27(Kip1) translocation and degradation. Cell Cycle. 2007;6:3015–20.

14 Guo Y, Sklar GN, Borkowski A, Kyprianou N. Loss of the cyclin-dependent kinase inhibitor p27(Kip1) protein in human prostate cancer correlates with tumor grade. Clin Cancer Res. 1997;3:2269–74.

15 Sowalsky AG, Ye H, Bubley GJ, Balk SP. Clonal progression of prostate cancers from Gleason grade 3 to grade 4. Cancer Res. 2013 Feb 1;73(3):1050–5.

16 Lotan TL, Carvalho FL, Peskoe SB, Hicks JL, Good J, Fedor HL, *et al.* PTEN loss is associated with upgrading of prostate cancer from biopsy to radical prostatectomy. Mod Pathol. 2015;28(1):128–37.

17 Serrano M. Cancer: A lower bar for senescence. Nature. 2010 Mar 18; 464(7287):363–4.

18 Bismar TA, Dolph M, Teng LH, Liu S, Donnelly B. ERG protein expression reflects hormonal treatment response and is associated with Gleason score and prostate cancer specific mortality. Eur J Cancer. 2012;48:538–46.

19 Berg KD, Vainer B, Thomsen FB, Røder MA3, Gerds TA, Toft BG, *et al.* ERG protein expression in diagnostic specimens is associated with increased risk of progression during active surveillance for prostate cancer. Eur Urol. 2014;66(5):851–60.

20 Lin D, Bayani J, Wang Y, Sadar MD, Yoshimoto M, Gout PW, *et al.* Development of metastatic and non-metastatic tumor lines from a patient's prostate cancer specimen-identification of a small subpopulation with metastatic potential in the primary tumor. Prostate. 2010;70(15):1636–44.

21 Tomlins SA, Mehra R, Rhodes DR, Cao X, Wang L, Dhanasekaran, SM, *et al.* Integrative molecular concept modeling of prostate cancer progression. Nat Genet. 2007;39:41–51.

22 True L, Coleman I, Hawley S, Huang CY, Gifford D, Coleman R, *et al.* A molecular correlate to the Gleason grading system for prostate adenocarcinoma. Proc Natl Acad Sci USA. 2006;103:10991–96.

23 Eggener S, Scardino P, Walsh P, Han M, Partin AW, Trock BJ, *et al.* Predicting 15 year prostate cancer specific mortality after radical prostatectomy. J Urol. 2011;185(3):869–75.

24 Scott Eggener, personal communication.

25 Ross HM, Kryvenko ON, Cowan JE, Simko JP, Wheeler TM, Epstein JI. Do adenocarcinomas of the prostate with gleason score (gs) < =6 have the potential to metastasize to lymph nodes? Am J Surg Pathol. 2012 Sep;36(9):1346–52.

26 Haffner M, Yegasubramanian S. The clonal origin of lethal prostate cancer. J Clin Invest. 2013 Nov 1;123(11):4918–22.

27 Haffner MC, De Marzo AM, Yegnasubramanian S, Epstein JI, Carter HB. Diagnostic challenges of clonal heterogeneity in prostate cancer. J Clin Oncol. 2015;33(7):e38–40.

28 Barbieri CE, Demichelis F, Rubin MA. The lethal clone in prostate cancer: Redefining the index. Eur Urol. 2014;66:395–7.

29 Cuzick J, Berney DM, Fisher G, the Transatlantic Prostate Group. Prognostic value of a cell cycle progression signature for prostate cancer death on conservatively managed needle biopsy cohort. Br J Cancer. 2012;106:1095–1099.

30 Knezevic D, Goddard AD, Natraj N, Cherbavaz DB, Clark-Langone KM, Snable J, *et al.* Analytical validation of the Oncotype DX prostate cancer assay—a clinical RT-PCR assay optimized for prostate needle biopsies. BMC Genomics. 2013 Oct 8;14:690.

31 Cooperberg MR, Davicioni E, Crisan A, Jenkins RB, Ghadessi M, Karnes RJ. Combined value of validated clinical and genomic risk stratification tools for predicting prostate cancer mortality in a high-risk prostatectomy cohort. Eur Urol. 2015;67:326–33.

32 Robinson K, Creed J, Reguly B, Powell C, Wittock R, Klein D, *et al.* Accurate prediction of repeat prostate biopsy outcomes by a mitochondrial DNA deletion assay. Prostate Cancer Prostatic Dis. 2013 Dec;16(4):398.

33 Bul M, Zhu X, Valdagni R, Pickles T, Kakehi Y, Rannikko A, *et al.* Active surveillance for low-risk prostate cancer worldwide: The PRIAS study. Eur Urol. 2013; 63:597.

34 Krakowsky Y, Loblaw A, Klotz L. Prostate cancer death of men treated with initial active surveillance: clinical and biochemical characteristics. J Urol. 2010 Jul; 184(1):131–5

35 Loblaw A, Zhang L, Lam A, Nam R, Mamedov A, Vesprini D, *et al.* Comparing prostate specific antigen triggers for intervention in men with stable prostate cancer on active surveillance. J Urol. 2010 Nov;184(5):1942–6

36 Vickers A. Systematic review of pretreatment psa velocity and doubling time as pca predictors. J Clin Oncol. 2008;27:398–403.

37 Vargas HA, Akin O, Afaq A, Goldman D, Zheng J, Moskowitz CS, *et al.* Magnetic resonance imaging for predicting prostate biopsy findings in patients considered for active surveillance of clinically low risk prostate cancer. J Urol. 2012 Nov; 188(5):1732–8.

38 Shakir NA, George AK, Siddiqui MM, Rothwax JT, Rais-Bahrami S, Stamatakis L, *et al.* Identification of threshold prostate specific antigen levels to optimize the detection of clinically significant prostate cancer by magnetic resonance imaging/ultrasound fusion guided biopsy. J Urol. 2014 Dec;192(6):1642–9.

39 Bratt O, Folkvaljon Y, Loeb S, Klotz L, Egevad L, Stattin P. Upper limit of cancer extent on biopsy defining very low risk prostate cancer. BJU Int. 2015;116(2):213–9.

40 Wolters T, Roobol M, Schröder F, van der Kwast T. A Critical analysis of the tumor volume threshold for clinically insignificant prostate cancer using a data set of a randomized screening trial. J Urol. 2011;185:121–5.

41 Jain S, Kattan M, Klotz L, Loblaw A. Gleason upgrading in a surveillance cohort: development of a risk calculator. AUA 2014

42 Sundi D, Faisal FA, Trock BJ, Landis PK, Feng Z, Ross AE, *et al.* Reclassification rates are higher among african american men than caucasians on active surveillance. Urology. 2015;85(1):55–60.

43 Sundi D, Ross AE, Humphreys EB, Han M, Partin AW, Carter HB, *et al.* African American men with very low-risk prostate cancer exhibit adverse oncologic outcomes after radical prostatectomy: should active surveillance still be an option for them? J Clin Oncol. 2013 Aug 20;31(24):2991–7.

44 Klotz L, Zhang L, Lam A, Nam R, Mamedov A, Loblaw A. Clinical results of long-term follow-up of a large, active surveillance cohort with localized prostate cancer. J Clin Oncol. 2010 Jan 1;28(1):126–31.

45 Klotz L, Vesprini D, Sethukavalan P, Jethava V, Zhang L, Jain S, *et al.* Long-term follow-up of a large active surveillance cohort of patients with prostate cancer. J Clin Oncol. 2015;33(3):272–7.

46 Dall'Era MA, Konety BR, Cowan JE, Shinohara K, Stauf F, Cooperberg MR, Meng MV *et al.* Active surveillance for the management of prostate cancer in a contemporary cohort. Cancer. 2008 Jun 15;112(12):2664–70.

47 Kakehi Y, Kamoto T, Shiraishi T, Ogawa O, Suzukamo Y, Fukuhara S, *et al.* Prospective evaluation of selection criteria for active surveillance in Japanese patients with stage T1cN0M0 prostate cancer. Jpn J Clin Oncol. 2008 Feb;38(2):122–8.

48 Tosoian JJ, Trock BJ, Landis P, Feng Z, Epstein JI, Partin AQ, *et al.* Active surveillance program for prostate cancer: An update of the Johns Hopkins experience. J Clin Oncol. 2011;29:2185–90.

49 Roemeling S, Roobol MJ, de Vries SH, Wolters T, Gosselaar C, van Leenders GJ, *et al.* Active surveillance for prostate cancers detected in three subsequent rounds of a screening trial: characteristics, PSA doubling times, and outcome. Eur Urol. 2007 May;51(5):1244–50.

50 Soloway MS, Soloway CT, Eldefrawy A, *et al.* Careful selection and close monitoring of low-risk prostate cancer patients on active surveillance minimizes the need for treatment. Eur Urol. 2010;58:831–5.

51 Patel MI, DeConcini DT, Lopez-Corona E, Ohori M, Wheeler T, Scardino PT. An analysis of men with clinically localized prostate cancer who deferred definitive therapy. J Urol. 2004 Apr;171(4):1520–4

52 Barayan GA, Brimo F, Bégin LR, Hanley JA, Liu Z, Kassouf W, *et al.* Factors influencing disease progression of prostate cancer under active surveillance: A Mcgill University health center cohort. BJU Int. 2014;114(6):E99–E104.

53 Rubio-Briones J, Iborra I, Ramírez M, Calatrava A, Collado A, Casanova J, *et al.* Obligatory information that a patient diagnosed of prostate cancer and candidate for an active surveillance protocol must know. Actas Urol Esp. 2014;38(9):559–65.

54 Godtman RA, Holmberg E, Khatami A, Stranne J, Hugosson J. Outcome following active surveillance of men with screen-detected prostate cancer. Results from the Göteborg randomised population-based prostate cancer screening trial. Eur Urol. 2013 Jan;63(1):101–7.

55 Thomsen FB, Røder MA, Hvarness H, Iversen P, Brasso K. Active surveillance can reduce overtreatment in patients with low-risk prostate cancer. Dan Med J. 2013 Feb;60(2):A4575.

56 Selvadurai ED, Singhera M, Thomas K, Mohammed K, Woode-Amissah R, Horwich A, *et al.* Medium-term outcomes of active surveillance for localised prostate cancer. Eur Urol. 2013;64:981–7.

57 Popiolek M, Rider JR, Andrén O, Andersson SO, Holmberg L, Adami HO, *et al.* Natural history of early, localized prostate cancer: a final report from three decades of follow-up. Eur Urol. 2013 Mar; 63(3):428–35.

58 Johansson JE, Andrén O, Andersson SO, Dickman PW, Holmberg L, Magnuson A, *et al.* Natural history of early, localized prostate cancer. JAMA. 2004 Jun 9; 291(22):2713–9.

59 Stephenson A, Klotz L. Comparative propensity analysis of active surveillance vs initial treatment. AUA 2013.

60 Hayes JH, Ollendorf DA, Pearson SD, Barry MJ, Kantoff PW, Stewart ST, *et al.* Active surveillance compared with initial treatment for men with low-risk prostate cancer: A decision analysis. JAMA. 2010 Dec 1;304(21):2373–80.

61 Reese AC, Cowan JE, Brajtbord JS, Harris CR, Carroll PR Cooperberg MR. The quantitative Gleason score improves prostate cancer risk assessment. Cancer. 2012 Dec 15;118(24):6046–54

62 Porten SP, Whitson JM, Cowan JE, Cooperberg MR, Shinohara K, Perez N, *et al.* Changes in prostate cancer grade on serial biopsy in men undergoing active surveillance. J Clin Oncol. 2011 Jul 10; 29(20):2795–800.

8

Tissue-Preserving Surgical Approaches in Urologic Oncology: The Therapeutic Mechanism for Tumor Ablation

Ganesh Kartha, MD,[1] and J. Stephen Jones, MD[2]

[1] The Glickman Urological and Kidney Institute, The Cleveland Clinic Foundation, Cleveland, OH, USA
[2] Department of Urology, Cleveland Clinic Department of Regional Urology, Cleveland, OH, USA

Introduction

Over the past two decades, imaging improvements with computed tomography (CT) scans and the incorporation of prostate-specific antigen (PSA) has increased the identification of small renal masses and low-volume, low-grade prostate cancers, respectively. This has caused a paradigm shift in management for these urologic cancers. New minimally invasive ablative therapies such as cryoablation offer patients a third option between surveillance and definitive surgical extirpation. Whether or not an incidentally discovered small renal mass or low-grade, low-volume prostate cancer needs to be treated can be debated. However, with the advent of new thermal ablative therapy that can now be delivered with minimal morbidity, treatment for these questionably insignificant cancers is being reconsidered.

In addition, we have a large aging population living with chronic comorbidities. Cryoablation can offer a relatively safe definite therapy for certain urologic neoplasms in patients in whom surgical therapy may be high risk. For small renal masses, percutaneous or laparoscopic cryoablation allows for nephron sparing without mobilization of the kidney and more importantly, without dissection and clamping of the hilum, which may cause ischemic injury. Elderly men diagnosed with low-volume, low-grade prostate cancer are increasingly being placed on active surveillance. Current opinion supports the concept that elderly men (especially those with chronic comorbid conditions) will likely die from other causes rather than their prostate cancer. However, life expectancy for the elderly is continuing to increase. The risk gap between death from chronic disease and death from prostate cancer may be shrinking over time.

Focal cryoablation techniques currently have a limited role in urologic neoplasms. Many of the current technologies have yet to be evaluated for long-term efficacy. Specifically, recurrence free survival has been questioned for many ablation techniques. As new technology and technique innovations develop, a new round of investigation is warranted. Ultimately, the goal of ablation therapies is to achieve similar, if not better, outcomes when compared with their surgical and medical counterparts. With improvement in imaging and therapeutic technique, the role of cryoablation therapy for urologic malignancies will become more prominent.

Management of Urologic Cancer: Focal Therapy and Tissue Preservation, First Edition.
Edited by Mark P. Schoenberg and Kara L. Watts.

Cryoablation: Extreme Cold for Tumor Necrosis

History

James Arnott, an English physician, was the first credited in using extreme cold temperature to treat medical conditions. Using a mixture of ice and salt, Arnott treated many lesions and tumors of the skin and cervix during the mid-1800s. Although the salt–ice mixture was able to achieve cold temperatures, definitive cell death, and effective tumor treatment was not observed. The cold achieved via this method was limited to a palliative role. It was not until the development of liquefied gasses (refrigerants) that extreme cold temperatures that cause tissue damage and cell death could be achieved. The thermodynamic principle that explains the extreme colds achieved by liquefied gasses (gasses under pressure) is the Joule-Thomson principle. Gasses under pressure cool when they are allowed to expansion. All ideal gasses exhibit this phenomenon. The exceptions to this principle are hydrogen and helium gas, which are heated when expanded at room temperature. Liquefied air and carbon dioxide were the first refrigerants readily available in the early 1900s and were used for treatment of many dermatologic conditions. The main drawback of cryotherapy during this area was its limited use for skin and superficial lesions and tumors. In 1963, a neurosurgeon named Irving Cooper developed the first closed loop cryoprobe [1]. The probe used liquid nitrogen as a refrigerant. The use of the cryoprobe allowed access to deeper tissues. First uses of the liquid nitrogen-based cryoprobe were for inoperable brain tumors.

In 1964, Gonder *et al.* described the use of cryo in urologic pathology with the first transurethral ablation of the prostate [2]. In the 1970s and 1980s, nitrogen-based cryoablation was introduced for prostate and renal neoplasms, but the technique never gained much favor in these early years. The main limitation of cryoablation at this time was lack of monitoring the expanding cryo field.

Physicians would palpate for the expanding ice ball to determine the extent of cryoablation. During this era, complications associated with cryoablation were common (i.e., urethral/bowel injury). In 1984, Onik *et al.* incorporated intraoperative ultrasound with cryoablation [3]. Physicians were then able to monitor the cryo field by visualizing the hyperechoic rim of the expanding ice ball. When further studies demonstrated that the visualized hyperechoic edge of the ice ball correlates with the zone of cell death the effectiveness, safety and popularity of cryoablation progressed [4,5].

Mechanism of Action

Cell death and injury using extreme cold temperatures from cryoablation is achieved through multiple mechanisms. The first mechanism of injury is related to a biochemical process related to an osmotic gradient created between the intracellular and extracellular tissue environments. In the initial phases of freezing, the extracellular fluid freezes [6,7]. Water in the extracellular environment begins to freeze at $0°C$, which increases the osmotic pressure of the unfrozen extracellular fluid. As fluid is drawn from within the cell to the extracellular space, intracellular dehydration and accumulation of toxins ensue. The change in intracellular pH leads to protein denaturation and cell organelle damage [8,9]. As the temperature continues to fall to $< -15°C$ most of the extracellular fluid is frozen and the intracellular fluid begins to crystallize [8,9]. The extensive freezing results in a second mechanism of cell damage, mechanical injury. As the freezing progresses, tissue trapping occurs and causes increased shear forces on cellular structure and destruction of cellular membranes. Together, the biochemical and mechanical mechanisms of injury cause direct cellular damage, which leads to cell death and fibrotic scar formation.

In addition to direct cellular injury from extreme cold, indirect mechanisms also play a role in the coagulative necrosis caused by cryoablation. Along with tissue damage, extreme cold also has an effect on the vasculature within the treatment field. Zacarian *et al.* demonstrated that extreme cold causes blood stasis and thrombosis within the microvasculature [10]. This in turn leads tissue hypoxia and ischemic necrosis. During the thaw phase after treatment, small damaged blood vessels dilate, resulting in hyperemic reperfusion injury and microthrombi formation [11,12]. Additionally during the thaw phase, extracellular fluid returns to the intracellular space further damaging organelles and cell membranes.

Studies have demonstrated that irreversible tissue injury occurs at temperatures between −20°C and −50°C [13-15]. The exact temperature to cause necrosis in the cryo field is tissue dependent. Different tissues have different thermal properties such as heterogeneity with calcifications and fibrosis. Vascular neoplasms tend to require a lower probe tip temperature because vascular networks can act as heat sinks. The heat sink created by vascular neoplasms and thermal resistance as a result of fibroblast deposition may explain why slightly colder temperatures are required for malignancies compared to normal target organ parenchyma. Tatsutani *et al.* demonstrated that a minimum of −40°C was required to irreversibly destroy prostate cells; thus, −40°C has become the standard minimum for adequate therapy for genitourinary malignancies [16].

Direct and indirect thermal damage during the freeze-thaw process occurs in the central zone of the cryofield. The central zone is adjacent to the distal end of the cryoprobe. The zone contains the irreversibly damaged cells showing evidence of coagulative necrosis and fibrotic scar formation histologically. Surrounding the central zone is the peripheral zone, which contains tissue showing evidence of cell injury without evidence of direct thermal damage. The injury that occurs in the peripheral zone occurs from cold temperatures above the therapeutic threshold for irreversible direct thermal damage. The mechanism of cell injury in the peripheral zone is via activation of the apoptosis cascade [8]. Although activation of the apoptosis cascade has been demonstrated, the exact mechanism and signaling pathway that initiates the cascade is currently unknown. The limit of the peripheral zone has been shown to correlate with the extent of the hyperechoic rim of the expanding ice ball on intraoperative ultrasound [4,5].

Current and Future Trends

There have been a few advancements in cryoablation that have increased the efficacy and shortened operative times. A major advancement has been the use of liquid argon gas to replace liquid nitrogen as a refrigerant. Argon has allowed for smaller probes and faster cooling rates. Faster cooling rates have been shown to be advantageous by increasing the efficacy of direct thermal damage. The rapid cooling allows intracellular crystals to form early, which increases the mechanical injury for organelle and cell membrane disruption as a result of increased shear forces [17]. Small probes and shorter operative times may also contribute to less morbidity from cryoablation.

Many cryoablation devices now incorporate helium gas for active thawing. There has been discrepancy in the literature regarding potentially negative therapeutic effects from active thawing when compared to passive thawing [13,18,19]. However, what has been definitely shown to increase cryoablation efficacy is repeating the freeze-thaw cycle [14,15]. A larger volume and significantly greater percentage of irreversible cell damage was noted in prostate neoplasms treated with two freeze-thaw cycles compared to one freeze thaw-cycle [20]. Post cryoablation of the prostate follow-up studies have shown decreased biochemical recurrence and positive biopsy rates in patients who underwent two freeze-thaw cycles [21–23]. Faster cooling rates with argon refrigerants and active thawing with helium make repeated freeze-thaw cycles possible with significantly shorter operative times.

Conclusion

Diagnoses of low-volume, low-grade urologic tumors are increasing with modern imaging and innovative biomarkers. This, in addition to a growing older patient population, has increased the role of focal therapy with cryoablation for treatment of urologic malignancies. Despite the growing popularity of cryoablation, there are still many limitations in its use for curative intent. New technological developments continue to push for increased efficacy and safety of ablation. Currently, most of the available data for these therapies are based on short follow-up and small patient cohorts. The challenge of conducting a good study with long-term follow-up is that the rate of technological advancement may outpace the study period.

The ultimate goal of any focal therapy is to achieve acceptable oncologic outcomes and safety while limiting side effects and increasing patient quality of life. Most of the efforts to improve current cryoablation technology center on more efficient energy delivery and better localization of the target lesion. Innovations in imaging have played a major role for real-time monitoring and target lesion identification. Fusion imaging with real-time ultrasound superimposed on a detailed magnetic resonance image (MRI) has shown promise in focal therapy for prostate cancer. MRI thermometry has also been investigated for detailed real-time monitoring of expanding thermal lesions. More accurate monitoring and targeting of the treatment lesion will aid in ensuring complete tumor necrosis while limiting injury to surrounding vulnerable structures (blood vessels, urethra, urothelium, bowel, etc.).

In addition to technologic advancement, a more in-depth understanding of therapeutic mechanisms and tumor biology may facilitate patient selection and posttherapy monitoring. Proper patient selection has not been standardized, and it is currently unclear which urologic patients benefit most from cryoablation over surgical or systemic medical treatment. Certain biologic characteristics of a tumor might make it more sensitive to certain therapeutic mechanisms. Tumor characteristic understanding may also shed light on multimodal or combination therapies. Individualization of a patients and tumors before treatment will aid in proper selection of management strategies for urologic malignancies.

Focal cryoablation with extreme cold temperature has been reserved as a low-morbidity alternative to surgical extirpation. The lack of technology and limited understanding of tumor biology have kept focal ablation as a secondary treatment option for curative intent. Unlike surgical excision, focal ablation does not provide pathologic evidence of successful treatment. Technologic advancements, novel imaging modalities and identification of new tumor biomarkers may close the gap between definitive evidence of treatment after surgery and post-ryoablation recurrence monitoring. By narrowing this gap, cryoablation may move from a low-morbidity palliative alternative to more of a curative option.

References

1 Cooper I. Cryogenic surgery: A new method for destruction or extirpation of benign or malignant tissues. New Engl J Med. 1963 Apr 4;268:743–9.

2 Gonder MJ, Soanes WA, Smith V. Experimental prostate cryosurgery. Invest Urol. 1964 May;1:610–9.

3 Onik G, Cooper C, Goldberg HI, Moss AA, Rubinsky B, Christianson M. Ultrasonic characteristics of frozen liver. Cryobiology.1984 Jun;21(3):321–8.

4 Weber SM, Lee FT, Jr., Warner TF, Chosy SG, Mahvi DM. Hepatic cryoablation: US monitoring of extent of necrosis in normal pig liver. Radiology.1998 Apr;207(1):73–7.

5 Steed J, Saliken JC, Donnelly BJ, Ali-Ridha NH. Correlation between thermosensor temperature and transrectal ultrasonography

during prostate cryoablation. Can Assoc Radiol J. 1997 Jun;48(3):186–90.

6 Whittaker DK. Mechanisms of tissue destruction following cryosurgery. Ann R Coll Surg Engl. 1984 Sep;66(5):313–8.

7 Gill W, Fraser J. A look at cryosurgery. Scott Med J. 1968 Aug;13(8):268–73.

8 Hoffmann NE, Bischof JC. The cryobiology of cryosurgical injury. Urology.2002 Aug; 60(2 Suppl 1):40–9.

9 Baust JG, Gage AA. The molecular basis of cryosurgery. BJU Int. 2005 Jun; 95(9):1187–91.

10 Zacarian SA, Stone D, Clater M. Effects of cryogenic temperatures on microcirculation in the golden hamster cheek pouch. Cryobiology. 1970 Jul–Aug; 7(1):27–39.

11 Kahlenberg MS, Volpe C, Klippenstein DL, Penetrante RB, Petrelli NJ, Rodriguez-Bigas MA. Clinicopathologic effects of cryotherapy on hepatic vessels and bile ducts in a porcine model. Ann Surg Oncol. 1998 Dec;5(8):713–8.

12 Weber SM, Lee FT, Jr., Chinn DO, Warner T, Chosy SG, Mahvi DM. Perivascular and intralesional tissue necrosis after hepatic cryoablation: results in a porcine model. Surgery. 1997 Oct;122(4):742–7.

13 Woolley ML, Schulsinger DA, Durand DB, Zeltser IS, Waltzer WC. Effect of freezing parameters (freeze cycle and thaw process) on tissue destruction following renal cryoablation. J Endourol. 2002 Sep; 16(7):519–22.

14 Neel HB, 3rd, Ketcham AS, Hammond WG. Requisites for successful cryogenic surgery of cancer. Arch Surg. 1971 Jan; 102(1):45–8.

15 Ravikumar TS, Steele G, Jr., Kane R, King V. Experimental and clinical observations on hepatic cryosurgery for colorectal

metastases. Cancer Res. 1991 Dec 1; 51(23 Pt 1):6323–7.

16 Tatsutani K, Rubinsky B, Onik G, Dahiya R. Effect of thermal variables on frozen human primary prostatic adenocarcinoma cells. Urology. 1996 Sep;48(3):441–7.

17 White WM, Kaouk JH. Ablative therapy for renal tumors. In: Wein AJ, Kavoussi LR, Novick AC, Partin AW, Peters CA, editors. Campbell-Walsh Urology. 10th ed. Philadelphia: Elsevier; 2012. p. 1670–82.

18 Desai MM, Gill IS. Current status of cryoablation and radiofrequency ablation in the management of renal tumors. Curr Opin Urol. 2002 Sep;12(5):387–93.

19 Klossner DP, Robilotto AT, Clarke DM, VanBuskirk RG, Baust JM, Gage AA, *et al.* Cryosurgical technique: Assessment of the fundamental variables using human prostate cancer model systems. Cryobiology. 2007 Dec;55(3):189–99.

20 Larson TR, Rrobertson DW, Corica A, Bostwick DG. In vivo interstitial temperature mapping of the human prostate during cryosurgery with correlation to histopathologic outcomes. Urology. 2000 Apr;55(4):547–52.

21 Shinohara K, Connolly JA, Presti JC, Jr., Carroll PR. Cryosurgical treatment of localized prostate cancer (stages T1 to T4): Preliminary results. J Urol. 1996 Jul; 156(1):115–20; discussion 20–1.

22 Pisters LL, von Eschenbach AC, Scott SM, Swanson DA, Dinney CP, Pettaway CA, *et al.* The efficacy and complications of salvage cryotherapy of the prostate. J Urol. 1997 Mar;157(3):921–5.

23 Babaian RJ, Donnelly B, Bahn D, Baust JG, Dineen M, Ellis D, *et al.* Best practice statement on cryosurgery for the treatment of localized prostate cancer. J Urol. 2008 Nov;180(5):1993–2004.

9

Focal Therapy for Prostate Cancer: An Evidence-Based Approach to Tissue-Preserving Strategies

Kara L. Watts, MD,[1] Yaalini Shanmugabavan, MD,[2] Victoria Chernyak, MD,[3] and Hashim Uddin Ahmed, MD, FRCS, PhD[2]

[1] *Department of Urology, Montefiore Medical Center, Albert Einstein College of Medicine, Bronx, NY, USA*
[2] *Division of Surgery & Interventional Sciences, University College Hospital, London, UK*
[3] *Department of Radiology, Montefiore Medical Center, Albert Einstein College of Medicine, Bronx, NY, USA*

Introduction

The treatment of prostate cancer (PCa) has shifted over the past two decades from traditional whole-gland therapies aimed at curative intent—namely surgical extirpation and radiation therapy—to a more complex milieu of therapeutic options. Rates of radical prostatectomy (RP), for example, have fallen as more conservative approaches, such as active surveillance, watchful waiting, radiotherapy, and more recently, focal ablation, have emerged. These changes have coincided with advances in our understanding of risk stratification for high- versus low-risk PCa, prostate cancer genomics, and our ability to more accurately identify PCa lesions within the prostate through advances in magnetic resonance imaging (MRI) and targeted prostate biopsy.

Evidence has demonstrated that RP for patients with high-risk disease may reduce their risk of PCa-related death by 5% over 10 to 15 years compared to watchful waiting, but the overall and PCa-specific survival does not significantly differ between RP and watchful waiting approaches in the low risk group [1–3]. Furthermore, functional outcomes after RP continue to be less than ideal,

despite technological and surgical advances, with rates of urinary incontinence after RP reported to be as high as 75% after surgery (average rates of 10–20%), and rates of impotence widely varying between 10% to greater than 50% even 2 years after surgery [4–6].

The concept of focal therapy (FT) has emerged as a therapeutic alternative to treat PCa in patients with localized disease with the aim of reducing collateral tissue damage that leads to genito-urinary toxicity, thus potentially affording better functional outcomes for the appropriate patient, while aiming to maintain disease control. Indeed, similar approaches have already been widely adapted in other organ systems, as witnessed by the widespread utilization and acceptance of partial mastectomy/lumpectomy, partial hepatectomy, partial nephrectomy, partial penectomy, and even partial pancreatectomy [7–9]. Despite this widespread acceptance in many other organ systems, it still largely lags behind in the treatment of PCa.

In PCa, the rationale for FT derives from the concept of treating the index lesion in men with localized disease. While current pathologic evidence from whole-gland RP specimens often reveals multiple foci of PCa, evidence suggests that the initial largest or highest-grade lesion, the *index lesion*, largely drives the natural history of the disease [10]. Furthermore, molecular evidence increasingly supports the concept that the index lesion is the one most likely to exhibit progression to local invasion or even metastasis [11–15]. It warrants mention here that PCa does not exist solely as a single lesion, but often as a multifocal disease on final whole-mount pathology in RP specimens (78% multifocal, 86% bilateral) [13]. However, it has also been demonstrated, for example, in a study of 100 whole-mount specimens that 99.4% of the no-index, satellite lesions were Gleason grade 6 or less and 87% smaller than 0.5 mL, or clinically insignificant disease [13]. The goal of focal ablation, therefore, is to deliver an ablative dose of energy to the index lesion while sparing the rest of the gland and avoiding the functional morbidity associated with whole-gland treatment.

The anatomic configurations of FT energy delivery vary by trial and include true "focal" therapy aimed solely at a lesion of interest, quadrant ablation (one quadrant of a prostate lobe), hemiablation (unilateral lobar ablation), hockey stick (hemiablation plus contralateral dog-leg), or multiple focal ablations of several lesions of interest. Multiple modalities have been investigated and used as a means of delivering ablative energy to a portion of the prostate containing a target lesion or lesions. These include, but are not limited to, cryoablation, high-intensity focused ultrasound (HIFU), laser interstitial thermal ablation (LITT), photodynamic therapy (PDT), radiofrequency interstitial tumor ablation (RITA), irreversible electroporation (IRE), among others.

In this chapter, we review the data available on the following focal therapies: cryotherapy, HIFU, IRE, focal radiation (namely, brachytherapy), and briefly, radiofrequency ablation (RFA), LITT, PDT. We also present an overview of the literature regarding proper patient selection for consideration for FT, including a brief description of current data surrounding the use of imaging and targeted biopsy as it pertains to PCa lesion identification and proper patient selection.

Key Concepts in FT for PCa

Patient Selection for FT

A growing body of literature has emerged with aims to refine the clinical criteria guiding patient selection for FT for PCa. There is currently no consensus with regard to the ideal age, clinical stage, or number of lesions in a patient considering FT. Several consensus meetings have been held over the years with the intention of defining these criteria, but controversy still exists. For example, in 2007 the International Task Force on PCa proposed criteria for selection that are akin to very low-risk PCA-based on National Comprehensive Cancer Network (NCCN) guidelines: prostate-specific antigen (PSA) <10 ng/mL, absence of Gleason grade 4 or 5, and very restrictive biopsy criteria among other factors [16]. The University College of London (UCL), on the other hand, identifies the index lesion amenable to FT by either of the following: (1) Gleason ≥4 + 3 and/or maximum core length ≥6 mm or (2) Gleason ≥3 + 4 and/or maximum core length ≥4 mm [17]. Further consensus meetings have since been held with recent reports reflecting the consideration of broader inclusion criteria to include patients with intermediate-risk and some higher-risk PCa as more data have emerged in this field [18–21].

PCa Lesion Detection for FT

Despite the ongoing controversies surrounding eligibility criteria for FT, the principle that underlies proper patient selection is the accurate detection and localization of *clinically significant* PCa lesions, or index lesions, as stated previously. The use of MRI, targeted fusion biopsy, and transperineal template mapping (TPM) studies has increased our ability to both detect and localize PCa lesions [22–26]. The use of MRI as both a screening and surveillance tool in the management of PCa has dramatically increased in the past two decades: some centers report almost 500% increase in prostate MRI use over the course of 2 years [27]. Such widespread use is a result of continuous technological advances that allow for improved detection and characterization of clinically significant PCa. Indeed, a recent systematic review of the use of MRI alone for the detection of clinically significant PCa lesions reported overall accuracy, sensitivity, and specificity values of MRI in the range of 44–87%, 58–96%, and 23–87%, respectively. In addition, the negative predictive value of MRI reaches 95% in some reports [23,28]. Furthermore, dominant lesion appearance on MRI is a biomarker predicting post-intervention disease-free survival, both after radical prostatectomy and after HIFU ablation [29–32].

Beyond screening and surveillance, MRI-fusion targeted biopsy is increasingly being used to optimize the detection and localization of PCa lesions. MRI-fusion biopsy has been shown to increase the detection of clinically significant lesions by at least 33% compared to standard transrectal ultrasound guided (TRUS) biopsy while reducing the detection of clinically insignificant PCa lesions [26,33–35]. In fact, a recent consensus statement from the American Urologic Association (AUA) and Society of Abdominal Radiology (SAR) concluded that PIRADS three to five lesions on prostate MRI in the setting of a prior negative prostate biopsy warrants an MRI-ultrasound fusion biopsy (rather than a standard TRUS biopsy), where available [36].

For true FT ablation—that is, with the goal of ablating a single index lesion—accurate localization of the latter is critical. TPM biopsies, which combine MRI, TRUS, and a transperineal template biopsy, boast sensitivity and negative predictive value (NPV) of up to 95% for lesions 0.5 cm^3 or greater in volume [20,37–39]. This technique is, therefore, suggested by most consensus groups as the gold standard for most accurate detection and localization of PCa lesions in patients undergoing FT [28,40,41]. However, this biopsy technique requires a general anesthetic, is time consuming, and is largely dependent on the skillset of the individual performing the biopsy. At present, it is not the current standard of care for the diagnosis of PCa, nor is it the standard biopsy approach in most studies on FT; it is largely reserved for clinical trials and large academic centers.

Follow up after FT

After a focal ablative energy in some form is delivered to a region of interest within the prostate, the ablated tissue and surrounding healthy tissue remain within the patient. Therefore, unlike surgical extirpation or whole-gland radiation, the oncologic efficacy of the therapy relies on a repeat biopsy of the treated area. Whereas the PSA can reliably be monitored after whole-gland therapy, there are no established PSA reference values or nadir after FT by which to reliably determine a curative treatment. Furthermore, the effect of each different ablative modality of FT on the PSA can vary, as can the area of the prostate tissue treated. Therefore, as important as accurate localization of a PCa lesion for FT ablation is, the same must be underscored for accurate posttherapeutic biopsy of a treated area to confirm efficacy of a treatment.

Tissue-Preserving FTs

As mentioned, there are a number of focal ablative modalities. The underlying principle behind each therapy is the delivery of a lethal dose of energy to a particular area of tissue, resulting in necrosis of that tissue while sparing the surrounding healthy tissue. Each therapy is considered minimally invasive, indeed against the comparative RP for PCa and can be delivered in the primary setting or as salvage therapy. In the remainder of this chapter, we review cryotherapy, HIFU, IRE, focal brachytherapy, and briefly RFA, PDT, and LITT.

Cryotherapy

Cryotherapy is one of the oldest focal ablative techniques that induces cell death by producing extreme hypothermia of the targeted tissue. It was originally developed in the 1960s and approved by the Food and Drug

Administration (FDA) in 1999 for primary treatment of PCa [42]. Under general anesthesia, probes are placed transperineally under TRUS guidance into an area of interest based on preoperative mapping or biopsy studies. The probes then generate two freeze-thaw cycles. During the freeze cycle, compressed argon gas freezes the tissue to a minimum of $-40°C$ (the lethal temperature for PCa cells is $-20°C$), resulting in irreversible cell death. Helium gas then warms the tissue in a cyclic manner to complete the freeze-thaw cycle. A warming urethral catheter is placed at the start of the procedure to protect the urethra and external sphincter [43]. The mechanism of action for cryotherapy appears to be a multifactorial; apoptosis, cytolysis, osmotic injury, and vascular damage are all thought to contribute.

The potential complications of cryotherapy include erectile dysfunction, incontinence, urethral stricture, and rectal injury. Although previous cryotherapy probes were large and afforded little to no intraoperative control, more recent third-generation devices have a number of features to minimize the morbidity associated with this treatment. For example, thin warming needles inserted between the prostate and rectum limit the potential for rectal injury. Furthermore, the probes consist of smaller gauge needles, resulting in smaller iceball formation, which is monitored through thermocouples inserted into the prostate, rectum, and occasionally near the sphincter.

Primary Focal Cryotherapy

Primary focal cryotherapy developed after the initial approval and use of whole-gland cryotherapy. Among the nearly dozen or so studies that have reported on focal cryotherapy, the anatomic zones of ablation include both hemiablation (unilateral lobar) and true "focal" cryotherapy. Systematic reviews, therefore, tend to lump these two approaches together when reporting overall outcomes for this approach.

Results from the largest series derive from a large database, the CRYO online database (COLD), in which 1,160 men underwent focal primary cryotherapy (both targeted and hemiablation) [44]. As evidence of a growing interest in FT for PCa, the study witnessed a significant increase in the percentage of patients enrolled who elected for FT (rather than whole-gland cryotherapy), increasing from 2.1% of participants at the start of the study to 38.2% and rising in the final 2 years of patient enrollment.

Mean age of this cohort was 67.8 years, mean follow up 21.1 months, and mean pretreatment PSA 9ng/mL (range <4–20+). Pretreatment Gleason score was 6 and 7 in 74% and 21% of patients, respectively. The biochemical disease-free survival (BDFS) using ASTRO criteria (3 PSA rises after nadir) at 12, 24, and 36 months postprocedure was 80.7%, 75.7%, and 75.7%, respectively. Among those men who underwent a postprocedural biopsy, positivity rate was 43%, representing 3.7% of the entire cohort [44]. Regarding functional outcomes, new onset urinary incontinence and erectile dysfunction (ED) were noted in 1.6% and 41.9% of men, respectively. It is important to note that the functional data are limited by a lack of standardized patient reported outcomes.

The second largest series reporting on focal cryotherapy for PCa was a matched comparison between 317 men with low-risk PCa (D'Amico criteria) who underwent focal cryotherapy (FC) to 317 men from the COLD database who underwent whole-gland (WG) cryotherapy [45]. Median age was 66.5 years and median follow-up was 58.3 months. Thirty percent and 17% of men receiving WG and FC, respectively, underwent a posttreatment biopsy, with positive biopsy results in 11.6% and 14.5%. Biochemical recurrent (BCR)-free survival rates at 60 months by Phoenix criteria were 80.1% and 73% in the WG and FC cohorts, respectively, and nearly identical by ASTRO criteria. Erectile function was preserved in 46.8% and 68.8%, respectively, of men in the WG and FC groups, and continence rates were 98.7% and 100%, respectively. Overall, this trial demonstrated comparable oncologic outcomes for low-risk PCa treated with FC compared to WG cryotherapy but with improved functional outcomes at a relatively long period of follow up.

In a recent report, 62 men with low-risk, organ-confined PCa (defined as Gleason 3 + 4 or less on TRUS biopsy, tumor burden <50%, and PSA <10 ng/dL) diagnosed on three-dimensional (3D) mapping biopsies underwent focal cryotherapy with median follow up of 28 months [46]. A posttreatment biopsy was performed in all patients at 1 year. From an oncologic standpoint, the 1-year posttreatment biopsy was negative in 81% of patients. Among those with a positive biopsy, the pathology revealed clinically insignificant disease, Gleason 6 in one or two cores. The median posttreatment change in PSA was a decrease of 3.0 ng/mL. There was no significant change in sexual function, no episodes of incontinence and no severe side effects post therapy.

Several smaller retrospective reviews (all with n <100 patients) have also reported their results with regard to FC for PCa [47–50]. The vast majority of patients included have had low- or intermediate-risk PCa, and the overwhelming majority of studies reported have included a hemiablation approach to FC. Among these studies, there is inconsistency about the requirement for a post-FC biopsy. However, when performed, rates of positivity for residual significant and any cancer remaining in the treated area ranged from 0–6.5% and 0–12.9%, respectively. Regarding functional outcomes, the data from the remaining studies is limited but tends toward high rates of potency preservation and continence post treatment.

Primary focal cryotherapy has demonstrated promising results for oncological control while limiting potential morbidity in comparison to conventional surgical approaches. However, as demonstrated by the data summarized here, there is a lack of large or randomized trials addressing the efficacy and oncologic outcomes for primary focal cryotherapy compared to other forms of FT or RP.

Salvage Focal Cryotherapy

Salvage focal cryotherapy has been employed as an alternative to WG cryotherapy to reduce the morbidity associated with the latter. Li et al. [51] reviewed 91 patients from the COLD database with biopsy proven radiorecurrent PCa who then underwent focal salvage cryotherapy. Median pretreatment PSA was 4.8 ng/dL (0–92.6 ng/dL) and median Gleason score was 7. Five-year BDFS rate was 46.5%. Postsalvage treatment biopsy positivity was detected in 4 of 14 (28.6%) patients had a positive biopsy. Five patients (5.5%) had de novo incontinence requiring the use of pads at 12 months, and 10 of 20 patients (50%) had preserved erectile function. Among major complications reported, there were three cases (3.3%) of rectourethral fistula.

In another small series, Abreu et al. [52] evaluated 25 patients each who underwent salvage FC or salvage WG cryotherapy for radiorecurrent PCa. In the FC cohort, median presalvage PSA was 2.8 ng/dL and Gleason score was 7. Median follow up was 31 months. Eight patients (32%) and three patients (12%) had biochemical failure (Phoenix criteria) in the FC and WG cohorts, respectively. Five-year BDFS rates were 54% and 86%, respectively. New onset incontinence was reported in 0 patients and 13%, and 2/7 and 0 patients retained their precryotherapy potency in the FC and WG arms, respectively. Similar results were reported by Eisenberg et al. [53] in a series of 19 men treated with salvage focal cryotherapy for radiorecurrent cancer. At 3 years follow up, BDFS rates were achieved by 50% and 79% by ASTRO and Phoenix criteria, respectively.

Overall, the series assessing focal salvage cryotherapy are limited in size and number. However, they highlight reasonable oncologic outcomes and decreased morbidity compared to salvage whole-gland therapies. There is again a need for prospective studies with long-term follow up to help delineate appropriate patient selection for this therapy.

HIFU

HIFU is a noninvasive technique that generates lethal thermal energy to temperatures above 60° C via high-intensity ultrasound waves. Ablation of targeted tissue—focal, hemiablation, or hockey stick (hemiablation plus dog-leg contralateral lobe) configuration—occurs due to a combination of coagulative necrosis and internal cavitation, which occurs as a result of the interaction of water and ultrasound in the cells [54]. Preoperative MRI with either MRI-ultrasound fusion biopsy or TPM biopsy identifies the lesion(s) of interest, and this is fused with real-time TRUS using HIFU software to confirm the zone of ablation (Figure 9.1). As ultrasound energy is converted to thermal energy high enough to cause coagulative necrosis, "popcorn" or Uchida changes of the targeted tissue are visualized on ultrasound imaging (Figure 9.2).

HIFU can be delivered to the prostate via a transurethral or a transrectal probe, using in-bore guidance and MRI-TRUS fusion to guide and localize the ablative energy, respectively. The transurethral form is investigational at the time of writing this chapter. Currently, there are two companies that market transrectal platforms for this technology: Sonacare, Inc., and EDAP TMS.

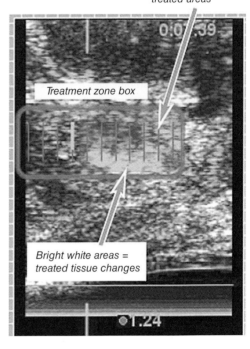

Figure 9.2 Sonablate 500 linear view displaying real time changes due to ablation induced by HIFU. Treated Tissue appears white, resembling popcorn [55].

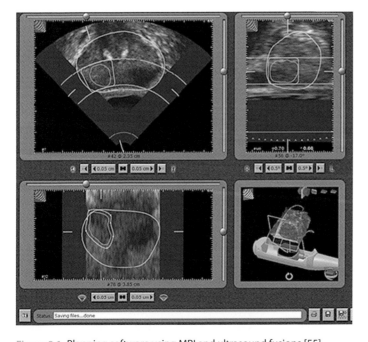

Figure 9.1 Planning software using MRI and ultrasound fusions [55].

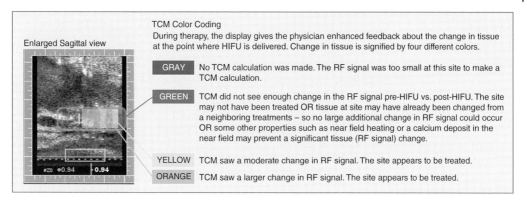

Figure 9.3 Tissue Change Monitor (TCM) from Sonablate 500 [55].

EDAP has created three generations of commercial devices: Ablatherm® Maxis (1993), Ablatherm® Integrated Imaging (2005), and Focal one® (2013) [38]. Sonacare has developed and marketed the Sonablate® 500 for prostate tissue ablation. Delivery of this therapy requires general anesthesia.

While the therapeutic principles behind Ablatherm® and Sonablate® 500 are the same, there are multiple technical differences between the two. In brief, Ablatherm® HIFU is a fully-automated device developed in 1993 for whole-gland treatment of localized prostate cancer in the primary or salvage setting. It does not require user input during the procedure and tends to complete an ablation faster than the Sonablate® 500. The Sonablate® 500, which recently received FDA 501K clearance for ablation of prostate tissue, requires user input throughout the procedure to adjust power settings and monitor the effect of the ablative procedure on prostate tissue, allowing for optimal operator control during a procedure [56,57].

HIFU delivery requires considerable expertise; a number of technical aspects and safety parameters must be considered. The "heat sink" effect refers to the inadequate propagation of ablative heat to a target lesion from the ultrasound transducer due to overheating of intervening tissue. This can occur in tissue with high water content (cysts or high vascularity) or calcifications. In addition, as the rectal wall lies between the transrectal transducer and the prostate, great caution must be exercised during the procedure to prevent overheating of this healthy structure, leading to potential rectourethral fistulae. The Sonablate® 500 includes a real-time tissue change monitor (TCM) to monitor and adjust the device settings throughout the procedure to minimize this effect (Figure 9.3).

In addition, prostate swelling and shift occurs throughout the procedure. Shoji *et al.* [58] discussed the implications of these changes on intraprocedural planning and monitoring. They found that the median 3D intraprostatic shift during a treatment session was 3.7 mm with a median total volume increase of 13%. In general, smaller glands experienced a greater proportion of swelling. As a result, the operator needs to monitor these changes and continuously modify the zone of ablation to ensure optimal ablation of the targeted tissue.

Primary Focal HIFU

More than a dozen studies have published outcomes of primary focal HIFU for PCa. The largest of these trials was recently published by Feijoo *et al.* [59], in which 71 men with unilateral clinically localized PCa underwent HIFU hemiablation using the Ablatherm system. PCa was diagnosed by a TRUS biopsy and preprocedural prostate MRI was performed in all participants. Posttreatment TRUS biopsies were performed at 1-year follow up. At a median follow-up of 12 months, 56/67 men had a negative post-treatment biopsy in the treated lobe. Six men had a newly detected cancer in the contralateral, untreated lobe. Median PSA concentration dropped by 43% at 3 months, and this persisted through the follow-up period. Continence was maintained in all patients and potency was maintained in 11/21 patient with preprocedural potency.

In 2011, a Phase I/II clinical trial reported on 20 men with unilateral PCa who underwent hemiablation using the Sonablate 500. One-quarter had low-risk disease and three-quarters had intermediate-risk disease localized to one lobe by either TRUS biopsy or MRI and TPM biopsy [60]. Posttreatment MRI was performed at 1 month and confirmatory biopsy of the treated side (and contralateral side if new lesion detected on MRI) at 6 months. At 12 months, 95% (19/20) of men with preoperative erections maintained sufficient rigidity for penetration, 90% were pad-free, and PSA decreased by 80% to a mean of 2.5 ng/dL. Therefore, 88% of the men achieved trifecta status at 12 months post therapy.

In 2012, Ahmed *et al.* [61] then reported their prospective data of 41 men with PCa treated with focal HIFU using the Sonablate 500. Seventy-three percent of the men had intermediate- or high-risk disease diagnosed by MRI and TPM biopsies. Up to two target lesions were ablated, permitting ablation of up to 60% of the prostate in each case. Targeted biopsies of the treated areas were performed at 6 months, and 30/39 men biopsied were negative in the treated zones. Only 3 men had clinically significant residual disease (Epstein criteria) and 4 received a second focal HIFU treatment. Of the 31 men with good baseline function, 26 achieved the trifecta: leak-free and pad-free continence, erections sufficient for intercourse, and no evidence of clinically significant disease on MRI at 12 months post ablation.

An interesting recent paper compared outcomes in 55 men with unilateral, clinically localized PCa after focal HIFU hemiablation to a matched-pair cohort after robotic-assisted laparoscopic prostatectomy (RALP)

[62]. At a median follow up of 36 months, there were no differences between the groups for salvage therapy, although 7/55 men in the HIFU arm required a second treatment for the contralateral lobe for a new cancerous lesion. In terms of functional outcomes, HIFU was associated with a better and faster recovery of continence, a significantly lower risk of de novo erectile dysfunction after treatment. Although small and non-randomized, this trial shows comparable oncologic control with unilateral focal HIFU to RALP for localized PCa control with significantly better functional outcomes.

As this section demonstrates, the literature pertaining to outcomes associated with primary focal HIFU for PCa comprises predominantly proof of concept or prospective development studies. These studies are small in number (majority fewer than 50 patients) and are nonrandomized, noncontrolled trials. Additionally, the data encompass both hemiablation and focal ablation, blurring the efficacy for each approach. Despite this, the evidence to support HIFU as focal therapy for PCa in the primary setting is promising.

Salvage Focal/Hemiablation HIFU

Salvage focal HIFU has been evaluated in a handful of small trials for patients with failure after primary radiotherapy (RT). As an alternative to salvage RP, which poses considerable surgical difficulty and potential morbidity, salvage HIFU has been evaluated as a less invasive and potentially less morbid alternative. Indeed, an acceptable alternative would be welcomed given that up to 63% of men with PCa recur after external beam radiation therapy (EBRT) and require some form of additional therapy [63].

Between 2009 and 2012, 48 men who developed biochemical failure (Phoenix criteria) after primary RT were prospectively enrolled in two European centers. Each patient had a positive MRI and >1 concordant positive core confined to one lobe [64].

They then underwent a salvage HIFU hemiablation. Disease progression occurred in one-third (16/48) of this high-risk population. Of these 16 patients, 4 developed recurrence in the untreated lobe, 4 bilaterally, and six men developed metastatic disease. Progression-free survival at 12, 18, and 24 months was 83%, 64%, and 52%, respectively. Seventy five percent of men were pad free and 17% required only one pad per day, demonstrating the feasibility of this therapeutic alternative with limited morbidity.

An additional small-scale study by Ahmed *et al.* [65] reported on 39 men with PCa who were treated with focal salvage HIFU for recurrence after EBRT. Progression-free survival was 69% and 49%, respectively, according to the Phoenix criteria at 1 and 2 years. Erectile function, assessed using International Index of Erectile Function (IIEF)-15 score, decreased by a median of 5 points. Pad-free and leak-free continence rates were 64% and 42% at 1 and 2 years, respectively.

Similar to the data on salvage focal cryotherapy, the data regarding focal salvage HIFU for PCa are quite limited. Although limited data suggest it has potential as an alternative in older patients who are poor surgical candidates and that it may be associated with improved functional outcomes, further studies are clearly needed.

IRE

IRE is a nonthermal ablative therapy using high-frequent electric pulses generated between electrodes which, above a certain electric threshold, induce nano-size pores in the cell membrane leading to apoptosis [66]. Under general anesthetic, needles are inserted transperineally using TRUS guidance for localization. The needles are placed around a lesion of interest and a series of electric pulses are delivered. Histopathologic slides of IRE demonstrate sharp demarcations between the treated and untreated tissue [67].

As Figure 9.4 depicts, each electrode generates an ablative current with a 5-mm

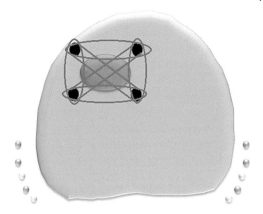

Figure 9.4 Schematic diagram of the prostate and anterior index lesion (red/central oval lesion). IRE needle probes (blue/small dark circles) generate an electric current (hollow grey ovals) around the lesion resulting in ablation.

circumferential margin around the electrode tip. Therefore, it is possible to accurately predict and map the therapeutic zone based on the placement of the electrodes in relation to the target tissue of interest.

Current literature regarding IRE for focal PCa ablation is limited. A small pilot study by Valerio *et al.* [68] evaluated the feasibility, safety and toxicity profile of primary focal IRE in 34 patients. With a mean age of 65 years, 71% of men had intermediate-risk PCA and 26% had low-risk PCa confined to an index lesion in one lobe. IRE was delivered using the Nanoknife™ system. According to the Common Terminology Criteria for Adverse Events (CTCE), 14 and 13 patients experienced a grade 1 and 2 adverse event, respectively. Twenty-eight patients were followed to a median 6 months; all were continent, and potency was preserved in 24 of the 25 who had good erectile function prior to treatment. The median ablation volume was 12 mL, and posttreatment MRI displayed residual disease in 6 (25%) men. Four (17%) of these underwent another form of local treatment. This study is limited by a short duration of follow up but, nonetheless, reports promising functional results in the short term.

This same group recently reported outcomes on 19 patients who underwent focal IRE for an index lesion that was diagnosed by

MRI imaging and TPM biopsy [69]. Sixteen patients were available for analysis at 1 year. All men were leak-free/pad-free, and 69% had erections sufficient for penetration from 75% pretreatment. On follow up biopsy, 61.1%, 5.6%, and 33.3%, respectively, had no residual disease, clinically insignificant disease, and clinically significant disease. This trial lends further support for the safety of focal IRE. However, given that one-third of patients had clinically significant residual cancer on repeat biopsy, the likelihood of needing an additional therapy must be taken into consideration.

At the time of writing this chapter, a large multicenter randomized controlled trial investigating IRE for localized PCa in a target population of 200 patients is enrolling patients (clinicaltrials.gov database registration number NCT01835977), which is substantially larger than the few limited studies published to date on this therapeutic approach.

Radiation

There are several modalities of delivering RT for the treatment of PCa; low-dose rate (LDR) brachytherapy, high-dose rate (HDR) brachytherapy, EBRT, immunomodulated radiation therapy (IMRT), and others. A handful of smaller case series have evaluated the former two in both the primary and salvage setting of focal therapy for PCa.

LDR brachytherapy involves the insertion of radioactive seeds into the prostate using TRUS guidance. The seeds then emit radiation to the surrounding prostatic tissue over a period of several weeks to months. Commonly used radioactive seeds include Iodine-125 (^{125}I), Palladium, and Cesium-131 (^{131}C), which have half-lives of 17, 60, and 10 days, respectively [70].

Focal LDR brachytherapy involves the transperineal insertion of radioactive seeds into prostatic tissue containing identified lesions while sparing the remainder of the gland and further reducing toxicity [71]. In HDR brachytherapy, a similar approach is used but with very high-dose radioactive seeds that are placed into a lesion of interest for a set amount of time and then removed at the same session.

Focal treatments with RT are gaining momentum in clinical trials due to the growing emphasis on functional preservation via tissue-sparing approaches [72]. There have been a number of technological advances over the last decade that make focal radiation therapy administered through external delivery systems a possibility. These include intensity-modulated radiotherapy (IMRT), helical IMRT, volumetric-modulated radiotherapy, image-guided radiotherapy (IGRT), and stereotactic body radiotherapy. In particular, stereotactic radiotherapy works by real-time tracking and robotic controlled radiation delivery systems that could treat focal areas of prostate. Robotic RT techniques (CyberKnife^{TM}) deliver high-dose hypofractionated, stereotactic RT using a robotic arm in combination with intrafractional prostate motion tracking.

Primary Focal Radiotherapy

In the largest trial on focal brachytherapy, Nguyen *et al.* [73] used ^{125}I for focal RT in 318 men with localized Gleason 6 (88%) or 3 + 4 = 7 (12%), T1c, PCa with a PSA less than 15 ng/mL. At 5 and 8 years post therapy, the PSA failure-free survival (based on nadir + 2) rates in the low-risk group were 95.1% and 80.4%, respectively.

Cosset *et al.* [74] also conducted a small pilot study for LDR focal brachytherapy with ^{125}I seeds in 21 patients with localized, low-risk PCa (Gleason <3 + 4, PSA < 10 ng/mL, unilateral disease) diagnosed by MRI and fusion biopsy. A posttreatment confirmatory biopsy revealed that only 1 patient (4.8%) had evidence of residual cancer; Gleason 6. At 6 months, urinary function and erectile function was preserved as evaluated by IPSS and IIEFF questionnaires. The group acknowledged that LDR focal brachytherapy had a lower toxicity with regard to urinary control and erectile function in comparison to previously reported whole-gland brachy-therapy at their institution (p = 0.04 and p = 0.014, respectively) [74].

Although these initial results for focal brachytherapy seem promising, there is a need to evaluate the feasibility and functional outcomes in a larger cohort with longer follow up.

Salvage Focal Radiotherapy

Focal brachytherapy, rather than WG RT, has also been evaluated in the salvage setting. The goal of this approach is to achieve the same oncologic outcomes as WG salvage RT while reducing the potential toxicities of the treatment. Peters *et al.* [75] evaluated 20 patients with locally radiorecurrent PCa, determined by MRI-fusion biopsy, who then underwent focal brachytherapy with ^{125}I seeds for a total focal dose of 144 Gy. Three patients subsequently had biochemical failure (Phoenix criteria) at 36 months follow up. De novo grade 1 urinary incontinence developed in 4 men (20%). Five men retained their potency postsalvage brachytherapy, and one patient developed a stricture that was successfully treated.

Kunogi *et al.* [76] also reviewed 12 patients with radiorecurrent PCa after primary brachytherapy who then underwent focal ^{125}I salvage brachytherapy. Focality was determined based on mapping biopsy. Although functional outcomes were not reported, the BDFS rate at 4 years post therapy was 78%. Similar rates were reported by Hsu *et al.* [77], who delivered salvage focal brachytherapy (^{125}I) to 15 patients with radiorecurrent PCa. At a median follow up of 23.3 months, 2 men (13%) developed a local recurrence. PFS rates by Phoenix criteria were 100% and 71.4%, respectively, at 1 and 3 years post therapy. Low rates of toxicity were reported, with 33% experiencing grade 2 urinary toxicities and 87% of men maintaining erections or reporting erections with pharmacologic medication.

Focal salvage brachytherapy seems technically feasible and oncological outcomes seem comparable to salvage WG treatment from the limited studies available [78]. The toxicity of salvage therapy, however, appears to be lower than the WG approach, where rates of severe (Grade 3) urinary toxicity can exceed 30% and erectile function impairment can exceed this [78,79]. Because there are currently no guidelines for salvage brachytherapy or, moreover, focal salvage brachytherapy, further studies are needed to validate these findings.

Additional Therapies

Several additional therapeutic approaches have been investigated for primary focal ablation of PCa; RFA, LITT, and PDT. Briefly, RFA is the percutaneous delivery of high frequency alternating current (range 350–500 Khz) across electrodes adjacent to a tissue of interest, resulting in heating and coagulative necrosis. It has been documented in many other organs such as liver, lung, and kidney, since the 1990s [80]. To date, there has been one small proof of concept trial in 15 patients evaluating focal RFA for PCa [81].

LITT is a form of thermal energy that uses transperineal laser fibers inserted directly into prostatic tissue that are directly heated to induce coagulative necrosis of the targeted tissue [54]. A handful of small studies (fewer than 100 patients total) have evaluated this therapy with very limited follow up (median 4.5 months). The presence of significant and insignificant cancer on posttreatment biopsy was 4.8% and 22.2%, respectively. The data are clearly limited and further studies are needed to determine the overall impact of this approach.

PDT, in comparison to LITT, is a technique that uses transperineal lasers to activate a vascular photosensitiviser, which is delivered intravenously, within a target area. This activation leads to the formation of reactive oxygen species, vessel thrombosis, necrosis, and apoptosis. A few small prospective development studies have been conducted with median follow-up of 6 months. Mandatory posttreatment biopsy has revealed an average of insignificant cancer in 45.9% of patients on repeat biopsy [54].

Implications for Research

There are a number of limitations based on the current literature available underscoring or lack of standards or consensus for the delivery of FT, either as a primary or salvage therapy, for PCa. Based on the literature available, there is a glaring lack of randomized controlled trials comparing any of the focal ablative therapeutic modalities to RP, RT, or even to each other. The published trials thus far largely comprise observational or small pilot studies. To better establish the efficacy of any of these therapies or to more clearly define the ideal patient for whom to use such a therapy, larger randomized controlled trials with longer follow up are needed.

There are several unique challenges facing researchers in designing future studies to assess focal therapy for PCa. First and foremost is the lack of standardization regarding a follow-up regimen for patients after focal therapy delivery. The literature supports the use of a targeted biopsy after ablative therapy and histologic review to establish oncologic efficacy and tumor ablation. That said, there are no clear guidelines regarding the optimal timing, focality, and frequency of this posttherapeutic biopsy. Furthermore, there is inconsistency among the currently available trials with regard to the uniformity of performing this.

Beyond the lack of standardization regarding a biopsy protocol, debate exists regarding what constitutes significant disease in the targeted lesion. It is known that focal ablation leads to distortion of the prostatic tissue and, therefore, prebiopsy templates or measurements that were used for the initial diagnostic and therapeutic biopsy likely will not be equally applicable in the postablation gland. There is yet no standard template for how to account for this discrepancy in the postablation gland.

Furthermore, as mentioned, the use of PSA as a surrogate to assess for such oncologic outcomes as biochemical recurrence rate

(BCR), as is standard after RP or radiation therapy, does not necessarily translate to equivalent use with focal therapy. Ablation of a portion of the prostate, rather than the, will not necessarily cause a PSA to decrease to zero and, therefore, may not be a reliable indicator of oncologic efficacy in focal ablation. The more likely use of PSA kinetics lies in a standardized PSA ratio that can be derived on a per-patient basis according to the pretreatment PSA, the proportion of prostate gland that was treated, and the posttreatment volume assessed [82].

Finally, as additional well-designed studies are needed to investigate the therapeutic modalities addressed in this chapter, other novel forms of focal therapy are also emerging. These include, but are not limited to, soluble vascular targeted photodynamic therapy (TOOKAD), IRE, RFA, water vapor ablation, injectable toxins, and magnetic nanoparticle heating [83,84]. The clinical utility and efficacy of these, and other forms of, focal ablative energy modalities remain to be better defined.

Conclusions

Despite the acceptance of tissue-sparing approaches for cancers in most other organ systems, the use of subtotal, or tissue-sparing, therapy for PCa continues to lag. In PCa, FT aims to deliver ablative energy via a variety of modalities targeted toward an index lesion while sparing surrounding healthy prostatic tissue. Based on the literature available, HIFU and cryotherapy have the most robust support through a variety of retrospective case series, registry cohorts, and prospective development trials.

It should be noted again that, whereas initial studies on FT included only men with low-risk PCa by NCCN guidelines, recent years have demonstrated inclusion of patients with higher risk and even multifocal PCa as more medium-term data with favorable outcomes are published. Focus on identification and ablation of the index lesion clearly underlies the foundation of FT and should serve as the basis for further studies going forward. As described previously, there are multiple and specific challenges facing clinicians and researchers with regard to understanding the long-term oncologic outcomes of these therapies, and their current use requires both an understanding of the potential benefit but also acceptance of these potential limitations. Further studies will help to elucidate and establish guidelines for optimal patient selection and therapeutic modality selection for focal ablation for PCa.

References

1 Wilt TJ, Brawer MK, Jones KM, Barry MJ, Aronson WJ, Fox S, *et al.* Radical prostatectomy versus observation for localized prostate cancer. New Engl J Med. 2012;367(3):203–13.

2 Bill-Axelson A, Holmberg L, Filen F, Ruutu M, Garmo H, Busch C, *et al.* Radical prostatectomy versus watchful waiting in localized prostate cancer: The Scandinavian prostate cancer group-4 randomized trial. J Natl Cancer Instit. 2008;100(16):1144–54.

3 Bill-Axelson A, Holmberg L, Ruutu M, Garmo H, Stark JR, Busch C, *et al.* Radical prostatectomy versus watchful waiting in early prostate cancer. New Engl J Med. 2011;364(18):1708–17.

4 Ficarra V, Novara G, Ahlering TE, Costello A, Eastham JA, Graefen M, *et al.* Systematic review and meta-analysis of studies reporting potency rates after robot-assisted radical prostatectomy. Eur Urol. 2012;62(3):418–30.

5 Ficarra V, Novara G, Rosen RC, Artibani W, Carroll PR, Costello A, *et al.* Systematic review and meta-analysis of studies reporting urinary continence recovery after robot-assisted radical prostatectomy. Eur Urol. 2012;62(3):405–17.

6 Holm HV, Fossa SD, Hedlund H, Schultz A, Dahl AA. How should continence and incontinence after radical prostatectomy be evaluated? A prospective study of patient ratings and changes with time. J Urol. 2014;192(4):1155–61.

7 Kennedy JE. High-intensity focused ultrasound in the treatment of solid tumours. Nat Rev Cancer. 2005;5(4):321–7.

8 Haar GT, Coussios C. High intensity focused ultrasound: physical principles and devices. Int J Hyperthermia. 2007;23(2):89–104.

9 Goldberg SN, Gazelle GS, Mueller PR. Thermal ablation therapy for focal malignancy: A unified approach to underlying principles, techniques, and diagnostic imaging guidance. AJR Am J Roentgenol. 2000;174(2):323–31.

10 Liu W, Laitinen S, Khan S, Vihinen M, Kowalski J, Yu G, *et al.* Copy number analysis indicates monoclonal origin of lethal metastatic prostate cancer. Nat Med. 2009;15(5):559–65.

11 Ahmed HU. The index lesion and the origin of prostate cancer. New Engl J Med. 2009;361(17):1704–6.

12 True L, Coleman I, Hawley S, Huang CY, Gifford D, Coleman R, *et al.* A molecular correlate to the Gleason grading system for prostate adenocarcinoma. Proc Natl Acad Sci USA. 2006;103(29):10991–6.

13 Karavitakis M, Winkler M, Abel P, Livni N, Beckley I, Ahmed HU. Histological characteristics of the index lesion in whole-mount radical prostatectomy specimens: Implications for focal therapy. Prostate Cancer Prostatic Dis. 2011;14(1):46–52.

14 Guo CC, Wang Y, Xiao L, Troncoso P, Czerniak BA. The relationship of TMPRSS2-ERG gene fusion between primary and metastatic prostate cancers. Human Pathol. 2012;43(5):644–9.

15 Mehra R, Tomlins SA, Yu J, Cao X, Wang L, Menon A, *et al.* Characterization of TMPRSS2-ETS gene aberrations in androgen-independent metastatic prostate cancer. Cancer Res. 2008;68(10):3584–90.

16 Eggener SE, Scardino PT, Carroll PR, Zelefsky MJ, Sartor O, Hricak H, *et al.* Focal therapy for localized prostate

cancer: A critical appraisal of rationale and modalities. J Urol. 2007;178(6):2260–7.

17 Bass EJ, Ahmed HU. Focal therapy in prostate cancer: A review of seven common controversies. Cancer Treat Rev. 2016;51:27–34.

18 Ahmed HU, Akin O, Coleman JA, Crane S, Emberton M, Goldenberg L, *et al.* Transatlantic Consensus Group on active surveillance and focal therapy for prostate cancer. BJU Int.. 2012;109(11):1636–47.

19 Bostwick DG, Waters DJ, Farley ER, Meiers I, Rukstalis D, Cavanaugh WA, *et al.* Group consensus reports from the Consensus Conference on Focal Treatment of Prostatic Carcinoma, Celebration, Florida, February 24, 2006. Urology. 2007;70(6 Suppl):42–4.

20 Donaldson IA, Alonzi R, Barratt D, Barret E, Berge V, Bott S, *et al.* Focal therapy: patients, interventions, and outcomes--a report from a consensus meeting. Eur Urol. 2015;67(4):771–7.

21 Postema AW, De Reijke TM, Ukimura O, Van den Bos W, Azzouzi AR, Barret E, *et al.* Standardization of definitions in focal therapy of prostate cancer: report from a Delphi consensus project. World J Urol. 2016;34(10):1373–82.

22 Turkbey B, Choyke PL. Multiparametric MRI and prostate cancer diagnosis and risk stratification. Curr Opin Urol. 2012;22(4):310–5.

23 Futterer JJ, Briganti A, De Visschere P, Emberton M, Giannarini G, Kirkham A, *et al.* Can clinically significant prostate cancer be detected with multiparametric magnetic resonance imaging? A systematic review of the literature. Eur Urol. 2015;68(6):1045–53.

24 Peng Y, Jiang Y, Yang C, Brown JB, Antic T, Sethi I, *et al.* Quantitative analysis of multiparametric prostate MR images: Differentiation between prostate cancer and normal tissue and correlation with Gleason score—computer-aided diagnosis development study. Radiology. 2013;267(3):787–96.

25 Arumainayagam N, Ahmed HU, Moore CM, Freeman A, Allen C, Sohaib SA, *et al.* Multiparametric MR imaging for detection of clinically significant prostate cancer: a validation cohort study with transperineal template prostate mapping as the reference standard. Radiology. 2013;268(3):761–9.

26 Porpiglia F, S DEL, Passera R, Manfredi M, Mele F, Bollito E, *et al.* Multiparametric-magnetic resonance/ultrasound fusion targeted prostate biopsy improves agreement between biopsy and radical prostatectomy Gleason score. Anticancer Res. 2016;36(9):4833–9.

27 Oberlin DT, Casalino DD, Miller FH, Meeks JJ. Dramatic increase in the utilization of multiparametric magnetic resonance imaging for detection and management of prostate cancer. Abdom Radiol (NY). 2016 Nov 17. [Epub ahead of print.]

28 Crawford ED, Rove KO, Barqawi AB, Maroni PD, Werahera PN, Baer CA, *et al.* Clinical-pathologic correlation between transperineal mapping biopsies of the prostate and three-dimensional reconstruction of prostatectomy specimens. Prostate. 2013;73(7):778–87.

29 Rosset R, Bratan F, Crouzet S, Tonoli-Catez H, Mege-Lechevallier F, Gelet A, *et al.* Can pre- and postoperative magnetic resonance imaging predict recurrence-free survival after whole-gland high-intensity focused ablation for prostate cancer? Eur Radiol. 2017;27(4):1768–75.

30 Yoon MY, Park J, Cho JY, Jeong CW, Ku JH, Kim HH, *et al.* Predicting biochemical recurrence in patients with high-risk prostate cancer using the apparent diffusion coefficient of magnetic resonance imaging. Invest Clin Urol. 2017;58(1):12–19.

31 Algarra R, Zudaire B, Tienza A, Velis JM, Rincon A, Pascual I, *et al.* Optimizing D'Amico risk groups in radical prostatectomy through the addition of magnetic resonance imaging data. Actas Urol Esp. 2014;38(9):594–99.

32 Jeong IG, Lim JH, You D, Kim MH, Choi HJ, Kim JK, *et al.* Incremental value of magnetic resonance imaging for clinically high risk prostate cancer in 922 radical prostatectomies. J Urol. 2013;190(6):2054–60.

33 Wegelin O, van Melick HH, Hooft L, Bosch JL, Reitsma HB, Barentsz JO, *et al.* Comparing three different techniques for magnetic resonance imaging-targeted prostate biopsies: A systematic review of in-bore versus magnetic resonance imaging-transrectal ultrasound fusion versus cognitive registration. Is there a preferred technique? Eur Urol. 2017;71(4):517–531.

34 Radtke JP, Schwab C, Wolf MB, Freitag MT, Alt CD, Kesch C, *et al.* Multiparametric magnetic resonance imaging (mri) and mri-transrectal ultrasound fusion biopsy for index tumor detection: correlation with radical prostatectomy specimen. Eur Urol. 2016;70(5):846–53.

35 Valerio M, Donaldson I, Emberton M, Ehdaie B, Hadaschik BA, Marks LS, *et al.* Detection of clinically significant prostate cancer using magnetic resonance imaging-ultrasound fusion targeted biopsy: A systematic review. Eur Urol. 2015;68(1):8–19.

36 Rosenkrantz AB, Verma S, Choyke P, Eberhardt SC, Eggener SE, Gaitonde K, *et al.* Prostate magnetic resonance imaging and magnetic resonance imaging targeted biopsy in patients with a prior negative biopsy: A consensus statement by AUA and SAR. J Urol. 2016;196(6):1613–8.

37 Ward JF, Pisters LL. Considerations for patient selection for focal therapy. Ther Adv Urol. 2013;5(6):330–7.

38 Reis LO, Billis A, Zequi SC, Tobias-Machado M, Viana P, Cerqueira M, *et al.* Supporting prostate cancer focal therapy: A multidisciplinary international consensus of experts ("ICE"). Aging Male. 2014;17(2):66–71.

39 Ahmed HU, Hu Y, Carter T, Arumainayagam N, Lecornet E, Freeman A, *et al.* Characterizing clinically significant prostate cancer using template prostate mapping biopsy. J Urol. 2011;186(2):458–64.

40 Scheltema MJ, Tay KJ, Postema AW, de Bruin DM, Feller J, Futterer JJ, *et al.* Utilization of multiparametric prostate magnetic resonance imaging in clinical practice and focal therapy: Report from a

Delphi consensus project. World J Urol. 2016 Sept 16 [ePub ahead of print].

41 Hossack T, Patel MI, Huo A, Brenner P, Yuen C, Spernat D, *et al.* Location and pathological characteristics of cancers in radical prostatectomy specimens identified by transperineal biopsy compared to transrectal biopsy. J Urol. 2012;188(3):781–5.

42 Babaian RJ, Donnelly B, Bahn D, Baust JG, Dineen M, Ellis D, *et al.* Best practice statement on cryosurgery for the treatment of localized prostate cancer. J Urol. 2008;180(5):1993–2004.

43 Hou AH, Sullivan KF, Crawford ED. Targeted focal therapy for prostate cancer: A review. Curr Opin Urol. 2009;19(3):283–9.

44 Ward JF, Jones JS. Focal cryotherapy for localized prostate cancer: A report from the national Cryo On-Line Database (COLD) Registry. BJU Int. 2012;109(11):1648–54.

45 Mendez MH, Passoni NM, Pow-Sang J, Jones JS, Polascik TJ. Comparison of outcomes between preoperatively potent men treated with focal versus whole gland cryotherapy in a matched population. J Endourol. 2015;29(10):1193–8.

46 Barqawi AB, Stoimenova D, Krughoff K, Eid K, O'Donnell C, Phillips JM, *et al.* Targeted focal therapy for the management of organ confined prostate cancer. J Urol. 2014;192(3):749–53.

47 Bahn D, de Castro Abreu AL, Gill IS, Hung AJ, Silverman P, Gross ME, *et al.* Focal cryotherapy for clinically unilateral, low-intermediate risk prostate cancer in 73 men with a median follow-up of 3.7 years. Eur Urol. 2012;62(1):55–63.

48 Hale Z, Miyake M, Palacios DA, Rosser CJ. Focal cryosurgical ablation of the prostate: A single institute's perspective. BMC Urol. 2013;13:2.

49 Durand M, Barret E, Galiano M, Rozet F, Sanchez-Salas R, Ahallal Y, *et al.* Focal cryoablation: a treatment option for unilateral low-risk prostate cancer. BJU Int. 2014;113(1):56–64.

50 Lian H, Zhuang J, Yang R, Qu F, Wang W, Lin T, *et al.* Focal cryoablation for unilateral low-intermediate-risk prostate cancer:

63-month mean follow-up results of 41 patients. Int Urol Nephrol. 2016;48(1):85–90.

51 Li YH, Elshafei A, Agarwal G, Ruckle H, Powsang J, Jones JS. Salvage focal prostate cryoablation for locally recurrent prostate cancer after radiotherapy: Initial results from the cryo on-line data registry. Prostate. 2015;75(1):1–7.

52 de Castro Abreu AL, Bahn D, Leslie S, Shoji S, Silverman P, Desai MM, et al. Salvage focal and salvage total cryoablation for locally recurrent prostate cancer after primary radiation therapy. BJU Int. 2013;112(3):298–307.

53 Eisenberg ML, Shinohara K. Partial salvage cryoablation of the prostate for recurrent prostate cancer after radiotherapy failure. Urology. 2008;72(6):1315–8.

54 Valerio M, Ahmed HU, Emberton M, Lawrentschuk N, Lazzeri M, Montironi R, et al. The role of focal therapy in the management of localised prostate cancer: A systematic review. Eur Urol. 2014;66(4):732–51.

55 Sonacare. Real-Time Tissue Change Monitoring System 2014. Available from www.ushifu.com.

56 Warmuth M, Johansson T, Mad P. Systematic review of the efficacy and safety of high-intensity focussed ultrasound for the primary and salvage treatment of prostate cancer. Eur Urol. 2010;58(6):803–15.

57 Uchida T, Tomonaga T, Kim H, Nakano M, Shoji S, Nagata Y, et al. Improved outcomes with advancements in high intensity focused ultrasound devices for the treatment of localized prostate cancer. J Urol. 2015;193(1):103–10.

58 Shoji S, Uchida T, Nakamoto M, Kim H, de Castro Abreu AL, Leslie S, et al. Prostate swelling and shift during high intensity focused ultrasound: implication for targeted focal therapy. J Urol. 2013;190(4):1224–32.

59 Feijoo ER, Sivaraman A, Barret E, Sanchez-Salas R, Galiano M, Rozet F, et al. Focal high-intensity focused ultrasound targeted hemiablation for unilateral prostate cancer: A prospective evaluation of oncologic and functional outcomes. Eur Urol. 2016;69(2):214–20.

60 Ahmed HU, Freeman A, Kirkham A, Sahu M, Scott R, Allen C, et al. Focal therapy for localized prostate cancer: A phase I/II trial. J Urol. 2011;185(4):1246–54.

61 Ahmed HU, Hindley RG, Dickinson L, Freeman A, Kirkham AP, Sahu M, et al. Focal therapy for localised unifocal and multifocal prostate cancer: A prospective development study. Lancet Oncol. 2012;13(6):622–32.

62 Albisinni S, Aoun F, Bellucci S, Biaou I, Limani K, Hawaux E, et al. Comparing high-intensity focal ultrasound hemiablation to robotic radical prostatectomy in the management of unilateral prostate cancer: A matched-pair analysis. J Endourol. 2017;31(1):14–9.

63 Agarwal PK, Sadetsky N, Konety BR, Resnick MI, Carroll PR. Treatment failure after primary and salvage therapy for prostate cancer: likelihood, patterns of care, and outcomes. Cancer. 2008;112(2):307–14.

64 Baco E, Gelet A, Crouzet S, Rud E, Rouviere O, Tonoli-Catez H, et al. Hemi salvage high-intensity focused ultrasound (HIFU) in unilateral radiorecurrent prostate cancer: a prospective two-centre study. BJU Int. 2014;114(4):532–40.

65 Ahmed HU, Cathcart P, McCartan N, Kirkham A, Allen C, Freeman A, et al. Focal salvage therapy for localized prostate cancer recurrence after external beam radiotherapy: A pilot study. Cancer. 2012;118(17):4148–55.

66 Scheltema MJ, van den Bos W, de Bruin DM, Wijkstra H, Laguna MP, de Reijke TM, et al. Focal vs extended ablation in localized prostate cancer with irreversible electroporation; a multi-center randomized controlled trial. BMC Cancer. 2016;16:299.

67 van den Bos W, de Bruin DM, Jurhill RR, Savci-Heijink CD, Muller BG, Varkarakis IM, et al. The correlation between the electrode configuration and histopathology of irreversible electroporation ablations in prostate cancer patients. World J Urol. 2016;34(5):657–64.

68 Valerio M, Stricker PD, Ahmed HU, Dickinson L, Ponsky L, Shnier R, et al. Initial assessment of safety and clinical feasibility of irreversible electroporation in the focal

treatment of prostate cancer. Prostate Cancer Prostatic Dis. 2014;17(4):343–7.

69 Valerio M, Dickinson L, Ali A, Ramachadran N, Donaldson I, McCartan N, *et al.* Nanoknife Electroporation Ablation Trial: A prospective development study investigating focal irreversible electroporation for localized prostate cancer. J Urol. 2017;197(3 Pt 1):647–54.

70 Moon DH, Efstathiou JA, Chen RC. What is the best way to radiate the prostate in 2016? Urol Oncol. 2017;35(2):59–68.

71 Tong WY, Cohen G, Yamada Y. Focal low-dose rate brachytherapy for the treatment of prostate cancer. Cancer Manage Res. 2013;5:315–25.

72 Kovacs G, Cosset JM, Carey B. Focal radiotherapy as focal therapy of prostate cancer. Curr Opin Urol. 2014;24(3):231–5.

73 Nguyen PL, Chen MH, Zhang Y, Tempany CM, Cormack RA, Beard CJ, *et al.* Updated results of magnetic resonance imaging guided partial prostate brachytherapy for favorable risk prostate cancer: Implications for focal therapy. J Urol. 2012;188(4):1151–6.

74 Cosset JM, Cathelineau X, Wakil G, Pierrat N, Quenzer O, Prapotnich D, *et al.* Focal brachytherapy for selected low-risk prostate cancers: a pilot study. Brachytherapy. 2013;12(4):331–7.

75 Peters M, Maenhout M, van der Voort van Zyp JR, Moerland MA, Moman MR, Steuten LM, *et al.* Focal salvage iodine-125 brachytherapy for prostate cancer recurrences after primary radiotherapy: a retrospective study regarding toxicity, biochemical outcome and quality of life. Radiother Oncol. 2014;112(1):77–82.

76 Kunogi H, Wakumoto Y, Yamaguchi N, Horie S, Sasai K. Focal partial salvage low-dose-rate brachytherapy for local recurrent prostate cancer after permanent prostate brachytherapy with a review of the literature. J Contemp Brachytherapy. 2016;8(3):165–72.

77 Hsu CC, Hsu H, Pickett B, Crehange G, Hsu IC, Dea R, *et al.* Feasibility of MR imaging/MR spectroscopy-planned focal partial salvage permanent prostate implant (PPI) for localized recurrence after initial PPI for prostate cancer. Int J Radiat Oncol Biol Phys. 2013;85(2):370–7.

78 Peters M, Moman MR, van der Poel HG, Vergunst H, de Jong IJ, Vijverberg PL, *et al.* Patterns of outcome and toxicity after salvage prostatectomy, salvage cryosurgery and salvage brachytherapy for prostate cancer recurrences after radiation therapy: A multi-center experience and literature review. World J Urol. 2013;31(2):403–9.

79 Kimura M, Mouraviev V, Tsivian M, Mayes JM, Satoh T, Polascik TJ. Current salvage methods for recurrent prostate cancer after failure of primary radiotherapy. BJU Int. 2010;105(2):191–201.

80 Okhunov Z, Roy O, Duty B, Waingankar N, Herati A, Morgenstern N, *et al.* Clinical evaluation of a novel bipolar radiofrequency ablation system for renal masses. BJU Int. 2012;110(5):688–91.

81 Zlotta AR, Djavan B, Matos C, Noel JC, Peny MO, Silverman DE, *et al.* Percutaneous transperineal radiofrequency ablation of prostate tumour: safety, feasibility and pathological effects on human prostate cancer. Br J Urol. 1998;81(2):265–75.

82 Marshall S, Taneja S. Focal therapy for prostate cancer: The current status. Prostate Int. 2015;3(2):35–41.

83 Azzouzi AR, Barret E, Bennet J, Moore C, Taneja S, Muir G, *et al.* TOOKAD(R) Soluble focal therapy: pooled analysis of three phase II studies assessing the minimally invasive ablation of localized prostate cancer. World J Urol. 2015;33(7):945–53.

84 79.Valerio M, Dickinson L, Ali A, Ramachandran N, Donaldson I, Freeman A, *et al.* A prospective development study investigating focal irreversible electroporation in men with localised prostate cancer: Nanoknife Electroporation Ablation Trial (NEAT). Contemp Clin Trials. 2014;39(1):57–65.

10

The Modern Basis for Nephron-Sparing Surgery in Patients with Renal Cancer: Biologic Heterogeneity, the Significance of Tumor Biopsy, and the Changing Roles of Partial Nephrectomy and Tumor Ablation

Jeffrey J. Tomaszewski, MD,[1] Robert G. Uzzo, MD, FACS,[2] and David Y.T. Chen, MD, FACS[2]

[1] Division of Urology, Department of Surgery, MD Anderson Cancer Center at Cooper, Rowan University School of Medicine, Camden, NJ, USA
[2] Department of Surgical Oncology, Division of Urologic Oncology, Fox Chase Center–Temple University Health System, Philadelphia, PA, USA

Introduction

The incidence of renal cell carcinoma (RCC) has been steadily rising over the past decade [1], in large part because of the increased detection of incidental small renal masses (SRMs) on cross-sectional abdominal imaging [2]. Nephron-sparing surgery (NSS) has become the standard of care for clinically localized T1a (<4cm) SRMs; however alternative treatment and management are accepted options in select comorbid or elderly patients [3-5]. Progress in technology has led to the adoption of minimally invasive surgical approaches for renal tumor excision instead of traditional open surgery, and includes applying laparoscopy and robotic-assisted surgery [6]. Likewise, in-situ alternatives to resection have arisen, including ATs such as radiofrequency ablation (RFA), cryoablation (CA), microwave ablation, laser ablation, radiosurgical ablation (CyberKnife), and high-intensity focused ultrasound (HIFU) ablation; these have been developed and administered by image-guided percutaneous access or via laparoscopic and minimally invasive surgical exposure. The optimal management approach should be based on clinical assessment of both patient comorbidities and tumor characteristics, but because SRMs represent a heterogeneous group of benign and malignant histologic entities, they may have a variability in clinical behavior that is not predictable by conventional imaging or clinical staging [7].

Traditionally, all localized solid renal masses had been presumed to be RCC and considered to have malignant potential, and they had been routinely treated with immediate surgical excision to address their risk for stage progression and metastatic dissemination [8]. However, RCC is now recognized as a heterogeneous disease process, with a number of distinct histopathological subtypes having substantial variance in biological aggressiveness [8], and the recent identification of significant intratumoral molecular level heterogeneity in clear-cell RCC [9] further makes difficult predicting tumor behavior based on histology alone. Importantly, 20–25% of SRMs suggestive for malignancy are benign [10], even though 5.2% of patients with a SRM 4cm or smaller present with metastases [11]. Because no specific computed tomography (CT) or magnetic resonance imaging (MRI) parameters can conclusively differentiate RCCs from benign tumors such as oncocytomas [12], renal mass biopsy (RMB) is increasingly recommended to help define RCC subtype and associated potential for aggressive behavior, allowing for a more rational treatment [8]. RMB is emerging as safe and useful for the preoperative identification of benign lesions to avoid unnecessary intervention, particularly in the older population [13]. Despite the excellent results following NSS of SRMs, RCC mortality has not improved [14], which has led some to suggest many SRMs may be clinically indolent and therefore overtreated; this concern for potentially unnecessary resection has spurred the development of alternative treatments for select patients with SRM having significant medical comorbidities, in particular, minimally invasive in-situ AT. Herein we review the modern basis for nephron preservation in patients with RCC, identify challenges posed by biologic heterogeneity, highlight the evolving role of RMB, and discuss the roles of partial nephrectomy (PN) and tumor ablation.

Principal Treatment Options for SRMs and the Basis for Nephron Preservation

Treatment options for SRMs include PN, radical nephrectomy (RN), minimally invasive AT, and active surveillance (AS; Table 10.1). Randomized controlled trials comparing the results of different treatment options for SRMs are lacking, and so the assessment of outcomes is based largely on observational studies [6]. Historically, RN was considered the gold standard treatment for patients with a SRM.

Table 10.1 Indications and Contraindications of Treatment Options for Small Renal Masses.

	Indications	Contraindications
Active Surveillance	• Severe renal dysfunction • Elderly, severe medical comorbidities, high surgical risk (limited life expectancy) • Refusal of active treatment • Biopsy confirmed benign disease (relative) • Consideration of initial AS for incidentally detected SRMs followed by treatment only for those that show progression (emerging)	• Unwillingness to comply with a strict radiologic follow-up • Healthy young patients (relative)
Ablative Therapy	• Elder, comorbid patients at high surgical risk who desire active treatment • Baseline renal dysfunction, solitary kidney • Informed younger patients who refuse surgery • Renal mass in a renal remnant (postsurgical)	• Healthy young patients (long-term oncologic efficacy data lacking) • Severe, irreversible coagulopathy • Hilar tumors close to collecting system, ureter • Infiltrative tumors • Irregularly shaped tumors • Unwillingness to comply with a strict radiologic follow-up
Partial Nephrectomy	• Enhancing solid/cystic renal mass when technically feasible • Young, healthy patients • Hilar tumors • Need for nephron preservation	• Severe, irreversible coagulopathy • Previous multiple abdominal surgeries (relative)
Radical Nephrectomy	• T1a renal mass for which PN is not technically feasible • ≥T1b renal mass (relative) • Comorbid patients at high surgical risk (relative)	• Solitary kidney (relative) • Healthy young patients with T1a renal mass amenable to PN

AS, active surveillance; PN, partial nephrectomy; SRMs, small renal masses.

However, over the last few years, accumulating evidence of oncologic equivalence, improved renal functional preservation, and acceptable morbidity have led to the increased use of PN instead of RN for localized unilateral RCC in a patient with a healthy contralateral kidney [6].

Comparative Effectiveness of Radical versus NSS

More frequent abdominal imaging has led to significant downward stage migration and smaller tumor size at diagnosis for patients presenting with localized RCC. In fact, incidental Stage Ia tumors now account for the vast majority of new RCC cases [2]. Observational studies from institutional and administrative data sets demonstrate equivalent oncological outcomes for SRMs treated either by RN or PN but suggest superior renal function and overall survival in cohorts undergoing PN [15,16]. Additionally, several large retrospective series report a correlation between improved renal function, reduced risk of cardiovascular events, and superior survival with renal preservation [16–20]. Because of this perceived benefit, current guidelines recommend PN for T1 tumors when technically feasible [3,4,21] and increasing NSS use reflects adoption of these management recommendations.

Impact of PN and RN on Survival

Chronic kidney disease (CKD) is currently defined as a glomerular filtration rate less than $60\,mL/minute/1.73\,m^2$ for more than 90 days. The development of CKD is associated with an increased risk of cardiovascular events and all-cause mortality in large population-based studies, even when controlling for measured and unmeasured confounders [22–24]. A systematic review and pooled meta-analysis comparing approximately 40,000 patients undergoing RN and PN revealed that in preselected patients PN is associated with a 19% lower risk of all-cause mortality, attributed to a 61% lower risk of development of severe CKD [25,26].

Despite numerous retrospective observational data suggesting superior outcomes for patients with SRM undergoing PN, the quality and validity of these data are questioned [25]. For instance, a meta-analysis of the available data reveals a paradoxical 29% cancer-specific survival (CSS) advantage to PN over RN, indicating significant selection bias is inherent within these cohorts [25]. Meanwhile, available Level-1 evidence demonstrates that RN is non-inferior to elective PN in patients with a normal contralateral kidney; the EORTC Phase III trial prospectively randomized 541 patients with a normal renal function and a 5 cm or less renal mass to PN or RN [27]. An unanticipated overall survival benefit for RN was observed at a median follow-up of 9.3 years on an intention-to-treat analysis. No significant difference was seen in CSS between PN and RN, so the observed survival advantage with RN could not be attributed to differences in kidney cancer mortality. Although NSS substantially reduced the incidence of moderate renal dysfunction (eGFR <60), the incidence of advanced kidney disease (estimated glomerular filtration rate [eGFR] <30) and kidney failure (eGFR <15) were essentially identical to that following RN [26]. Furthermore, in these patients with a normal contralateral renal unit, initial GFR decline after surgery was followed by stabilization of renal function, such that moderate renal dysfunction arising from surgery in these patients was not found to be clinically meaningful or progressive to increasing levels of CKD [26,28].

The EORTC trial (30904) has been criticized, and specific study concerns deserve mention. First, the trial was initially designed as a noninferiority study and powered to show a 10% difference in overall survival at 5 years between groups; however, accrual was slow and the trial was ultimately closed early because of poor enrollment. Second, the design of a noninferiority trial is complex and is founded on assumptions that are difficult to verify directly [29]. Third, the intention-to-treat analysis is typically preferred as the more robust analytical framework in a superiority trial but can be biased toward non-inferiority in the setting of considerable patient crossover between treatment arms [29]. And fourth, there were considerable disparities in baseline comorbidities and loss to follow-up, which can increase the similarity between groups and bias results toward non-inferiority [26]. Limitations notwithstanding, the EORTC trial provides important Level-I evidence regarding the significance of nephron preservation in patients with a normal contralateral kidney undergoing surgical treatment for SRMs, and clinicians should not ignore the important implications of the trial because it is unlikely a similar randomized trial will be repeated [26].

Rationale for Ablative Therapies

The current versions of both the European Association of Urology (EAU) and the American Urological Association (AUA) SRM guidelines recommend NSS as the standard treatment for solitary renal tumors up to a diameter of 7 cm, whenever technically feasible [3,4]. Given the morbidity associated with PN, it may not represent the ideal treatment for all patients, especially among the elderly and infirm. Several ablative technologies have been investigated, including CA, RFA, microwave thermotherapy [30], HIFU [31], irreversible electroporation [32], and histotripsy [33]. Only the first two modalities have achieved widespread use with published reports of short- to intermediate-term results; HIFU and the other techniques for ATs remain experimental.

The rationale of AT is to effectively treat SRMs in patients at high surgical risk but with potentially reduced treatment-associated morbidity. Many ATs can be performed percutaneously in an outpatient setting, and ideal candidates are the elderly and infirm who desire active treatment [3]. Patients at risk of complete renal loss with surgery, such as those with SRM in a solitary kidney and baseline renal dysfunction, are also candidates for ablation, although long-term radiographic surveillance is required [4]. Contraindications to AT include tumors with a low chance of

successful treatment because of size more than 3 cm or location, healthy young patients (75 years or younger), the presence of multiple tumors, and irreversible coagulopathy [4]. Large tumors (more than 3 cm), hilar tumors close to the proximal ureter or central collecting system, or tumors with an irregular shape and infiltrative appearance should not be recommended for AT because of the increased likelihood of incomplete treatment and risk of local recurrence [3,4].

CA and RFA

CA is a thermal ablative technique that relies on the Joule Thomson phenomenon, whereby a highly compressed liquid (argon) expanding through a restricted orifice rapidly changes to a gaseous state and creates extreme cooling (Figure 10.1) [34]. During CA, the extracellular fluid freezes causing increased osmotic pressure in the extracellular compartment; the resulting fluid shift causes cellular dehydration, accumulation of toxins within the cells, change in pH, and protein denaturation [34]. Ice-ball formation also produces mechanical disruption of cellular membranes and blood vessel walls [35], leading to crystallization of the intracellular fluid, as well as endothelial damage, which indirectly triggers ischemia, thrombosis, and coagulative necrosis and these effects synergize to result in cell death [34]. Modern probes are capable of creating ice balls of widely varied sizes (3.1×3.6 cm to

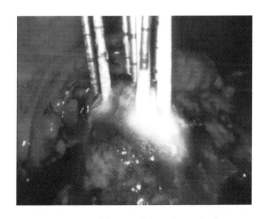

Figure 10.1 Cryoablation of a renal mass [59].

4.5 × 6.4 cm), but the −40 °C isotherm, the zone of lethal treatment, is generally smaller [35]. Therefore in clinical practice an ice ball formed during CA is usually extended 5–10 mm beyond the tumor edge to ensure coverage of the target area falls sufficiently within the −40 °C isotherm. A double freeze-thaw cycle is associated with greater clinical efficacy compared to a single cycle [36], and renal CA can be performed either laparoscopically or percutaneously.

Like CA, RFA is performed percutaneously or laparoscopically, and the approach depends on the condition of the patient, tumor location, and provider preference [37]. Currently there is insufficient evidence to indicate one approach as the ideal method. RFA uses high-frequency monopolar alternating current delivered directly to the target tissue to generate thermal damage by converting radiofrequency waves into heat [38]. When tissue reaches temperatures >60 °C, thermal dessication and coagulative necrosis lead to cell death through irreversible protein denaturation and cross-linking [38]. The effectiveness of RFA depends on both the temperature and duration of treatment [35]. A wide variety of RFA probes are available, with single-needle probes for small lesions, multiprobe array electrodes for larger areas (3–5 cm), and internally cooled electrodes to create the largest ablation volumes [39].

Follow-up of Renal Ablation

Although no standard post-CA protocol has been universally adopted, CT and MRI are commonly used for follow-up imaging. Initially after treatment tumor size may increase as a result of peritumoral hemorrhage, but tumor periphery can be hard to differentiate from surrounding fibrosis and stranding [34]. Post-CA, any enhancement 10 HU or higher or an interval increase in tumor size is suspicious for inadequate tumor ablation and local recurrence. On T1-weighted MRI, 61% of adequately treated tumors are isointense to renal parenchyma, whereas 95% are hypointense on T2 [34,40].

Post-RFA, imaging plays an important role in tumor localization, real-time monitoring of the ablation zone, and follow-up. RFA is typically monitored during therapy with ultrasound, and ablation zones are seen as hyperechogenic areas created by vaporization of interstitital fluid. A follow-up contrast-enhanced CT or MRI is typically used after RFA to ensure a lack of enhancement within the targeted region, and a thin enhancing rim representing either inflammation or hemorrhagic granulation tissue may be seen in early follow-up [41]. Given the difficulty in determining the extent of the coagulation zone, the goal of RFA is to ablate a 1-cm margin of normal tissue surrounding the tumor on all sides; however the concurrent aim for preservation of normal surrounding renal parenchyma limits margin size [37]. Radiologic absence of disease recurrence may not serve as a surrogate for clinical cure; 3.6% of post-RFA biopsies are positive 6 months following treatment [42].

Outcomes of Renal Ablation

Although some have suggested follow-up for CA, the series is too limited to draw meaningful conclusions about oncological efficacy [43]. Intermediate-term oncologic outcomes after CA with follow-up ranging from 9 to 36 months report excellent local control (95–100%) and CSS (95–100%) in patients undergoing treatment of a solitary SRM (Table 10.2) [44–46]. Following RFA, short- and intermediate-term oncologic outcomes reveal recurrence-free rates of 90–96.8 % in patients with mean tumor volumes of 2.0–3.2 cm [44]. In the 2009 AUA guidelines for the management of clinically localized stage I RCC, a meta-analysis revealed total recurrence-free survival of 87.6% and 85.2%, respectively, for CA and RFA with a mean follow-up of 26.2 months and 39.3 months, respectively [44]. A recent meta-analysis of 20 studies with a total of 457 cases revealed a pooled proportion of clinical efficacy of 89% (95% CI 0.83–0.94) for CA and 90% (95% CI 0.86–0.93) for RFA [44].

Table 10.2 Summary of Patient and Tumor Characteristics and Outcomes of Kidney Mass Ablation.

Study	Approach	Patients (n)	Mean Tumor Size (cm)	Mean Follow-Up (months)	Outcome	Complications
Psutka et al. [47]	Perc RFA	185	3.0	76	Residual disease (13%) 5-year CSS (99.4%) 5-year disease-free survival (87.6%) 5-year overall survival (73.3%)	None reported
Hegarty et al. [48]	Lap CA	161	2.6	36	Residual tumor (1.9%)	Urine leak (0.6%) MI (0.6%) Pneumothorax (2.4%) Blood transfusion (2.4%) CHF (0.6%)
Matsumoto et al. [49]	Perc/Lap RFA	109	2.4	19.4	Residual tumor (2.8%)	Major (2.8%) Minor (9%)
Hiraoka et al. [50]	Perc RFA	40	2.4	16	Residual tumor (15%)	Major (0%) Minor (3.9%; hematuria, perinephric hematoma)
Schwartz et al. [51]	Lap CA	85	2.6	10	Complete lesion resolution (97.3%)	Bleeding (2.4%)
Bandi et al. [52]	Perc/Lap CA	78	2.6	19	Overall survival (88.5%) CSS (100%) RFS (98.7%)	Perinephric bleeding (2.8%) Bowel injury (1.3%) Persistent disease (5.1%)
Desai et al. [53]	Lap CA	78	2.1	24.6	Complete lesion resolution (97%)	Pulmonary (5.1%) Bleeding (1.3%) Biopsy-proven recurrence (3%)
Levinson et al. [54]	Perc/Lap RFA	31	2.0	60.5	Residual tumor (9.7%)	Overall (20.6%) Mortality (3.2%) Perirenal hematoma (12.9%)

CA, cryoablation; CHF, congestive heart failure; CSS, cancer-specific survival; Lap, laparoscopic; MI, myocardial infarction; Perc, percutaneous; RFA, radiofrequency ablation; RFS, recurrence-free survival.

From a review of 2104 tumors, reported overall complication rates range from 0.9% to 16.2% [34], with hemorrhage (1.1–16.2%), perinephric hematoma (1.6–4.4%), and urine leak (1.2–7.1%) the most commonly reported. Increasing anatomic tumor complexity and "nearness" to the renal hilum as objectified by R.E.N.A.L. nephrometry score [55] is associated with an increased risk of complications following CA [56]. Following RFA, the most-common minor complication is pain and paresthesias at the percutaneous probe insertion site, whereas most major complications are secondary to thermal injury to the renal collecting system (e.g., ureteropelvic junction obstruction, urinary extravasation). A meta-analysis of 11 studies revealed a complication rate of 19.0% (95% CI 0.12–0.27) [43], and renal function following RFA is generally unchanged [57].

Unfortunately no prospective trial has compared results for RFA compared with CA [58]. As opposed to RFA, CA has been shown to also be effective in the treatment of tumors larger than 3 cm in greatest dimension [59]. One potential limitation of RFA is in the treatment of central renal masses, where thermal sink effects originating in the highly vascular renal hilum can interfere with uniform tissue heating [60]. Specifically, conductive tissue cooling can occur at the margin of the zone of ablation, and local failures can occur in as much as a third of such masses [61].

A recent large series demonstrates no clear differences between the technologies with regard to complication and local recurrence-free rates [43,60]. The debate about which technology is more effective is essentially over, with RFA and CA demonstrating equal efficacy and morbidity [62]. Long-term data on oncological efficacy and more rigorous head to head trials are needed to establish any different role of CA and RFA in the management of small renal tumors.

Other Ablative Techniques

Several recent studies have assessed the safety and efficacy of emerging ablation techniques for treatment of SRMs. Microwave ablation performed substantially worse than would be expected following CA or RFA and should not be used routinely for ablation of SRMs when these other established techniques are available [63,64]. Laser-induced thermal therapy is also experimental, and there are currently no long-term experiences regarding its use for ablation of renal tumors [63]. Irreversible electroporation (IRE) is a non-thermal ablative technique using direct electrical pulses to induce apoptosis and ultimately cell death in the exposed area [65]. Although preliminary results suggest IRE induces effective necrosis and is safe in humans [65,66], more data on efficacy is required before IRE can be endorsed for the treatment of SRMs. HIFU is a technique of thermal ablation using focused ultrasound waves that can achieve a temperature sufficient for immediate thermal destruction of all tissue within the target zone [6,63]. Limited clinical data on extracorporeal HIFU of SRM show generally unsatisfactory results with suboptimal outcomes compared with other thermal ablative techniques, and there is still no reliable real-time monitoring during the procedure [6,63,65]. Although there have been no serious side effects from HIFU, it appears to be inadequate, in its current state, for treatment of RCC, and it also needs to be further evaluated and validated in prospective clinical studies before widespread application.

Treatment Trends for Stage I RCC

Increased early detection of low-stage renal tumors has decreased the proportion of tumors diagnosed at advanced stages but has not altered the age adjusted incidence rate of advanced disease [2,67]. With acceptance of the oncological safety of NSS and appreciation of the importance of renal preservation, a recent analysis of the National Cancer Database revealed rates of NSS continue to increase [68]. The rate of PN increased more than fourfold between 1993–1995 and

2005–2007, from 6.3% to 32.2%, whereas the use of total nephrectomy decreased from 88.3% to 57.7% over the same period [68]. A contemporary analysis of the Surveillance, Epidemiology and End Result (SEER) database also documented an increase in the PN rate as of 2006, up to 45% of cases of 2- to 4-cm lesions [55]. The use of focal ablation has also increased from 1.0% to 6.8% [68], and the use of AS varied from 2.9% to 5.1%, with no consistent trend in application over time. However, management decisions reflect patient and tumor characteristics that are poorly captured using secondary data sources, and contemporary studies using administrative or registry data to assess national practice patterns inadequately reflect case mix and may give biased results [69]. Examination of institutional level data reveals a decrease in the use of ATs, likely because they have been partly supplanted by AS in recognition of the limited biologic aggressiveness of most SRMSs [69,70].

The Role of RMB

Traditionally, RMB has been used in specific clinical scenarios in which a tissue diagnosis would obviate surgery, such as renal lymphoma, metastatic carcinoma, infection/ abscess, or performed concurrent with ATs [8,71]. However, concerns regarding RMB safety, diagnostic yield, accuracy, and the limited impact of RMB on treatment decisions, based on the perception that all solid SRMs have malignant potential and should be removed with surgery upfront, have limited the widespread adoption of RMB. However, increasing detection of incidental SRMs, development of management alternatives in select patients, and the discovery of several effective biologically targeted drugs for metastatic disease, have raised the awareness that pretreatment tumor histology can be useful and necessary to individualize treatment decisions [7]. Increased expertise in biopsy performance and pathological interpretation of RMB, use of modern biopsy

techniques, and increasing confidence of urologists in using biopsy results to support treatment decisions have helped to overcome the traditional limitations of RMB and fuel a renewed interest in RMB as a routine diagnostic tool [7,8,72].

The role of RMB has expanded to include the evaluation of complex cystic lesions, SRMs 4 cm or smaller, and determination of tumor subtype (Table 10.3) [8,73,74]. Because clinicians cannot rely on imaging alone to differentiate benign from malignant SRM [75], RMB can define oncological risk. The largest increase in incidentally detected SRMs has occurred among patients 70–89 years of age, in whom comorbidities are more frequent and the risk of competing-cause mortality is higher [76]. Competing-cause mortality increases with older patient age, regardless of tumor size [77], and increased comorbidity (as measured by Charlson Comorbidity Index) is associated with worse overall survival after standard surgical tumor resection [19,78]. For patients who are candidates for a wide range of treatment options ranging from AS to AT to PN or RN, RMB can be useful in the management of any solid, contrast-enhancing SRMs when the histologic diagnosis has the potential of impacting the choice of treatment [8]. Importantly, for young and healthy patients, RMB is not routinely recommended because long-term oncologic outcomes of nonsurgical therapies are not available, and there may be a risk of histologic transformation with a renal tumor under prolonged observation [7].

RMB: Safety

RMB is a safe procedure with minimal morbidity. Contemporary series reveal overall complications rates ranging from 1.4% [8,78–86] to 4.7% [71,87–93], with major complications reported in 0.46% [8,79,80,94]. Potential complications of RMB include bleeding, tumor seeding, infection, pneumothorax, and arteriovenous fistula [7,8,92]. Most RMB-related complications are minor and related to bleeding, but clinically significant bleeding is unusual

Table 10.3 Current Indications and Contraindications for Renal Mass Biopsy.

Indications	
Absolute	• Indeterminate SRM on abdominal imaging
	• Suspicious renal mass and known extrarenal malignancy
	• Incidentaloma in candidates for AS or ablative therapy
	• Suspected lymphoma
	• Confirm histologic success and monitor for recurrence following thermal ablation
	• Renal mass and febrile UTI, possible abscess
	• Metastatic renal tumor, to select optimal biologic systemic therapy
	• Unresectable retroperitoneal tumors involving the kidney
Relative	• Uni-/bilateral multifocal tumors
	• Solitary kidney
	• Medically unfit
Emerging	• Enhancing SRM
	• Indeterminate cystic lesions
	• Determine histologic subtype in metastatic RCC
Contraindications	• Coagulopathy (uncorrected)
	• Patients who are not candidates for any type of therapy (surgery, ablation, medical therapy) given limited life expectancy

AS, active surveillance; RCC, renal cell carcinoma; SRM, small renal mass; UTI, urinary tract infection.

and almost always self-limiting. The overall estimated risk of tract seeding is<0.01% [7,95], and with only a handful of case reports documenting its occurrence and no reported cases since 1994, tumor seeding should be considered anecdotal [74].

RMB: Diagnostic Accuracy for Malignancy

The ultimate benefit of RMB is to better and more appropriately pair tumor biology to treatment, so its value is dependent upon the clinical scenario encountered and the accuracy of RMB in determination of malignancy and tumor grade. Among recent series, diagnostic yield of RMB ranges from 78% to 100%, while sensitivity and specificity for the diagnosis of malignancy are 86–100% and 100%, respectively (Table 10.4) [13,79,80,83,84,86,90,96,97]. In a review of 2474 recent RMB results, PPV and NPV for the diagnosis of malignancy were 97.5% and 82%, respectively, with an overall sensitivity of 92.1% and specificity of 89.7% [71].

Although the rate of nondiagnostic biopsy remains in the range of 10–20%, in patients with an initially nondiagnostic biopsy, the diagnostic rate on rebiopsy is high, from 75–100% [79,82,84,86,94,96,98,99].

RMB: Inaccuracy

Inaccurate RMB, including false-negative and false-positive results, represents the most concerning outcome for clinicians. Fortunately the rate of false-negative RMB (excluding noninformative RMB) among modern series ranges from 0% to 3.8% [8,83,109]. Sampling error, tumor necrosis, and tumor heterogeneity are responsible for most false-negative biopsy results [88]. Smaller tumors can be more difficult to visualize and target [92], but larger tumors are prone to sampling error given the greater incidence of necrosis [88,98]. In a series of 115 core RMBs, the false-negative rate was lowest for tumors 4–6 cm in diameter (2.3%), compared with small (1–3 cm; 13%) and large (>6 cm; 12%) tumors [88]. In a larger series of

Table 10.4 Contemporary Outcomes from Renal Mass Biopsy Series.

Series	Tumors (n)	Accuracy (%)				Complications (%)
		Diagnosis	Malignancy	RCC Subtype	Grade	
Lebret *et al.* [100]	119	79	86	86	74*	0
Richter *et al.* [101]	205	62.4	38.3	NA	NA	NA
Dechet *et al.* [102]	100	100	76	NA	NA	NA
Shannon *et al.* [103]	235	78	100	98	NA	0.9
Volpe *et al.* [104]	100	84	100	100	75*	1.0
Veltri *et al.* [105]	103	100	NA	93.2	NA	5.3
Leveridge *et al.* [106]	345	80.6	99.7	88	63.5	0.3
Veltri *et al.* [105]	150	100	NA	93.2	NR	0
Maturen *et al.* [107]	152	96	Sensitivity 97.7 Specificity 100	NA	NA	1.3
Wang *et al.* [108]	110	90.9	100	96.6	NR	1.8

Restricted to series with at least 100 biopsies performed for brevity

* Classified as low- (Fuhrman) grade I/II or high- (Fuhrman) grade III/IV.
RCC, renal cell carcinoma.

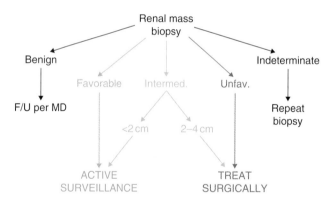

Figure 10.2 Simplified biopsy directed management algorithm designating active surveillance compared with treatment based on mass size and histological risk category. Reproduced with permission from Elsevier[102].

345 RMBs, the odds ratio for a diagnostic result was 2.3 (95% CI, 1.5–6.3) for each 1-cm increase in tumor size [13].

Concern for a coexisting malignancy in otherwise benign tumors is also a significant barrier to RMB acceptance, undermining the validity of RMB and likely deterring its routine use [71,110]. Hybrid tumor rates as high as 27.1% have been reported [110], but this discrepancy stems from the pathological criteria used to classify the malignant component, and importantly, hybrid tumors are believed to be generally nonaggressive [110,111].

Collectively, these data suggest that uncertainty regarding hybrid malignant pathology coexisting with benign pathological components should not deter RMB in efforts to minimize overtreatment of SRMs, especially in frail and comorbid populations [111]. Finally, the accuracy of grading renal cell cancers with percutaneous biopsy is controversial and largely unreliable, with reported accuracy for grading ranging from 43% to 75% [75,84,90,96,112,113]. Accepting these limitations, a RMB-directed management algorithm has been proposed (Figure 10.2).

Challenges Posed by Intratumoral Heterogeneity

A potential challenge in the imagined future of oncology is its underestimation of tumor heterogeneity—not just heterogeneity between tumors, which is a central feature of the concept of personalized medicine, but heterogeneity within an individual tumor [114]. Gerlinger *et al* [9] performed unbiased whole-exome sequencing of multiple primary and metastatic RCC tumor sites in several different patients to map genetic heterogeneity within a single tumor. A majority of somatic mutations were not present ubiquitously within a tumor, and branched evolutionary tumor development was evident [9]. Approximately two-thirds of the mutations (including point mutations, allelic imbalance, and ploidy) that were found in single biopsies were not uniformly detectable throughout all the sampled regions of the same patient's tumor [9]. "Favorable" and "unfavorable" prognostic gene profiles were expressed in different regions of the same tumor. Unlike previous studies using next-generation sequencing of a single index lesion per patient and targeted sequencing of the mutated genes in other sites, the author's independently sequenced and validated mutant gene expression and altered function throughout primary and metastatic sites.

Further, there were widespread alterations in the total number of tumor cell chromosomes (aneuploidy) and detection of many allelic imbalances at the chromosomal level, in which one allele of a gene pair was lost [9,114]. These imbalances can be the result of chromosome loss or gene imprinting and may also alter gene expression [114]. Convergent evolution was also evident, with different tumor regions containing different mutations within the same genes. This article underscores the importance of dynamic tumor-cell functions as the tumor expands and evolves [9,114]. Tumor heterogencity presents a considerable therapeutic challenge because treatment choices based on a biomarker present in a single biopsy specimen may not be uniformly valid [115], and genomics analyses from single tumor-biopsy specimens may underestimate the mutational burden of heterogeneous tumors [9]. Thus, a single tumor biopsy, the standard of tumor diagnosis and the cornerstone of personalized medicine decisions, might not be representative of the entire landscape of genomic abnormalities. Given that selective gene activation and inactivation occurs to guarantee tumor survival, the genes that are affected by convergent evolution may be suitable targets for functional inhibition or restoration. However, the concept of directing therapy on the basis of genetic tumor markers is probably too simple. Reconstructing tumor clonal architectures and the identification of common mutations located in the trunk of the phylogenetic tree may be needed, to lead to more robust biomarkers and therapeutic approaches [9].

Conclusions

The increased use of imaging has led to an increase in the incidence of asymptomatic SRMs. Surgical removal with nephron preservation when technically feasible remains the standard of care for management of the T1 renal mass. Increased recognition that a significant proportion of SRMs are benign or low grade with an indolent clinical course has resulted in development and increased use of less invasive and potentially less morbid treatments. ATs such as CA and RFA are an option for treatment of the SRM in older patients with significant medical comorbidities who are poor candidates for standard extirpative surgical approaches. ATs may offer potentially curative outcomes while conferring several advantages over extirpative surgery, including improved patient procedural tolerance, faster recovery, better preservation of renal function, and reduction in the risk of intraoperative and postsurgical complications, but until longer-term efficacy data are available, AT should be considered a restricted treatment option only for the patient at high surgical risk who desires active treatment. Patients considering ATs should be informed regarding the risks of local recurrence, the potential need for re-intervention, the lack of consensus regarding radiographic and pathologic parameters for treatment success, and for the potential for difficult surgical salvage if tumor recurrence or progression subsequently occurs.

Novel ATs are emerging, but most remain investigational and further study is required before they can be advocated for routine clinical use. Advances in the understanding of the limited biological potential of many SRMs, expanding treatment and surveillance options for RCC, improved biopsy techniques, and the integration of molecular factors into

prognostic and therapeutic algorithms have led to renewed interest in RMB. RMB of SRMs can be useful in select patients at high surgical risk to support treatment decisions and avoid unnecessary surgery. Intratumoral heterogeneity presents a considerable therapeutic challenge because treatment choices based on a biomarker present in a single biopsy specimen may not be entirely valid, and genomics analyses from single tumor-biopsy specimens may underestimate the mutational burden of heterogeneous tumors. Future studies should be directed at the long-term oncologic efficacy of AT and address reliability of radiographic-based metrics as outcome measures.

References

1 Ljungberg B, Campbell SC, Choi HY, Jacqmin D, Lee JE, Weikert S, *et al.* The epidemiology of renal cell carcinoma. Eur Urol. 2011 Oct;60(4):615–21.

2 Kane CJ, Mallin K, Ritchey J, Cooperberg MR, Carroll PR. Renal cell cancer stage migration: Analysis of the National Cancer Data Base. Cancer. 2008 Jul 1;113(1):78–83.

3 Campbell SC, Novick AC, Belldegrun A, Blute ML, Chow GK, Derweesh IH, *et al.* Guideline for management of the clinical T1 renal mass. J Urol. 2009 Oct;182(4):1271–9.

4 Ljungberg B, Cowan NC, Hanbury DC, Hora M, Kuczyk MA, Merseburger AS, *et al.* EAU guidelines on renal cell carcinoma: The 2010 update. Eur Urol. 2010 Sep; 58(3):398–406.

5 Gill IS, Aron M, Gervais DA, Jewett MA. Clinical practice. Small renal mass. New Engl J Med. 2010 Feb 18;362(7):624–34.

6 Volpe A, Cadeddu JA, Cestari A, Gill IS, Jewett MA, Joniau S, *et al.* Contemporary management of small renal masses. Eur Urol. 2011 Sep;60(3):501–15.

7 Volpe A, Finelli A, Gill IS, Jewett MA, Martignoni G, Polascik TJ, *et al.* Rationale for percutaneous biopsy and histologic characterisation of renal tumours. Eur Urol. 2012 Sep;62(3):491–504.

8 Samplaski MK, Zhou M, Lane BR, Herts B, Campbell SC. Renal mass sampling: An enlightened perspective. Int J Urol. 2011 Jan;18(1):5–19.

9 Gerlinger M, Rowan AJ, Horswell S, Larkin J, Endesfelder D, Gronroos E, *et al.* Intratumor heterogeneity and branched evolution revealed by multiregion sequencing. New Engl J Med. 2012 Mar 8; 366(10):883–92.

10 Frank I, Blute ML, Cheville JC, Lohse CM, Weaver AL, Zincke H. Solid renal tumors: An analysis of pathological features related to tumor size. J Urol. 2003 Dec; 170(6 Pt 1):2217–20.

11 Nguyen MM, Gill IS. Effect of renal cancer size on the prevalence of metastasis at diagnosis and mortality. J Urol. 2009 Mar; 181(3):1020–7; discussion 1027.

12 Choudhary S, Rajesh A, Mayer NJ, Mulcahy KA, Haroon A. Renal oncocytoma: CT features cannot reliably distinguish oncocytoma from other renal neoplasms. Clin Radiol. 2009 May;64(5):517–22.

13 Leveridge MJ, Finelli A, Kachura JR, Evans A, Chung H, Shiff DA, *et al.* Outcomes of small renal mass needle core biopsy, nondiagnostic percutaneous biopsy, and the role of repeat biopsy. Eur Urol. 2011 Sep;60(3):578–84.

14 Hollingsworth JM, Miller DC, Daignault S, Hollenbeck BK. Rising incidence of small renal masses: A need to reassess treatment effect. J Natl Cancer Instit. 2006 Sep 20; 98(18):1331–4.

15 Miller DC, Schonlau M, Litwin MS, Lai J, Saigal CS, Urologic Diseases in America P. Renal and cardiovascular morbidity after partial or radical nephrectomy. Cancer. 2008 Feb 1;112(3):511–20.

16 Thompson RH, Boorjian SA, Lohse CM, Leibovich BC, Kwon ED, Cheville JC, *et al.* Radical nephrectomy for pT1a renal masses may be associated with decreased overall survival compared with partial nephrectomy. J Urol. 2008 Feb;179(2): 468–71; discussion 472–3.

17 Motzer RJ, Agarwal N, Beard C, Bolger GB, Boston B, Carducci MA, *et al.* NCCN clinical practice guidelines in oncology: Kidney cancer. J Natl Compr Canc Netw. 2009 Jun;7(6):618–30.

18 Weight CJ, Larson BT, Fergany AF, Gao T, Lane BR, Campbell SC, *et al.* Nephrectomy induced chronic renal insufficiency is associated with increased risk of cardiovascular death and death from any cause in patients with localized cT1b renal masses. J Urol. 2010 Apr;183(4):1317–23.

19 Lane BR, Abouassaly R, Gao T, Weight CJ, Hernandez AV, Larson BT, *et al.* Active treatment of localized renal tumors may not impact overall survival in patients aged 75 years or older. Cancer. 2010 Jul 1; 116(13):3119–26.

20 Sun M, Trinh QD, Bianchi M, Hansen J, Hanna N, Abdollah F, *et al.* A non-cancer-related survival benefit is associated with partial nephrectomy. Eur Urol. 2012 Apr;61(4):725–31.

21 Sun M, Bianchi M, Hansen J, Trinh QD, Abdollah F, Tian Z, *et al.* Chronic kidney disease after nephrectomy in patients with small renal masses: A retrospective observational analysis. Eur Urol. 2012 Oct;62(4):696–703.

22 Go AS, Chertow GM, Fan D, McCulloch CE, Hsu CY. Chronic kidney disease and the risks of death, cardiovascular events, and

hospitalization. New Engl J Medi. 2004 Sep 23;351(13):1296–305.

23 Levey AS, Coresh J. Chronic kidney disease. Lancet. 2012 Jan 14;379(9811):165–80.

24 Tan HJ, Norton EC, Ye Z, Hafez KS, Gore JL, Miller DC. Long-term survival following partial vs radical nephrectomy among older patients with early-stage kidney cancer. JAMA. 2012 Apr 18;307(15):1629–35.

25 Kim SP, Murad MH, Thompson RH, Boorjian SA, Weight CJ, Han LC, *et al.* Comparative effectiveness for survival and renal function of partial and radical nephrectomy for localized renal tumors: A systematic review and meta-analysis. J Urol. 2012 Oct 18. pii: S0022-5347(12)05254-8.

26 Tomaszewski JJ SM, Uzzo RG, Kutikov A. Is radical nephrectomy a legitimate therapeutic option in patients with renal masses amenable to nephron-sparing surgery? BJU Int. 2015 Mar;115(3):357–63.

27 Van Poppel H, Da Pozzo L, Albrecht W, Matveev V, Bono A, Borkowski A, *et al.* A prospective, randomised EORTC intergroup phase 3 study comparing the oncologic outcome of elective nephron-sparing surgery and radical nephrectomy for low-stage renal cell carcinoma. Eur Urol. 2011 Apr;59(4):543–52.

28 Scosyrev E, Messing EM, Sylvester R, Campbell S, Van Poppel H. Renal Function After Nephron-sparing Surgery Versus Radical Nephrectomy: Results from EORTC Randomized Trial 30904. Eur Urol. 2014;65(2):372–7.

29 Piaggio G, Elbourne DR, Altman DG, Pocock SJ, Evans SJ, Group C. Reporting of noninferiority and equivalence randomized trials: An extension of the CONSORT statement. JAMA. 2006 Mar 8;295(10):1152–60.

30 Yoshimura K, Okubo K, Ichioka K, Terada N, Matsuta Y, Arai Y. Laparoscopic partial nephrectomy with a microwave tissue coagulator for small renal tumor. J Urol. 2001 Jun;165(6 Pt 1):1893–6.

31 Watkin NA, Morris SB, Rivens IH, ter Haar GR. High-intensity focused ultrasound ablation

of the kidney in a large animal model.
J Endourol. 1997 Jun;11(3):191–6.

32 Olweny EO, Kapur P, Tan YK, Park SK, Adibi M, Cadeddu JA. Irreversible electroporation: Evaluation of nonthermal and thermal ablative capabilities in the porcine kidney. Urology. 2013 Mar;81(3): 679–84.

33 Winterroth F, Xu Z, Wang TY, Wilkinson JE, Fowlkes JB, Roberts WW, *et al.* Examining and analyzing subcellular morphology of renal tissue treated by histotripsy. Ultrasound Med Biol. 2011 Jan;37(1):78–86.

34 Kapoor A, Touma NJ, Dib RE. Review of the efficacy and safety of cryoablation for the treatment of small renal masses. Can Urol Assoc J.2013 Jan;7(1):E38–44.

35 Vricella GJ, Ponsky LE, Cadeddu JA. Ablative technologies for urologic cancers. Urol Clin North Am. 2009 May;36(2): 163–78, viii.

36 Woolley ML, Schulsinger DA, Durand DB, Zeltser IS, Waltzer WC. Effect of freezing parameters (freeze cycle and thaw process) on tissue destruction following renal cryoablation. J Endourol. 2002 Sep;16(7):519–22.

37 Friedman M, Mikityansky I, Kam A, Libutti SK, Walther MM, Neeman Z, *et al.* Radiofrequency ablation of cancer. Cardiovasc Interven Radiol. 2004 Sep–Oct;27(5):427–34.

38 Corwin TS, Lindberg G, Traxer O, Gettman MT, Smith TG, Pearle MS, *et al.* Laparoscopic radiofrequency thermal ablation of renal tissue with and without hilar occlusion. J Urol. 2001 Jul;166(1):281–4.

39 Shah DR, Green S, Elliot A, McGahan JP, Khatri VP. Current oncologic applications of radiofrequency ablation therapies. World J Gastrointest Oncol. 2013 Apr 15;5(4):71–80.

40 Remer EM, Weinberg EJ, Oto A, O'Malley CM, Gill IS. MR imaging of the kidneys after laparoscopic cryoablation. AJR Am J Roentgenol. 2000 Mar;174(3):635–40.

41 Atwell TD, Farrell MA, Leibovich BC, Callstrom MR, Chow GK, Blute ML, *et al.*

Percutaneous renal cryoablation: Experience treating 115 tumors. J Urol. 2008 Jun;179(6):2136–40; discussion 2140–1.

42 Mirza AN, Fornage BD, Sneige N, Kuerer HM, Newman LA, Ames FC, *et al.* Radiofrequency ablation of solid tumors. Cancer J. 2001 Mar-Apr;7(2):95–102.

43 El Dib R, Touma NJ, Kapoor A. Cryoablation vs radiofrequency ablation for the treatment of renal cell carcinoma: A meta-analysis of case series studies. BJU Int. 2012 Aug;110(4):510–6.

44 Lehman DS, Hruby GW, Phillips CK, McKiernan JM, Benson MC, Landman J. First Prize (tie): Laparoscopic renal cryoablation: Efficacy and complications for larger renal masses. J Endourol. 2008 Jun;22(6):1123–7.

45 Johnson DB, Solomon SB, Su LM, Matsumoto ED, Kavoussi LR, Nakada SY, *et al.* Defining the complications of cryoablation and radio frequency ablation of small renal tumors: A multi-institutional review. J Urol. 2004 Sep;172(3):874–7.

46 Finley DS, Beck S, Box G, Chu W, Deane L, Vajgrt DJ, *et al.* Percutaneous and laparoscopic cryoablation of small renal masses. J Urol. 2008 Aug;180(2):492–8; discussion 498.

47 Psutka SP, Feldman AS, McDougal WS, McGovern FJ, Mueller P, Gervais DA. Long-term oncologic outcomes after radiofrequency ablation for T1 renal cell carcinoma. Eur Urol. 2013 Mar;63(3):486–92.

48 Hegarty NJ, Gill IS, Desai MM, Remer EM, O'Malley CM, Kaouk JH. Probe-ablative nephron-sparing surgery: Cryoablation versus radiofrequency ablation. Urology. 2006 Jul;68(1 Suppl):7–13.

49 Matsumoto ED, Johnson DB, Ogan K, Trimmer C, Sagalowsky A, Margulis V, *et al.* Short-term efficacy of temperature-based radiofrequency ablation of small renal tumors. Urology. 2005 May; 65(5):877–81.

50 Hiraoka K, Kawauchi A, Nakamura T, Soh J, Mikami K, Miki T. Radiofrequency ablation

for renal tumors: Our experience. Int J Urol. 2009 Nov;16(11):869–73.

51 Schwartz BF, Rewcastle JC, Powell T, Whelan C, Manny T, Jr., Vestal JC. Cryoablation of small peripheral renal masses: A retrospective analysis. Urology. 2006 Jul;68(1 Suppl):14–8.

52 Bandi G, Wen CC, Hedican SP, Moon TD, Lee FT, Jr., Nakada SY. Cryoablation of small renal masses: Assessment of the outcome at one institution. BJU Int. 2007 Oct;100(4):798–801.

53 Desai MM, Aron M, Gill IS. Laparoscopic partial nephrectomy versus laparoscopic cryoablation for the small renal tumor. Urology. 2005 Nov;66(5 Suppl):23–8.

54 Levinson AW, Su LM, Agarwal D, Sroka M, Jarrett TW, Kavoussi LR, *et al.* Long-term oncological and overall outcomes of percutaneous radio frequency ablation in high risk surgical patients with a solitary small renal mass. J Urol. 2008 Aug;180(2):499–504; discussion 504.

55 Kutikov A, Uzzo RG. The R.E.N.A.L. nephrometry score: A comprehensive standardized system for quantitating renal tumor size, location and depth. J Urol. 2009 Sep;182(3):844–53.

56 Sisul DM, Liss MA, Palazzi KL, Briles K, Mehrazin R, Gold RE, *et al.* RENAL nephrometry score is associated with complications after renal cryoablation: A multicenter analysis. Urology. 2013 Apr; 81(4):775–80.

57 Lucas SM, Stern JM, Adibi M, Zeltser IS, Cadeddu JA, Raj GV. Renal function outcomes in patients treated for renal masses smaller than 4 cm by ablative and extirpative techniques. J Urol. 2008 Jan;179(1):75–9; discussion 9–80.

58 Meng MV. Commentary on "Radiofrequency ablation of incidental benign small renal mass: Outcomes and follow-up protocol." Tan YK, Best SL, Olweny E, Park S, Trimmer C, Cadeddu JA, Department of Urology, University of Texas Southwestern Medical School, Dallas, Texas, TX. Urologic Oncol. 2013 Jan;31(1):132–3.

59 Atwell TD, Farrell MA, Callstrom MR, Charboneau JW, Leibovich BC, Frank I, *et al.* Percutaneous cryoablation of large renal masses: Technical feasibility and short-term outcome. AJR Am J Roentgenol. 2007 May;188(5):1195–200.

60 Atwell TD, Schmit GD, Boorjian SA, Mandrekar J, Kurup AN, Weisbrod AJ, *et al.* Percutaneous ablation of renal masses measuring 3.0 cm and smaller: Comparative local control and complications after radiofrequency ablation and cryoablation. AJR Am J Roentgenol. 2013 Feb; 200(2):461–6.

61 Gervais DA, McGovern FJ, Arellano RS, McDougal WS, Mueller PR. Radiofrequency ablation of renal cell carcinoma: Part 1, Indications, results, and role in patient management over a 6-year period and ablation of 100 tumors. AJR Am J Roentgenol. 2005 Jul;185(1):64–71.

62 Cadeddu JA. Re: Percutaneous ablation of renal masses measuring 3.0 cm and smaller: Comparative local control and complications after radiofrequency ablation and cryoablation. J Urol. 2013 Jul;190(1):63.

63 Klatte T, Shariat SF, Remzi M. systematic review and meta-analysis of perioperative and oncologic outcomes of laparoscopic cryoablation versus laparoscopic partial nephrectomy for the treatment of small renal tumors. 2014 May;191(5): 1209–17.

64 Castle SM, Salas N, Leveillee RJ. Initial experience using microwave ablation therapy for renal tumor treatment: 18-month follow-up. Urology. 2011 Apr;77(4):792–7.

65 Zagoria RJ, Childs DD. Update on thermal ablation of renal cell carcinoma: Oncologic control, technique comparison, renal function preservation, and new modalities. Current urology reports. 2012 Feb;13(1):63–9.

66 Deodhar A, Monette S, Single GW, Jr., Hamilton WC, Jr., Thornton R, Maybody M, *et al.* Renal tissue ablation with irreversible electroporation: Preliminary results in a porcine model. Urology. 2011 Mar;77(3):754–60.

67 Hock LM, Lynch J, Balaji KC. Increasing incidence of all stages of kidney cancer in the last 2 decades in the United States: An analysis of surveillance, epidemiology and end results program data. J Urol. 2002 Jan; 167(1):57–60.

68 Cooperberg MR, Mallin K, Kane CJ, Carroll PR. Treatment trends for stage I renal cell carcinoma. J Urol. 2011 Aug; 186(2):394–9.

69 Smaldone MC, Churukanti G, Simhan J, Kim SP, Reyes J, Zhu F, *et al.* Clinical characteristics associated with treatment type for localized renal tumors: Implications for practice pattern assessment. Urology. 2013 Feb;81(2):269–75.

70 Campbell SC, Mir C. Editorial comment. Urology. 2013 Feb;81(2):275–6; discussion 276.

71 Lane BR, Samplaski MK, Herts BR, Zhou M, Novick AC, Campbell SC. Renal mass biopsy—a renaissance? J Urol. 2008 Jan;179(1):20–7.

72 Klatte T. The contemporary role of renal tumor biopsy. Eur Urol. 2012 Sep;62(3):505–6.

73 Sahni VA, Silverman SG. Biopsy of renal masses: When and why. Cancer Imaging. 2009;9:44–55.

74 Silverman SG, Gan YU, Mortele KJ, Tuncali K, Cibas ES. Renal masses in the adult patient: The role of percutaneous biopsy. Radiology. 2006 Jul;240(1):6–22.

75 Millet I, Doyon FC, Hoa D, Thuret R, Merigeaud S, Serre I, *et al.* Characterization of small solid renal lesions: Can benign and malignant tumors be differentiated with CT? AJR Am J Roentgenology. 2011 Oct; 197(4):887–96.

76 Chow WH, Devesa SS, Warren JL, Fraumeni JF, Jr. Rising incidence of renal cell cancer in the United States. JAMA. 1999 May 5;281(17):1628–31.

77 Hollingsworth JM, Miller DC, Daignault S, Hollenbeck BK. Five-year survival after surgical treatment for kidney cancer: A population-based competing risk analysis. Cancer. 2007 May 1;109(9):1763–8.

78 Santos Arrontes D, Fernandez Acenero MJ, Garcia Gonzalez JI, Martin Munoz M, Paniagua Andres P. Survival analysis of clear cell renal carcinoma according to the Charlson comorbidity index. J Urol. 2008 Mar;179(3):857–61.

79 Shannon BA, Cohen RJ, de Bruto H, Davies RJ. The value of preoperative needle core biopsy for diagnosing benign lesions among small, incidentally detected renal masses. J Urol. 2008 Oct;180(4):1257–61; discussion 1261.

80 Maturen KE, Nghiem HV, Caoili EM, Higgins EG, Wolf JS, Jr., Wood DP, Jr. Renal mass core biopsy: Accuracy and impact on clinical management. AJR Am J Roentgenol. 2007 Feb;188(2):563–70.

81 Reichelt O, Gajda M, Chyhrai A, Wunderlich H, Junker K, Schubert J. Ultrasound-guided biopsy of homogenous solid renal masses. Eur Urol. 2007 Nov;52(5):1421–6.

82 Somani BK, Nabi G, Thorpe P, N'Dow J, Swami S, McClinton S, *et al.* Image-guided biopsy-diagnosed renal cell carcinoma: Critical appraisal of technique and long-term follow-up. Eur Urol. 2007 May; 51(5):1289–95; discussion 1296–7.

83 Schmidbauer J, Remzi M, Memarsadeghi M, Haitel A, Klingler HC, Katzenbeisser D, *et al.* Diagnostic accuracy of computed tomography-guided percutaneous biopsy of renal masses. Eur Urol. 2008 May;53(5):1003–11.

84 Volpe A, Mattar K, Finelli A, Kachura JR, Evans AJ, Geddie WR, *et al.* Contemporary results of percutaneous biopsy of 100 small renal masses: A single center experience. J Urol. 2008 Dec;180(6):2333–7.

85 Masoom S, Venkataraman G, Jensen J, Flanigan RC, Wojcik EM. Renal FNA-based typing of renal masses remains a useful adjunctive modality: Evaluation of 31 renal masses with correlative histology. Cytopathology. 2009 Feb;20(1):50–5.

86 Wang R, Wolf JS, Jr., Wood DP, Jr., Higgins EJ, Hafez KS. Accuracy of percutaneous core biopsy in management of small renal masses. Urology. 2009 Mar;73(3):586–90; discussion 90–1.

87 Johnson PT, Nazarian LN, Feld RI, Needleman L, Lev-Toaff AS, Segal SR, *et al.*

Sonographically guided renal mass biopsy: Indications and efficacy. J Ultrasound Med. 2001 Jul;20(7):749–53; quiz 55.

88 Rybicki FJ, Shu KM, Cibas ES, Fielding JR, vanSonnenberg E, Silverman SG. Percutaneous biopsy of renal masses: Sensitivity and negative predictive value stratified by clinical setting and size of masses. AJR Am J Roentgenol. 2003 May;180(5):1281–7.

89 Eshed I, Elias S, Sidi AA. Diagnostic value of CT-guided biopsy of indeterminate renal masses. Clin Radiol. 2004 Mar;59(3):262–7.

90 Neuzillet Y, Lechevallier E, Andre M, Daniel L, Coulange C. Accuracy and clinical role of fine needle percutaneous biopsy with computerized tomography guidance of small (less than 4.0 cm) renal masses. J Urol. 2004 May;171(5):1802–5.

91 Hara I, Miyake H, Hara S, Arakawa S, Hanioka K, Kamidono S. Role of percutaneous image-guided biopsy in the evaluation of renal masses. Urol Int. 2001;67(3):199–202.

92 Volpe A, Kachura JR, Geddie WR, Evans AJ, Gharajeh A, Saravanan A, et al. Techniques, safety and accuracy of sampling of renal tumors by fine needle aspiration and core biopsy. J Urol. 2007 Aug;178(2):379–86.

93 Caoili EM, Bude RO, Higgins EJ, Hoff DL, Nghiem HV. Evaluation of sonographically guided percutaneous core biopsy of renal masses. AJR Am J Roentgenol. 2002 Aug;179(2):373–8.

94 Vasudevan A, Davies RJ, Shannon BA, Cohen RJ. Incidental renal tumours: The frequency of benign lesions and the role of preoperative core biopsy. BJU Int. 2006 May;97(5):946–9.

95 Herts BR, Baker ME. The current role of percutaneous biopsy in the evaluation of renal masses. Semin Urol Oncol. 1995 Nov;13(4):254–61.

96 Lebret T, Poulain JE, Molinie V, Herve JM, Denoux Y, Guth A, et al. Percutaneous core biopsy for renal masses: Indications, accuracy and results. J Urol. 2007 Oct;178 (4 Pt 1):1184–8; discussion 1188.

97 Veltri A, Garetto I, Tosetti I, Busso M, Volpe A, Pacchioni D, et al. Diagnostic accuracy and clinical impact of imaging-guided needle biopsy of renal masses. Retrospective analysis on 150 cases. Eur Radiol. 2011 Feb;21(2):393–401.

98 Lechevallier E, Andre M, Barriol D, Daniel L, Eghazarian C, De Fromont M, et al. Fine-needle percutaneous biopsy of renal masses with helical CT guidance. Radiology. 2000 Aug;216(2):506–10.

99 Wood BJ, Khan MA, McGovern F, Harisinghani M, Hahn PF, Mueller PR. Imaging guided biopsy of renal masses: Indications, accuracy and impact on clinical management. J Urol. 1999 May;161(5):1470–4.

100 Lebret T, Poulain JE, Molinie V, Herve JM, Denoux Y, Guth A, et al. Percutaneous core biopsy for renal masses: Indications, accuracy and results. J Urol. 2007 Oct; 178(4 Pt 1):1184–8; discussion 1188.

101 Richter F, Kasabian NG, Irwin RJ, Jr., Watson RA, Lang EK. Accuracy of diagnosis by guided biopsy of renal mass lesions classified indeterminate by imaging studies. Urology. 2000 Mar; 55(3):348–52.

102 Dechet CB, Zincke H, Sebo TJ, King BF, LeRoy AJ, Farrow GM, et al. Prospective analysis of computerized tomography and needle biopsy with permanent sectioning to determine the nature of solid renal masses in adults. J Urol. 2003 Jan;169(1):71–4.

103 Shannon BA, Cohen RJ, de Bruto H, Davies RJ. The value of preoperative needle core biopsy for diagnosing benign lesions among small, incidentally detected renal masses. J Urol. 2008 Oct; 180(4):1257–61; discussion 1261.

104 Volpe A, Mattar K, Finelli A, Kachura JR, Evans AJ, Geddie WR, et al. Contemporary results of percutaneous biopsy of 100 small renal masses: A single center experience. J Urol. 2008 Dec;180(6):2333–7.

105 Veltri A, Garetto I, Tosetti I, Busso M, Volpe A, Pacchioni D, et al. Diagnostic accuracy and clinical impact of imaging-guided needle biopsy of renal masses. Retrospective analysis on 150 cases. Eur Radiol. 2011 Feb;21(2):393–401.

106 Leveridge MJ, Finelli A, Kachura JR, Evans A, Chung H, Shiff DA, *et al.* Outcomes of small renal mass needle core biopsy, nondiagnostic percutaneous biopsy, and the role of repeat biopsy. Eur Urol. 2011 Sep;60(3):578–84.

107 Maturen KE, Nghiem HV, Caoili EM, Higgins EG, Wolf JS, Jr., Wood DP, Jr. Renal mass core biopsy: Accuracy and impact on clinical management. AJR Am J Roentgenol. 2007 Feb;188(2):563–70.

108 Wang R, Wolf JS, Jr., Wood DP, Jr., Higgins EJ, Hafez KS. Accuracy of percutaneous core biopsy in management of small renal masses. Urology. 2009 Mar; 73(3):586–90; discussion 90–1.

109 Beland MD, Mayo-Smith WW, Dupuy DE, Cronan JJ, DeLellis RA. Diagnostic yield of 58 consecutive imaging-guided biopsies of solid renal masses: Should we biopsy all that are indeterminate? AJR Am J Roentgenol. 2007 Mar; 188(3):792–7.

110 Waldert M, Klatte T, Haitel A, Ozsoy M, Schmidbauer J, Marberger M, *et al.* Hybrid renal cell carcinomas containing histopathologic features of chromophobe renal cell carcinomas and oncocytomas have excellent oncologic outcomes. Eur Urol. 2010 Apr;57(4):661–5.

110 Ginzburg S, Uzzo R, Al-Saleem T, Dulaimi E, Walton J, Corcoran A, *et al.* Coexisting hybrid malignancy in a solitary sporadic solid benign renal mass: Implications for treating patients following renal biopsy. J Urol. 2014 Feb; 191(2):296–300.

112 Blumenfeld AJ, Guru K, Fuchs GJ, Kim HL. Percutaneous biopsy of renal cell carcinoma underestimates nuclear grade. Urology. 2010 Sep;76(3):610–3.

113 Ficarra V, Brunelli M, Novara G, D'Elia C, Segala D, Gardiman M, *et al.* Accuracy of on-bench biopsies in the evaluation of the histological subtype, grade, and necrosis of renal tumours. Pathology. 2011 Feb; 43(2):149–55.

114 Longo DL. Tumor heterogeneity and personalized medicine. New Engl J Med. 2012 Mar 8;366(10):956–7.

115 Halverson SJ, Kunju LP, Bhalla R, Gadzinski AJ, Alderman M, Miller DC, *et al.* Accuracy of determining small renal mass management with risk stratified biopsies: Confirmation by final pathology. J Urol. 2013 Feb;189(2):441–6.

11

Bladder-Preserving Strategies in the Treatment of Urothelial Cancer: The Disease Spectrum and the Dawn of Molecular Surgical Guidance

Stephan Kruck, MD, and Arnulf Stenzl, MD

Department of Urology, University Hospital Tuebingen, Tuebingen, Germany

Bladder cancer is one of the most frequently diagnosed tumor types and accounts for up to 70,000 new cancer cases per year and approximately 14,000 deaths annually in the United States and an estimated number of about 166,000 newly diagnosed cases and about 59,000 deaths as a result of the disease in Europe in 2012 [1,2]. Approximately 70% of patients initially present with superficial pTa or pT1 tumors. Nonmuscle-invasive bladder cancer (NMIBC) is associated with a high recurrence risk, in part because of persistence of lesions following initial transurethral resection of bladder tumor (TURBT). Furthermore up to 15% of these tumors progress to a muscle-invasive stage, depending on risk stratification, which is associated with a limited 5-year survival rate [3]. Only early diagnosis and complete TURBT can potentially prevent progression to a muscle-invasive stage, which is associated with aforementioned increase in mortality [4]. Therefore NMIBC is one of the main health problems for modern urology.

Diagnosis, management, and long-term follow-up of NMIBC requires noninvasive imaging and invasive endoscopic monitoring. Healthcare costs associated with follow-up endoscopy and TURBT represent about 71% of bladder cancer expenditures [5]. Additionally, these procedures are a substantial burden on patients and to healthcare systems, contributing to one of the highest lifetime costs among the all human cancers [6]. These costs are mainly driven low- and intermediate-risk tumors with a high recurrence rate within the first 2 years but a low progression rate and, fortunately, a high overall 5- and 10-year survival rate [7]. Today the diagnostic and therapeutic work-up of NMIBC is mainly based on macroscopic imaging derived from conventional white light cystoscopy (WLC). Conventional WLC using rigid or flexible endoscopes is currently the gold standard and will remain a fundamental diagnostic tool for the detection and surveillance of patients with bladder cancer, especially in the outpatient setting.

Precise tumor delineation under WLC from normal urothelium is often difficult in endophytic and especially in flat tumors [3,8]. Conventional WLC TURBT has been estimated to overlook 10–20% of papillary and 50% of flat bladder carcinoma in situ (CIS) lesions [9,10]. Additionally, false-positive results are significantly more frequent under WLC resection. Consequently, the goal of future endoscopic imaging should be to define more specific biological targets, which are highly relevant for bladder cancer oncogenesis and to obtain detailed bladder tumor information. In this scenario, the ideal endoscopic modality should be able to distinguish between different (benign and

Management of Urologic Cancer: Focal Therapy and Tissue Preservation, First Edition.
Edited by Mark P. Schoenberg and Kara L. Watts.
© 2017 John Wiley & Sons Ltd. Published 2017 by John Wiley & Sons Ltd.

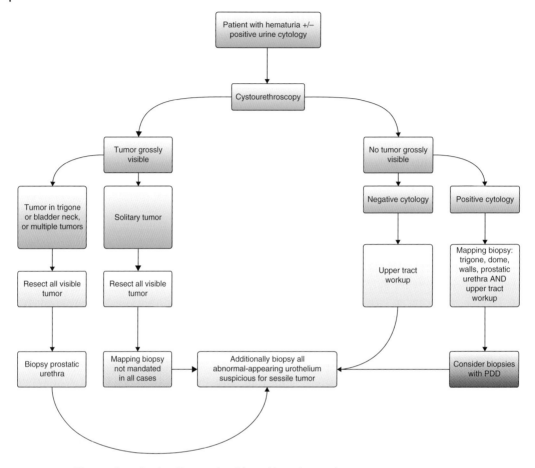

Figure 11.1 Diagnostic evaluation: Hematuria with positive urine cytology.

malignant) lesions, as well as to characterize grade and stage. In the context of maximum bladder preservation, adequate visualization of the primary tumor and an accurate differentiation of normal from tumor infiltrated anatomical layers is urgently needed. Several newly developed technologies show promise in addressing the acknowledged shortcomings of WLC (Figure 11.1).

Augmented Cystoscopy

Macroscopic imaging techniques, such as photodynamic diagnosis (PDD) and narrow band imaging (NBI) were developed to improve TURBT performance. PDD detects fluorescent signals from neoplastic tissue

after selective accumulation of intravesical administrated photoactive porphyrins. Exogenous administration of the hexylesther (hexaminolevulinate, HAL, HEXVIX®) of the photosensitizing agent 5-aminolevulinic acid (5-ALA) induces a transient rise in the cellular concentration of the fluorescent protoporphyrin IX (PpIX), which is more pronounced in urothelial carcinoma. Increased intratumoral neovascularization may explain the observed accumulation of PpIX in bladder tumors; and this hypothesis raises the possibility that photodynamic targeting may someday be used therapeutically [11]. PpIX biosynthesis by 5-ALA is closely linked to potential metabolic targets to the Warburg effect [12]. Today, HAL offers more enhanced fluorescence in shorter time and at lower concentrations compared to its predecessor 5-ALA and is the only approved intravesical photosensitizer by the European Union and the U.S. Food and Drug Administration (FDA). PDD studies have demonstrated improved cancer detection, decreased residual tumor rates, and increased recurrence-free survival [13–16]. A large prospective randomized Phase III trial enrolled 814 patients with NMIBC and showed a relative reduction in cancer recurrence of 16% during the 9-month follow-up in the fluorescence arm and in 16% of patients at least one additional tumor was detected only with PDD guidance [16]. In accordance a recent meta-analysis, including 12 prospective trials, confirmed an improved additional PDD detection rate of 20% for all NMIBC and of 39% for CIS lesions [17]. Based on these positive results PDD is recommended by the European Association of Urology for the detection of CIS [8,18].

Conventional TURBT violates the fundamental oncologic surgical principle of removing en-bloc tumor resection with a safety margin. One of the most promising endosurgical innovations uses transurethral en-bloc water-jet dissection in combination with PDD to clearly define tumor and safety margins. A 30-bar high-pressure water-jet injection needle is used to raise the bladder mucosa and tumor. In this plane, the created liquid cushion enables complete and safe en-bloc electro-resection. The first prospective clinical with 17 included patients underlined the technically feasibility and safety of tumor resection [19]. The currently recruiting HybridBlue-study will compare conventional and hydro-dissection with regard to pathological validity and residual tumor rate [20].

NBI is based on an improved contrast between abnormal and normal tissue. NBI is based on a specific light source that consists of two bandwidths (415 nm [blue] and 540 nm [green]), enhancing the contrast between the light absorption of hemoglobin in capillaries and nonabsorbing mucosa. Because hypervascularity and distinct angiogenic pathways also differ between normal bladder urothelium and superficial and invasive tumors, NBI endoscopy may provide enhanced visualization without the application of an intravesical exogenous contrast agent. NBI is only based on the premise of an enhanced angiogenesis compared to the surrounding normal bladder. Unlike, the contrast-media–enhanced tumor delineation of PDD, the interpretation of NBI images relies on the surgeon's ability to recognize changes in the bladder vasculature. The literature on NBI is less robust than that available for PDD [21]. Recent trials of NBI in the detection of bladder cancer reported additional tumor detection in up to 41% of patients studied [22] and a false-positive rate of 32% compared to WL-TURBT [21–24].

Fiber-Optic Probe Technology

Both PDD and NBI are biased by the fact that not only tumors, but also regenerating and inflammatory cells, show increased angiogenesis or metabolic changes, leading to false-positive findings. In particular patients with concomitant inflammation or scarring after surgery often show mucosal lesions mimicking urothelial tumors that limit preservation of normal urothelium.

More detailed information on cellular morphology of suspicious lesions can be provided by three new technical innovations: optical coherence tomography (OCT), confocal laser endomicroscopy (CLE), and Raman spectroscopy (RS). OCT, CLE, and RS are based on specialized fiber-optic probes. For image acquisition, the endoscopic probe placement depends on WLC or advanced cystoscopic image guidance to identify areas of interest for further characterization.

OCT

OCT uses high-resolution cross-sectional imaging by measuring the intensity of back-reflected infrared light between bladder urothelium, lamina propria, and muscularis. This technique allows noninvasive examination of bladder mucosal surface tissue at microscopic (10–20 μm) resolution [25]. Small nonrandomized studies showed promising results for optical "in vivo biopsy," particularly for three-dimensional (3D) OCT, with sensitivity and specificity rates as high as 92–95% [26].

A small retrospective study reported a 100% sensitivity and 90% specificity in the detection of muscle-invasion in seven lesions of 32 patients with bladder cancer [25].

CLE

CLE is also a probe-based imaging technology that enables real-time in vivo microscopy. CLE has the highest resolution (2–5 μm) in microarchitecture and cellular imaging. CLE technique requires an exogenous contrast agent. Fluorescein, which is an FDA-approved dye for ophthalmic applications is most commonly used intravenously or intravesically. The CLE probe uses a low-power laser light to illuminate tissue by direct contact and records reflected light as video sequences. CLE is currently approved for clinical use in the gastrointestinal and respiratory tracts. In bladder imaging, intravesically administered Fluorescein rapidly stains the extracellular matrix with minimal systemic toxicity [27]. The largest feasibility study included 66 patients and demonstrated distinct differences between normal mucosa and bladder cancer tissue [28].

RS

RS is based on the Raman Effect or inelastic scattering that examines the interaction of

light with molecular bonds. Raman molecular imaging (RMI) combines the molecular chemical analysis of Raman spectroscopy with high-definition digital microscopy allowing the visualization of physical and molecular tissue architecture [29,30]. Initial studies demonstrated high sensitivity and specificity rates of RMI for bladder cancer detection [30]. RS also diagnosed bladder cancer with a high sensitivity (up to 100% in high-grade tumors), and specificity in epithelial cells separated from urine samples obtained from 340 patients, including 116 patients without bladder cancer, 92 patients with low-grade, and 132 high-grade cancer [30]. Additional promising technologies such as ultraviolet auto-fluorescence, multiphoton microscopy, or scanning fiber endoscopy may further expand this growing armamentarium of novel diagnostic and therapeutic tools [31].

Conclusion

The development of adjuncts to diagnostic endoscopy presents both physicians and patients with the tantalizing possibility that the age of molecular surgical guidance has arrived. Concerns related to cost of implementation as well as efficacy and comparative effectiveness will require the execution of robust clinical trials designed to determine whether the promise of early experience will translate into the much hoped for medical and social benefits of improved bladder cancer care.

References

1 Kohler BA, Ward E, McCarthy BJ, Schymura MJ, Ries LA, Eheman C, *et al.* Annual report to the nation on the status of cancer, 1975–2007, featuring tumors of the brain and other nervous system. J Natl Cancer Instit. 2011;103(9):714–36.

2 International Agency for Research on Cancer. Globocan 2012: Estimated cancer incidence and prevalence worldwide in 2012.

3 Stenzl A, Cowan NC, De Santis M, Kuczyk MA, Merseburger AS, Ribal MJ, *et al.* Treatment of muscle-invasive and metastatic bladder cancer: Update of the EAU guidelines. Eur Urol. 2011;59(6):1009–18.

4 Millan-Rodriguez F, Chechile-Toniolo G, Salvador-Bayarri J, Palou J, Algaba F, Vicente-Rodriguez J. Primary superficial bladder cancer risk groups according to

progression, mortality and recurrence. J Urol. 2000;164(3 Pt 1):680–4.

5 Grossman HB SA, Moyad MA, Droller. Bladder cancer: Chemoprevention, complementary approaches and budgetary considerations. Scand J Urol Nephrol Suppl. 2008(218):213–33.

6 Sievert KD, Amend B, Nagele U, Schilling D, Bedke J, Horstmann M, *et al.* Economic aspects of bladder cancer: What are the benefits and costs? World J Urol. 2009;27(3):295–300.

7 Sylvester RJ, van der Meijden AP, Oosterlinck W, Witjes JA, Bouffioux C, Denis L, *et al.* Predicting recurrence and progression in individual patients with stage Ta T1 bladder cancer using EORTC risk tables: A combined analysis of 2596 patients from seven EORTC trials. Eur Urol. 2006;49(3):466–5; discussion 75–7.

8 Babjuk M, Oosterlinck W, Sylvester R, Kaasinen E, Bohle A, Palou-Redorta J. EAU guidelines on non-muscle-invasive urothelial carcinoma of the bladder. Eur Urol. 2008;54(2):303–14.

9 Jichlinski P LH. Fluorescence cystoscopy in the management of bladder cancer: a help for the urologist! Urol Int. 2005;74(2):97–101.

10 Soloway MS MW, Rao MK, Cox C. Serial multiple-site biopsies in patients with bladder cancer. J Urol. 1978;120(1):57–9.

11 Bader MJ, Stepp H, Beyer W, Pongratz T, Sroka R, Kriegmair M, *et al.* Photodynamic therapy of bladder cancer - a phase I study using hexaminolevulinate (HAL). Urol Oncol. 2013;31(7):1178–83.

12 Sugiyama Y, Hagiya Y, Nakajima M, Ishizuka M, Tanaka T, Ogura S. The heme precursor 5-aminolevulinic acid disrupts the Warburg effect in tumor cells and induces caspase-dependent apoptosis. Oncol Rep. 2014;31(3):1282–6.

13 Schmidbauer J, Witjes F, Schmeller N, Donat R, Susani M, Marberger M. Improved detection of urothelial carcinoma in situ with hexaminolevulinate fluorescence cystoscopy. J Urol. 2004;171(1):135–8.

14 Fradet Y, Grossman HB, Gomella L, Lerner S, Cookson M, Albala D, *et al.* A comparison of hexaminolevulinate fluorescence cystoscopy and white light cystoscopy for the detection of carcinoma in situ in patients with bladder cancer: A phase III, multicenter study. J Urol. 2007;178(1):68–73; discussion

15 Grossman HB, Gomella L, Fradet Y, Morales A, Presti J, Ritenour C, *et al.* A phase III, multicenter comparison of hexaminolevulinate fluorescence cystoscopy and white light cystoscopy for the detection of superficial papillary lesions in patients with bladder cancer. J Urol. 2007;178(1):62–7.

16 Stenzl A, Burger M, Fradet Y, Mynderse LA, Soloway MS, Witjes JA, *et al.* Hexaminolevulinate guided fluorescence cystoscopy reduces recurrence in patients with nonmuscle invasive bladder cancer. J Urol. 2010;184(5):1907–13.

17 Kausch I, Sommerauer M, Montorsi F, Stenzl A, Jacqmin D, Jichlinski P, *et al.* Photodynamic diagnosis in non-muscle-invasive bladder cancer: A systematic review and cumulative analysis of prospective studies. Eur Urol. 2010;57(4):595–606.

18 Stenzl A, Kruck S. Should photodynamic diagnosis be standard practice for bladder cancer? Expert Rev Anticancer Ther. 2009;9(6):697–9.

19 Fritsche HM, Otto W, Eder F, Hofstadter F, Denzinger S, Chaussy CG, *et al.* Water-jet-aided transurethral dissection of urothelial carcinoma: A prospective clinical study. J Endourol. 2011;25(10):1599–603.

20 https://drks-neu.uniklinik-freiburg.de/drks_web/navigate.do?navigationId=trial.HTML&TRIAL_ID=DRKS00004414.

21 Zheng C, Lv Y, Zhong Q, Wang R, Jiang Q. Narrow band imaging diagnosis of bladder cancer: systematic review and meta-analysis. BJU Int. 2012;110(11b):E680–E7.

22 Bryan RT, Billingham LJ, Wallace DM. Narrow-band imaging flexible cystoscopy in the detection of recurrent urothelial cancer of the bladder. BJU Int. 2008;101(6):702–5; discussion 705–6.

23 Cauberg EC, Kloen S, Visser M, de la Rosette JJ, Babjuk M, Soukup V, *et al.* Narrow band imaging cystoscopy improves the detection of non-muscle-invasive bladder cancer. Urology. 2010;76(3):658–63.

24 Naselli A, Introini C, Bertolotto F, Spina B, Puppo P. Narrow band imaging for detecting residual/recurrent cancerous tissue during second transurethral resection of newly diagnosed non-muscle-invasive high-grade bladder cancer. BJU Int. 2010;105(2):208–11.

25 Goh AC, Tresser NJ, Shen SS, Lerner SP. Optical coherence tomography as an adjunct to white light cystoscopy for intravesical real-time imaging and staging of bladder cancer. Urology. 2008;72(1):133–7.

26 Kamat AM, Hegarty PK, Gee JR, Clark PE, Svatek RS, Hegarty N, *et al.* ICUD-EAU International Consultation on Bladder Cancer 2012: Screening, diagnosis, and molecular markers. Eur Urol. 2013;63(1):4–15.

27 Chang TC, Liu JJ, Liao JC. Probe-based confocal laser endomicroscopy of the urinary tract: The technique. J Vis Exp. 2013(71):e4409.

28 Wu K, Liu JJ, Adams W, Sonn GA, Mach KE, Pan Y, *et al.* Dynamic real-time microscopy of the urinary tract using confocal laser endomicroscopy. Urology. 2011;78(1):225–31.

29 Draga RO, Grimbergen MC, Vijverberg PL, van Swol CF, Jonges TG, Kummer JA, *et al.* In vivo bladder cancer diagnosis by high-volume Raman spectroscopy. Anal Chem. 2010;82(14):5993–9.

30 Shapiro A, Gofrit ON, Pizov G, Cohen JK, Maier J. Raman molecular imaging: A novel spectroscopic technique for diagnosis of bladder cancer in urine specimens. Eur Urol. 2011;59(1):106–12.

31 Lopez A, Liao JC. Emerging endoscopic imaging technologies for bladder cancer detection. Curr Urol Rep. 2014;15(5):406.

12

Image-Guided Thermal Ablation of Adrenal Malignancies

Kyungmouk Steve Lee, MD,[1] Bradley B. Pua, MD,[1] and Stephen B. Solomon, MD[2]

[1] *Department of Radiology, Division of Interventional Radiology, New York-Presbyterian Hospital/Weill Cornell Medical Center, New York, NY, USA*
[2] *Interventional Radiology Service, Memorial Sloan-Kettering Cancer Center, New York, NY, USA*

Introduction

Adrenal masses are common and may be seen in up to 10% of elderly patients undergoing diagnostic imaging studies [1]. Although the vast majority of these adrenal lesions are benign, the probability of malignancy rises exponentially if an extra-adrenal malignancy is identified [2–4]. The most-common malignant neoplasm of the adrenal gland is metastatic tumor, usually from lung carcinoma, renal cell carcinoma, gastrointestinal tumors, or melanoma. Although local surgical treatment of adrenal metastasis remains controversial, in selected patients with isolated adrenal metastatic disease, adrenalectomy has shown improved survival [5–7]. The most-common primary adrenal neoplasm is nonfunctioning adenoma, with other primary adrenal tumors being myelolipomas, cortisol-producing adenomas, aldosteronomas, pheochromocytomas, and adrenocortical carcinomas. Although nonfunctioning adenoma and myelolipomas generally require no treatment, functional adrenal tumors and adrenal cortical carcinoma are typically treated with surgical resection. Adrenal cortical carcinoma is a rare tumor that responds poorly to chemotherapy or radiation therapy, and therefore surgery is the preferred method of treatment; unfortunately, repeat surgery is often needed because of local recurrence and metastases [8].

Although surgical resection is the current standard treatment for both primary and selected metastatic adrenal tumors, patients who are not operative candidates or who have failed surgery may undergo alternative treatments including arterial embolization, ethanol ablation, and thermal ablation. The focus of this chapter will be on percutaneous image-guided thermal ablation of adrenal malignancies.

Clinical Results

Image-guided percutaneous thermal ablation is a minimally invasive procedure that is used in the treatment of selected adrenal malignancies. Many studies in the literature have demonstrated the effectiveness and safety of percutaneous adrenal tumor ablation in the management of both primary and metastatic adrenal tumors. The earliest studies of thermal ablation in adrenal malignancies were performed using radiofrequency ablation (RFA) or cryoablation, and more recently, microwave ablation.

The first reported study of thermal ablation of the adrenal tumors was in 2003 when Wood *et al.* used RFA to treat 15 adrenocortical carcinoma recurrences or metastases with a mean tumor size of 4.3 cm (range of 1.5–9 cm) [9]. After a mean follow-up of 10.3 months, only 3 of the 15 ablated tumors demonstrated interval growth. Further studies by Mayo-Smith *et al.* [10] and Carrafiello *et al.* [11] corroborated the effectiveness of percutaneous image-guided RFA for the treatment of adrenal metastases (see Table 12.1). In the largest reported single-institution study of image-guided thermal ablation of adrenal metastases, Welch *et al.* treated 36 tumors with a curative intent and one 8.2-cm tumor with planned cryoablation debulking for palliation [12]. In the Welch *et al.* study, the adrenal metastases had a mean size of 3.0 cm with range of 0.8–8.2 cm. Percutaneous computed tomography (CT)-guided cryoablation was performed in 27 tumors and RFA in 10 tumors. Technical success was achieved in 35 (97%) tumors. After a mean follow-up of 22.7 months, local recurrence occurred in only 8.8% of tumors. Among the thermal ablations performed in the 12 patients with solitary metastatic disease (only adrenal gland), there was no local tumor recurrence, and furthermore 6 of 12 patients were cured of their overall disease at a mean follow-up of 29.8 months.

Early clinical results for microwave ablation of adrenal malignancies are also promising [13–15]. In the study by Li *et al.*, CT-guided percutaneous microwave ablation resulted in local control in 9 of 10 tumors after a mean follow-up of 11.3 months [13]. One case of residual tumor at 1-month follow-up was successfully retreated with repeat microwave ablation. Wolf *et al.* reported microwave ablation and radiofrequency ablation in 20 adrenal metastases and three hyperfunctioning adrenal tumors, with a 83% local recurrence-free survival at 45-month mean follow-up [14]. Additional long-term clinical trials are needed to properly evaluate the role of the various thermal ablative modalities (i.e., RFA, microwave ablation, and cryoablation) in the treatment of adrenal malignancies.

Preprocedural Evaluation

A multidisciplinary team comprising of surgeons, oncologists, endocrinologists, and interventional radiologists is required to properly evaluate a patient before percutaneous image-guided thermal ablation of adrenal malignancies. The indications for ablation include patient medical comorbidities, patient's refusal to undergo surgery, unresectable tumors, and recurrent tumors that have failed multiple surgical resections. Preprocedural cross-sectional imaging with contrast-enhanced CT or magnetic resonance imaging (MRI) is obtained to assess the tumor size, tumor location, and optimal approach to the tumor. A thorough history and physical examination as well as pertinent blood work, including internalized normalized ratio (which should be less than 1.5) and platelet count (which should be greater than 50×10^9/L), as well as serum and urine biochemical assays should be performed for functioning tumors.

Preprocedural biopsy may be indicated depending on the clinical scenario. In cases of new or enlarging adrenal lesions or positive positron emission tomography (PET)/CT findings, image-guided ablation without a biopsy may be reasonable [16]. Alternatively, because adrenal tissue is not removed during an ablation, preablation biopsy may be needed to avoid unnecessary treatment of a benign lesion. However, the biopsy itself can induce a hypertensive crisis, especially in the case of a suspected pheochromocytoma. As such, it would be prudent in the work-up of an uncertain adrenal mass to obtain urine biochemical assay because a positive catecholamine would preclude a biopsy.

Patients undergoing adrenal thermal ablation may release catecholamines during the procedure leading to a hypertensive crisis. To prepare the patient for a potential hypertensive issue during an adrenal ablation, consultation with an endocrinologist is helpful to consider preprocedural adrenergic blockade with alpha-blockers [17,18]. Because alpha-blockade is associated with tachycardia,

Table 12.1 Selected Studies of Image-Guided Thermal Ablation of Primary and Metastatic Adrenal Malignancies.

Study	Thermal Ablation Type	Tumor Type	Tumor Size Mean [Range] (cm)	Mean Follow-Up (months)	Local Residual and Recurrence Rate (%)	Complication
Wood et al. [9]	RFA	15 adrenocortical carcinoma recurrences or metastases	4.3 [1.5–9.0]	10.3	20	No major complications
Mayo-Smith et al. [10]	RFA	11 metastases, 1 pheochromocytoma, 1 aldosteronoma	3.9 [1.0–8.0]	11.2	15.3	1 small hematoma; no hypertensive crisis
Carrafiello et al. [11]	RFA	6 metastases	2.9 [1.5–4.0]	21	0	1 hypertensive crisis
Li et al. [13]	Microwave	8 metastases, 1 primary adrenocortical carcinoma	3.8 [2.1–6.1]	11.3	10	1 hypertensive crisis
Wolf et al. [14]	Microwave, RFA	20 metastases, 3 hyperfunctioning tumors	4.2 [1.0–8.0]	45.1	17	2 hypertensive crises
Welch et al. [12]	Cryoablation, RFA	37 metastases	3.0 [0.8–8.2]	22.7	9	16 hypertensive crises, 1 hemothorax, 1 pleural effusion, 1 splenic hemorrhage

RFA, radiofrequency ablation.

many patients require beta-blockers after initiation of alpha-blockers. The premedication protocol typically consists of an alpha-blocker (e.g., phenoxybenzamine) with titration of a beta-blocker (e.g., atenolol) 10–14 days before the adrenal ablation [19]. Additional premedication to inhibit catecholamine synthesis (e.g., alpha-methyl–paratyrosine) may be administered before ablation [18]. However, many patients who are scheduled for adrenal ablation may be normotensive and may be unable to have preprocedure alpha blockade without developing symptoms. Because of the risk of intraprocedural hypertensive crisis, preprocedural consultation with an anesthesiologist is also necessary as most adrenal tumor ablations are performed under general anesthesia with continuous blood pressure monitoring using a radial arterial catheter.

Technical Considerations

Imaging guidance during percutaneous adrenal ablation is usually provided by CT imaging, although ultrasound is sometimes used. CT fluoroscopy is also available to guide real-time insertion of ablation probes. MR fluoroscopy is a less established technique that has the advantage of superior soft-tissue contrast and no radiation dose to the operator. Percutaneous adrenal ablation is often performed with the patient in the ipsilateral decubitus or prone position. When the patient is in the ipsilateral decubitus position, the ablation probe is inserted from the posterior approach to access the adrenal tumor. The ipsilateral decubitus position compresses the ipsilateral lung, which helps avoid pulmonary transgression during probe placement; this position also minimizes the craniocaudal motion of the ipsilateral adrenal gland from respiratory motion [16]. When percutaneous access to the adrenal gland cannot be attained without pulmonary transgression, the patient may be placed in the prone position. In rare cases, when the lung or colon obstructs direct access to the

adrenal gland, a transhepatic approach may be used with caution [20]. To avoid nontarget thermal injury to adjacent critical organs (i.e., kidneys, stomach, colon, liver, pancreas), hydrodissection may be used. During hydrodissection, a percutaneous needle is used to instill fluid between the adrenal gland and the critical organ, providing a thermal buffer. Nonionic fluid (e.g., 5% dextrose) is used for hydrodissection during radiofrequency ablation, whereas normal saline should be avoided because of its electroconductive properties. Contrast may also be mixed with the instilled fluid to differentiate the imaging appearance of the fluid from the ablation zone [21].

Currently, the thermal ablative techniques used in the treatment of adrenal tumors are RFA, cryoablation, and microwave ablation. As the first thermal ablative therapy to be widely used, RFA is the most studied.

RFA

RFA uses electromagnetic energy of a specific range, usually 375–500 kHz, to generate electric current directly to induce thermal destruction of tumor [22]. In the monopolar form of RFA, an active electrode is placed into the tumor under image guidance. A grounding electrode is placed on the thigh to complete the closed circuit. A radiofrequency generator is connected to the active and grounding electrodes, and a voltage gradient is applied, resulting in an oscillating electric field to produce frictional heat [23]. Tissue heating to a temperature greater than 60°C leads to immediate cell death secondary to coagulation necrosis (see Figure 12.1) [22].

There are a varying number of RFA devices currently on the market. These devices vary by utilization of local temperatures or impedance as the endpoint of ablation. Configuration and probe design also varies with some designs, such as the Starburst (Angiodynamics, Latham, NY) that deploy multiple tines from the main electrode shaft, to single shaft designs. Other devices, such as

(a)   (b)   (c)

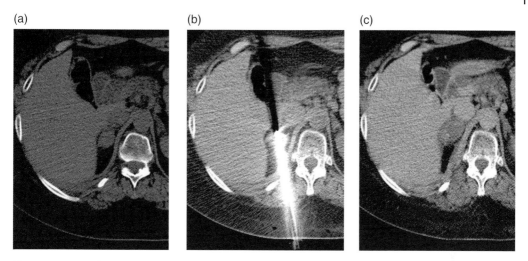

Figure 12.1 Radiofrequency ablation. (a) Preablation images demonstrate the target adrenal mass in close proximity to the right hepatic lobe. (b) Intraprocedural images demonstrate the ablation probe within the lesion. (c) Postablation images, 1 week after ablation, demonstrate heterogeneous density of the target adrenal lesion and decreased density in the abutting liver representing the ablation margin. Increased size of the lesion in the immediate post-ablation setting should not be misinterpreted as treatment failure but attributed to local inflammation.

the Cool-tip device (Covidien, Boulder, CO) uses a single or "triple" cluster electrode that is perfused with cold saline or water pumped internally; this mechanism is thought to distribute tissue heating to reduce charring.

A stepwise RFA protocol for pheochromocytoma metastases has been described by Venkatesan *et al.* using a Covidien ablation device and may be used to help control the release of catecholamines to prevent a hypertensive crisis [24]. The key to the stepwise protocol is time separation of 10–60 seconds between steps. In response to RFA-associated hemodynamic changes, this brief pause allows the physicians to make pharmacologic adjustments (e.g., nitroprusside drip, labetalol, nitroglycerine); therefore, close communication between the operator and the anesthesiologist is required throughout the procedure. The stepwise RFA protocol is as follows: place the RFA probe into the tumor; after a pause of 10–60 seconds, apply an initial 0.1 Amp (A) current for a duration of 10 seconds; after a pause of 10–60 seconds, gradual increase the current until a continuous current of approximately 0.1 A is tolerated by the patient without arterial pressures

increases greater than 200 mm Hg systolic. Next, current increases in 0.1 A increments are applied; each separated by pauses of 10–60 seconds to allow for evaluation of hemodynamic changes and pharmacologic manipulations. This incremental process of gradually increasing the current is immediately terminated if the mean arterial pressure increases 10–20 mm Hg greater than the baseline. The endpoint is reached when the patient tolerates a continuous current of 2 A for 12 minutes. Postablation intratumoral temperature may be measured at the electrode tip to ensure that adequate coagulation necrosis has occurred [24]. Because ablation of any normal adrenal parenchyma has the potential for adrenergic crisis, use of this step-wise protocol should not be limited to treatment of pheochromocytoma.

Microwave Ablation

Microwave ablation uses electromagnetic energy at a much higher frequency range (generally 900–2450 MHz) compared to RFA and is thought to create a larger zone of coagulation necrosis more rapidly [25]. Unlike RFA, microwave ablation does not generate electric current directly but induces alternating electric fields that cause highly polar water molecules to spin rapidly resulting in tissue heating. Compared to RFA, microwave ablation can achieve higher temperatures faster and therefore requires less time to treat a tumor; some believe less ablation time decreases stimulation of the adrenal gland and thereby reduces the risk of hypertensive crisis [13]. However, others believe more rapid elevation of ablative temperatures may make it more difficult to control excessive catecholamine release and associated hemodynamic changes [26]. Six microwave ablation devices are available for use, those that are based on a 2450-MHz generator (Amica, Hospital Service, Rome, Italy; Acculis MTA, Microsulis, AngioDynamics Latham NY; Certus 140, Neuwave, Madison, WI) and those based on a 915-MHz generator (Avecure, Medwaves, San Diego, CA; Evident, Covidien, Mansfield, MA; MicrothermX, BSD Medical, Salt Lake City, UT). The microwave antennae are straight applicators with active tips measuring 0.6–4.0 cm in length with smallest available needle measuring 17-gauge. The proximal portion of the antennae is cooled with room-temperature fluid or carbon dioxide to minimize damage of skin and tissues.

Cryoablation

Cryoablation uses rapid freezing and thawing to cause tumor destruction. Highly pressurized argon gas is used to attain extremely cold temperatures as low as −140°C based on the Joule-Thomson principle. At temperatures less than −40°C, cryogenic tissue destruction occurs as a result of protein denaturation, cell rupture from osmotic water shifts across cell membranes, and microvascular thrombosis-induced ischemia [27]. A key advantage of cryoablation is the easy visualization of the ice ball on CT, MRI, or even ultrasound. The ability to visualize the cryoablative zone with respect to tumor margin allows for treatment of tumors close to vital structures [28]. One limitation of cryoablation may be the lack of control of catecholamine release once the thaw process begins.

Each cryoprobe undergoes a freeze-thaw-freeze cycle to induce thermal coagulation while minimizing bleeding. The thaw portion of the cycle is achieved using helium and the cryoprobe is allowed to reach approximately 20°C. A typical cryoablation protocol consists of a 10-minute freeze of the tumor, followed by an 8-minute thaw, and then a 10-minute freeze. Two cryoablation devices are available: Cryocare (Endocare, Irvine, CA) and Precise (Galil Medical, Arden Mills, MN). A cryoprobe measures 1.5–2.4 mm in diameter. One to 15 cryoprobes may be placed in a single session with each probe achieving thermocoagulation after a single freeze-thaw-freeze cycle.

Complications

Hypertensive crisis is defined as systolic blood pressure greater than 180 mm Hg or diastolic blood pressure greater than 120 mm Hg [29]. During adrenal tumor ablation, hypertensive crisis occurs because of the release of catecholamines [17] and has been reported to occur in up to 43% of cases [12]. In the Welch *et al.* study of 37 adrenal metastases (no pheochromocytomas), all 16 cases of hypertensive crisis were treated successfully and resulted in no major complications; other complications in this study included one case of hemothorax, one case of pleural effusion in a patient who received concurrent treatment of bilateral adrenal metastases, and one case of splenic hemorrhage in a patient who received warfarin. Other studies have reported lower rates of hypertensive crises (see Table 12.1). During cryoablation of adrenal tumors, intraprocedural hypertension tends to occur during the thaw phase possibly because of the release of catecholamines from lysed cells [17,28]. In contradistinction, catecholamine release tends to occur during the heating phase for RFA and microwave ablation. This distinction is important as reversal of the ablation energy can often temporize the problem. For instance, if hypertensive crisis occurs during the active thaw phase of cryoablation, rapid refreezing can often limit the problem allowing time for pharmacologic intervention [30]. In a reported rare life-threatening complication during cryoablation of an adrenal gland metastasis from lung carcinoma, a patient experienced hypertensive crisis at the beginning of the thaw phase and was eventually diagnosed with Takotsubo cardiomyopathy left ventricular dysfunction syndrome [31]. Additional uncommon complications include pneumothorax, hemothorax, infection, pain, and small retroperitoneal hematoma [10,32,33]. Adrenal function is compromised when greater than 90% of the adrenal tissue is destroyed. Therefore, adrenal insufficiency is an uncommon complication of image-guided ablation [10,16,34]. There has not been any mortality attributed to adrenal ablation in the literature.

Follow-up

Although there is currently no standardized follow-up imaging protocol after adrenal ablation, most practitioners generally adhere to established algorithms used in other organs [35–37]. Baseline imaging with contrast-enhanced CT or MRI is performed within 1 month post ablation with subsequent follow-up imaging at 3- and 6- month intervals or 6-month and 12-month intervals depending on the tumor type (Figure 12.2). Nodular enhancement or interval growth represents residual disease or local tumor progression, and early detection of recurrence is important for potential repeat intervention. The short-interval postablation imaging appearance can be heterogeneous as reported by Brook *et al.* who described the CT appearance of 14 tumors after RFA. There is variability in the ablation zone size response, and the ablated tumor demonstrates slightly increased attenuation immediately after the ablation that eventually decreases on long-term follow-up [38]. Air bubbles and fat stranding are often seen in the postablation setting and should not be interpreted as super-infection [38]. For patients with functioning tumors, postablation serum hormone and catecholamine levels should be obtained. Clinical and laboratory follow-up, in conjunction with imaging findings, can confirm local tumor control and guide hormone replacement therapy as needed.

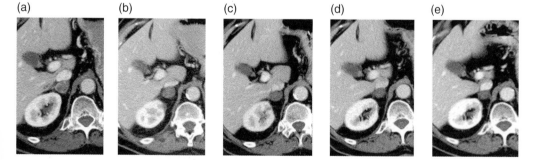

(a) (b) (c) (d) (e)

Figure 12.2 CT follow-up after thermal ablation. (a) Preablation images demonstrate a minimally enhancing right adrenal nodule a biopsy proven lung metastasis. (b) Contrast-enhanced CT 1 month after the ablation demonstrates a lesion, which is heterogenous in attentuation owing to postablation change. (c) Three-month follow-up imaging shows slight decrease in size of the lesion. (d) Eight-month follow-up CT shows continued decrease size of the lesion with no enhancement. (e) Twelve-month follow-up imaging demonstrates a non-enhancing lesion that is further decreased in size. CT, computed tomography.

Conclusion

Image-guided thermal ablation is safe and effective for the local control of primary or metastatic adrenal malignancy. Although minimally invasive, thermal ablation of adrenal tumors does carry the risk of hypertensive crisis, so patients may require pre-procedural adrengergic blockade, general anesthesia, and intraprocedural arterial blood pressure monitoring (such as a radial arterial line). Despite these drawbacks, percutaneous thermal ablation remains an attractive treatment option for patients who are high-risk surgical candidates and cannot undergo adrenalectomy. Image-guided ablation can provide local tumor eradication with decreased morbidity, and early data suggest survival benefit similar to surgery. In a recent study of adrenal metastases, image-guided ablation was associated with a median survival of 34.5 months and local, recurrence-free survival of 88% at 36 months [12]. Future clinical studies with long-term follow-up are warranted to compare the oncologic outcomes among each ablative technique and between adrenal ablation and adrenalectomy.

References

1 Kloos RT, Gross MD, Francis IR, Korobkin M, Shapiro B. Incidentally discovered adrenal masses. Endocr Rev. 1995 Aug;16(4):460–84.

2 Song JH, Chaudhry FS, Mayo-Smith WW. The incidental adrenal mass on CT: Prevalence of adrenal disease in 1,049 consecutive adrenal masses in patients with no known malignancy. AJR Am J Roentgenol. 2008 May;190(5):1163–8.

3 Young WFJ. Clinical practice. The incidentally discovered adrenal mass. N Engl J Med. 2007 Feb 8;356(6):601–10.

4 Lenert JT, Barnett CCJ, Kudelka AP, Sellin RV, Gagel RF, Prieto VG, *et al.* Evaluation and surgical resection of adrenal masses in patients with a history of extra-adrenal malignancy. Surgery. 2001 Dec; 130(6):1060–7.

5 Paul CA, Virgo KS, Wade TP, Audisio RA, Johnson FE. Adrenalectomy for isolated adrenal metastases from non-adrenal cancer. Int J Oncol. 2000 Jul;17(1):181–7.

6 Lo CY, van Heerden JA, Soreide JA, Grant CS, Thompson GB, Lloyd RV, *et al.* Adrenalectomy for metastatic disease to the adrenal glands. Br J Surg. 1996 Apr; 83(4):528–31.

7 Kim SH, Brennan MF, Russo P, Burt ME, Coit DG. The role of surgery in the treatment of clinically isolated adrenal metastasis. Cancer. 1998 Jan 15;82(2):389–94.

8 Pommier RF, Brennan MF. An eleven-year experience with adrenocortical carcinoma. Surgery. 1992 Dec;112(6):963–70; discussion 970–71.

9 Wood BJ, Abraham J, Hvizda JL, Alexander HR, Fojo T. Radiofrequency ablation of adrenal tumors and adrenocortical carcinoma metastases. Cancer. 2003 Feb 1; 97(3): 554–60.

10 Mayo-Smith WW, Dupuy DE. Adrenal neoplasms: CT-guided radiofrequency ablation—preliminary results. Radiology. 2004 Apr;231(1):225–30.

11 Carrafiello G, Lagana D, Recaldini C, Giorgianni A, Ianniello A, Lumia D, *et al.* Imaging-guided percutaneous radiofrequency ablation of adrenal metastases: Preliminary results at a single institution with a single device. Cardiovasc Intervent Radiol. 2008 Aug;31(4):762–7.

12 Welch BT, Callstrom MR, Carpenter PC, Wass CT, Welch TL, Boorjian SA, *et al.* A single-institution experience in image-guided thermal ablation of adrenal gland metastases. J Vasc Interv Radiol JVIR. 2014 Apr;25(4):593–8.

13 Li X, Fan W, Zhang L, Zhao M, Huang Z, Li W, *et al.* CT-guided percutaneous microwave ablation of adrenal malignant carcinoma: Preliminary results. Cancer. 2011 Nov 15;117(22):5182–8.

14 Wolf FJ, Dupuy DE, Machan JT, Mayo-Smith WW. Adrenal neoplasms: Effectiveness and safety of CT-guided ablation of 23 tumors in 22 patients. Eur J Radiol. 2012 Aug;81(8):1717–23.

15 Wang Y, Liang P, Yu X, Cheng Z, Yu J, Dong J. Ultrasound-guided percutaneous microwave ablation of adrenal metastasis: Preliminary results. Int J Hyperth Off J Eur Soc Hyperthermic Oncol North Am Hyperth Group. 2009;25(6):455–61.

16 Uppot RN, Gervais DA. Imaging-guided adrenal tumor ablation. AJR Am J Roentgenol. 2013 Jun;200(6):1226–33.

17 Yamakado K, Takaki H, Yamada T, Yamanaka T, Uraki J, Kashima M, et al. Incidence and cause of hypertension during adrenal radiofrequency ablation. Cardiovasc Intervent Radiol. 2012 Dec; 35(6):1422–7.

18 Sudheendra D, Wood BJ. Appropriate premedication risk reduction during adrenal ablation. J Vasc Interv Radiol JVIR. 2006 Aug;17(8):1367–8.

19 Welch BT, Atwell TD, Nichols DA, Wass CT, Callstrom MR, Leibovich BC, et al. Percutaneous image-guided adrenal cryoablation: Procedural considerations and technical success. Radiology. 2011 Jan; 258(1):301–7.

20 Kuehl H, Stattaus J, Forsting M, Antoch G. Transhepatic CT-guided radiofrequency ablation of adrenal metastases from hepatocellular carcinoma. Cardiovasc Intervent Radiol. 2008 Dec;31(6):1210–4.

21 Gervais DA, Arellano RS, McGovern FJ, McDougal WS, Mueller PR. Radiofrequency ablation of renal cell carcinoma: part 2, Lessons learned with ablation of 100 tumors. AJR Am J Roentgenol. 2005 Jul;185(1).

22 Nahum Goldberg S, Dupuy DE. Image-guided radiofrequency tumor ablation: Challenges and opportunities–part I. J Vasc Interv Radiol JVIR. 2001 Sep; 12(9):1021–32.

23 Organ LW. Electrophysiologic principles of radiofrequency lesion making. Appl Neurophysiol. 1976 1977;39(2).

24 Venkatesan AM, Locklin J, Lai EW, Adams KT, Fojo AT, Pacak K, et al. Radiofrequency ablation of metastatic pheochromocytoma. J Vasc Interv Radiol JVIR. 2009 Nov;20(11):1483–90.

25 Simon CJ, Dupuy DE, Mayo-Smith WW. Microwave ablation: principles and applications. Radiogr Rev Publ Radiol Soc N Am Inc. 2005 Oct;25 Suppl 1.

26 Venkatesan AM, Locklin J, Dupuy DE, Wood BJ. Percutaneous ablation of adrenal tumors. Tech Vasc Interv Radiol. 2010 Jun;13(2).

27 Gage AA, Baust J. Mechanisms of tissue injury in cryosurgery. Cryobiology. 1998 Nov;37(3):171–86.

28 Hinshaw JL, Lee FTJ, Laeseke PF, Sampson LA, Brace C. Temperature isotherms during pulmonary cryoablation and their correlation with the zone of ablation. J Vasc Interv Radiol JVIR. 2010 Sep;21(9):1424–8.

29 Chobanian AV, Bakris GL, Black HR, Cushman WC, Green LA, Izzo JLJ, et al. The Seventh Report of the Joint National Committee on Prevention, Detection, Evaluation, and Treatment of High Blood Pressure: the JNC 7 report. JAMA. 2003 May 21;289(19):2560–72.

30 Atwell TD, Wass CT, Charboneau JW, Callstrom MR, Farrell MA, Sengupta S. Malignant hypertension during cryoablation of an adrenal gland tumor. J Vasc Interv Radiol JVIR. 2006 Mar; 17(3):573–5.

31 Tsoumakidou G, Buy X, Zickler P, Zupan M, Douchet M-P, Gangi A. Life-threatening complication during percutaneous ablation of adrenal gland metastasis: Takotsubo syndrome. Cardiovasc Intervent Radiol. 2010 Jun;33(3):646–9.

32 Mendiratta-Lala M, Brennan DD, Brook OR, Faintuch S, Mowschenson PM, Sheiman RG, et al. Efficacy of radiofrequency ablation in the treatment of small functional adrenal neoplasms. Radiology. 2011 Jan;258(1):308–16.

33 Arima K, Yamakado K, Suzuki R, Matsuura H, Nakatsuka A, Takeda K, et al. Image-

guided radiofrequency ablation for adrenocortical adenoma with Cushing syndrome: outcomes after mean follow-up of 33 months. Urology. 2007 Sep; 70(3):407–11.

34 Williams G, Dluhy R. Diseases of the adrenal cortex. In: Isselbacher KJ, Braunwaald EJ, Wildson JD, Martin JB, Fauci AS, Kasper DL, eds. Harrison's principles of internal medicine. 13th ed. New York, NY: McGraw-Hill; 1994. p. 1953–76.

35 Zagoria RJ. Percutaneous image-guided radiofrequency ablation of renal malignancies. Radiol Clin North Am. 2003 Sep;41(5):1067–75.

36 Rose SC, Dupuy DE, Gervais DA, Millward SF, Brown DB, Cardella JF, *et al.* Research reporting standards for percutaneous thermal ablation of lung neoplasms. J Vasc Interv Radiol JVIR. 2009 Jul;20 (7 Suppl):S474–485.

37 Pua BB, Thornton RH, Solomon SB. Radiofrequency ablation: treatment of primary lung cancer. Semin Roentgenol. 2011 Jul;46(3):224–9.

38 Brook OR, Mendiratta-Lala M, Brennan D, Siewert B, Faintuch S, Goldberg SN. Imaging findings after radiofrequency ablation of adrenal tumors. AJR Am J Roentgenol. 2011 Feb; 196(2):382–8.

13

Managing Penile Cancer: Integrating Tissue Preservation, Energy-Based Therapeutics, and Surgical Reconstruction

Arthur L. Burnett, MD, MBA, FACS

Department of Urology, Johns Hopkins Medical Institutions, Baltimore, MD, USA

Introduction

Although cancer of the penis is a rare genitourinary malignancy, it frequently presents a clinical management dilemma for the urologist. Factors traditionally influencing this effect include delays in clinical presentation, diagnostic error, and ambiguous treatment in terms of efficacy compared with morbidity. Furthermore, the disease itself is recognized as having an adverse health and survival risk profile. Notwithstanding therapeutic intent, prognosis is largely dictated by the pathologic stage of the disease, including extent of lymph node metastasis, coupled with histologic features of the primary tumor [1–5]. Reported 5-year survival rates are 60–80% for patients with inguinal lymph node progression [1,6,7] and 0–15% when pelvic nodal metastases exist [1,8].

Various clinical developments surrounding penile cancer have yielded an improved prognostic outcome for this disease. Advances in staging in such areas as imaging techniques, lymphatic mapping, and surgical biopsy procedures have improved staging accuracy and guided treatment planning. Advances in therapeutic modalities have also been auspicious. Owing to biomedical and technological progress, therapeutic advancements have occurred or are in progress across all modalities of surgery, radiation, and chemotherapy for this disease.

Surgery is well situated in the management of penile cancer, serving several important clinical roles. It facilitates successful diagnosis and staging, by way of excisional or deep biopsy, which are preferable to shave or incisional biopsy. For purposes of definitive treatment, an array of surgical options offer potential ways to eradicate both the primary tumor and its spread to regional lymph nodes. It is acknowledged that controlled clinical trials comparing different treatment modalities for treatment of the primary tumor are lacking. Nonetheless, surgical management occupies a central place in treatment, increasingly aimed toward objectives of reducing morbidity and preserving function of the penis. Although surgical amputation of the primary tumor represents the oncologic gold standard for the treatment of primary penile cancer, emerging opinion holds that organ-preserving treatment is acceptable and should be sought when oncologically feasible to retain quality of life and maximize sexual function. Further support for this conservative strategy derives from analyses indicating that local disease recurrence exerts little influence on long-term survival [9]. Innovative organ-preserving surgery, as well as novel reconstructive strategies, comprise this paradigm shift in management.

This chapter serves to present contemporary surgical approaches for managing penile cancer, with an emphasis on recent surgical

Management of Urologic Cancer: Focal Therapy and Tissue Preservation, First Edition.
Edited by Mark P. Schoenberg and Kara L. Watts.
© 2017 John Wiley & Sons Ltd. Published 2017 by John Wiley & Sons Ltd.

innovations. New developments in schemes and techniques of surgery are presented. Technological advancements that are implemented in combination with surgical procedures are also presented.

Description

Penile cancer comprises benign and malignant tumors of the penis. Squamous cell carcinoma of the penis represents the most common type of malignant neoplasm (48–65% of cases) [10,11]. Its degree of invasiveness distinguishes the invasive form from its superficial counterpart, termed *superficial carcinoma in situ* (i.e., erythroplasia of Queyrat, Bowen disease of the penis, or intraepithelial neoplasia grade III). Penile cancer may also present as a low-grade noninvasive malignancy, commonly termed *verrucous carcinoma*. Other rare types of penile cancer include adeno- and adenosquamous carcinoma, basal cell carcinoma, melanoma, sarcomas, Kaposi sarcoma, neuroendocrine (small-cell) undifferentiated carcinoma, sebaceous gland carcinoma, and metastases from other possible sites (e.g., prostate, bladder, colon, or kidney).

Penile cancer features several commonly associated precursors or risk factors, including phimosis, poor penile hygiene, presence of foreskin, genital viral infections (i.e., human papilloma virus 16, 18, and 33; human immunodeficiency virus), conditions (e.g., leukoplakia, cutaneous horn, Bowenoid papulosis, lichen sclerosis [balanitis xerotica obliterans]), and premalignant lesions (i.e., Giant condylomata [Buschke-Lowenstein] and Paget's disease) [10,11]. Such penile lesions must also be noted in the differential diagnosis of penile cancer. The presence of smegma, desquamated epithelial cells accumulating commonly beneath the prepuce in uncircumcised males, represents a risk factor, although it is not a carcinogen.

Squamous cell carcinoma of the penis arises at various possible locations of the organ: glans, 34.5%; prepuce, 13.2%; shaft, 5.3%; overlapping, 4.5%; unspecified, 42.5% [12]. Its disease course adheres to a predictable pattern of progression. Invasive disease represents disease advancement from superficial carcinoma in situ. Thereafter, the cancer grows into the skin locally and has the potential to invade the corporal bodies before subsequently extending into the regional lymphatic and nodal system, from superficial to deep inguinal lymph nodes and then to pelvic lymph nodes, and usually late in the course of the disease, it may advance as distant metastatic disease. Common metastatic sites for penile cancer include lung, bone, and liver. The extent or stage of disease is currently defined by the unified Union Internationale Contre le Cancer (UICC) and American Joint Committee on Cancer (AJCC) TNM clinical classification system, which describes the primary tumor, regional lymph nodes, and distant metastasis (Table 13.1) [5,13,14]. This system is advantageous in including clinical and pathologic nodal staging descriptors that enable an improved prediction of prognosis and guidance of definitive therapy.

Diagnosis and Staging

As for the evaluation of any disease state, careful clinical history taking and performance of physical examination are fundamental aspects of initial management [10,11]. Besides basic queries of the clinical presentation, such as onset and duration of the condition, it is paramount to explore the descriptive characteristics of the penile lesion including its location and its appearance (e.g., induration, erythema, nodularity, bleeding), as well as presence of pain associated with it. Precipitating features such as prior genital lesions, irritation or trauma, or infections should also be explored. Additional inquiries as to possible risk factors for penile cancer such as presence or absence of foreskin (i.e., whether circumcision has been performed), sexual practices and number of partners, and history of cigarette smoking may also be

Table 13.1 NCCN Guidelines Version 1.2014: Penile Cancer.

NCCN — National Comprehensive Cancer Network®	NCCN Guidelines Version 1.2014 Penile Cancer	NCCN Guidelines Index Penile Cancer TOC Discussion

American Joint Committee on Cancer (AJCC)

TNM Staging System for Penile Cancer (7th ed., 2010)

Primary Tumor (T)

		ANATOMIC STAGE/PROGNOSTIC GROUPS		
TX	Primary tumor cannot be assessed	**Stage 0**	Tis	N0	M0
T0	No evidence of primary tumor		Ta	N0	M0
Ta	Noninvasive verrucous carcinoma*				
Tis	Carcinoma in situ	**Stage I**	T1a	N0	M0
T1a	Tumor invades subepithelial connective tissue without lymph vascular invasion and is not poorly differentiated (i.e., grade 3-4)	**Stage II**	T1b	N0	M0
T1b	Tumor invades subepithelial connective tissue with lymph vascular invasion or is poorly differentiated		T2	N0	M0
			T3	N0	M0
T2	Tumor invades corpus spongiosum or cavernosum				
T3	Tumor invades urethra	**Stage IIIA**	T1-3	N1	M0
T4	Tumor invades other adjacent structures				
Note: Broad pushing penetration (invasion) is permitted; destructive invasion is against the diagnosis		**Stage IIIB**	T1-3	N2	M0

Regional Lymph Nodes (N)

		Stage IV	T4	Any N	M0
Clinical Stage Definition*			Any T	N3	M0
cNX	Regional lymph nodes cannot be assessed		Any T	Any N	M1

cN0 No lymph node metastasis

cN1 Palpable mobile unilateral inguinal lymph node

cN2 Palpable mobile multiple or bilateral inguinal lymph nodes

cN3 Palpable fixed inguinal nodal mass or pelvic lymphadenopathy unilateral or bilateral

Pathologic Stage Definition*

pNX Regional lymph nodes cannot be assessed

pN0 No regional lymph node metastasis

pN1 Metastasis in a single inguinal node

pN2 Metastasis in multiple or bilateral inguinal lymph nodes

pN3 Extranodal extension of lymph node metastasis or pelvic lymph node(s) unilateral or bilateral

*Note: Pathologic stage definition based on biopsy or surgical excision.

Distant Metastasis (M)

M0 No distant metastasis

M1 Distant metastasis

(*Continued*)

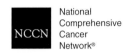

National
Comprehensive **NCCN Guidelines Version 1.2014**
Cancer **Penile Cancer**
Network®

NCCN Guidelines Index
Penile Cancer TOC
Discussion

Edge SB, Byrd DR, Compton CC, *et al.* AJCC cancer staging manual. 7th ed. New York: Springer; 2010.

informative. Baseline urinary (e.g., obstruction, dysuria, hematuria) and sexual (e.g., erection ability, penile sensation) functions should also be ascertained to reveal possible consequences of the condition on lower genitourinary tract function before implementing clinical management that may also affect this function. Prior clinical evaluations and treatments should also be documented.

Physical examination should involve thorough inspection of the penis including the glans and urethral meatus and entire penile shaft. Circumcision status should be noted, and careful evaluation beneath the prepuce is recommended to identify a possible obscure penile cancer lesion. When necessary in the presence of phimosis, dorsal slit may be performed to fully assess the lesion. The concerning penile lesions should be identified by number, size and location, and appearance (e.g., induration, erythema, nodularity, ulceration, bleeding, purulence). The inguinal regions should be inspected and palpated bilaterally to assess for abnormalities (e.g., presence and number of masses, induration, degree of fixation, tenderness) that may be consistent with regional adenopathy.

Basic serum laboratory testing, urinalysis, and culture may be done, although results are often normal and thus non-specific for penile cancer. Various serologic examinations,

cultures, or specialized histologic techniques are available for evaluating penile lesions included in the differential diagnosis of penile cancer. Imaging tests offer a particularly useful role in the diagnosis and staging of this disease. Penile ultrasound or contrast-enhanced magnetic resonance imaging (MRI), which may be done with a medically induced artificial erection, may inform the possibility of corporal infiltration [15,16], and their utility is likely most considerable when deliberating on organ-preserving management. Computed tomography (CT) of the pelvis is commonly done for assessing involvement of regional lymph nodes, although its success in detecting local spread of disease in the absence of palpable adenopathy has been questioned [17]. It is recognized that all current imaging techniques (e.g., CT, ultrasound, MRI), or investigational F18 fluorodeoxyglucose positron emission tomography/CT (^{18}F-FDG-PET/CT scans) are unreliable in detecting micro-metastatic disease that may be present as much as 25% of the time in clinically normal inguinal lymph nodes [18–20]. Lymphangiography has been used historically in attempts to identify microscopic inguinal and pelvic nodal metastases and to direct needle biopsy [21]. However, with the emergence of CT and MRI for clinical staging, lymphangiography has become obsolete for this role in penile cancer. Lymphotropic nanoparticle-enhanced MRI is a relatively new technology under evaluation for detecting nodal micrometastatic disease in penile cancer that requires further study [22]. Abdominopelvic CT and chest radiography or CT serve for evaluating the presence and extent of systemic disease [23,24]. Radionuclide bone scintigraphy also may be used for staging purposes [21].

Despite the oftentimes physical conspicuousness of penile cancer, penile biopsy is mandatory to verify the histology and assess the stage of the cancer. Small lesions may be excised in entirety where possible, whereas large lesions may be locally sampled. An excisional biopsy is preferable rather than an incisional or punch biopsy because this strategy best serves to assess depth of invasion, and it may achieve local disease eradication. Pathologic description should include the histologic type or variant, grade, perineural and lymphovascular invasion, and surgical margin status, all of which are prognostically relevant. Perineural, lymphatic, and vascular invasion [5,25,26] and high grade [3,5,25,27] represent high-risk pathologic features, as is the finding of high-risk variants [28]. Studies in penile cancer have explored its molecular biology, although current data predicting poor biologic behavior remain limited. Alterations in the chromosomal locus 8q24 [29], epigenetic alterations of CpG island methylation in CDKN2A [30], and allelic loss of the p53 gene [31] are promising markers of poor prognosis. Fine-needle aspiration with cytopathology of palpably enlarged inguinal nodes or fine-needle biopsy of pelvic adenopathy suggested by CT is an optional procedure for determining positive pathologic nodal status [17], although definitive surgical staging is usually performed in this clinical setting.

Treatment

In general, the treatment of penile cancer is determined by the pathological stage of the disease, with focus given toward the primary tumor and regional lymph nodes in early stage disease and toward distant metastatic disease in later stages. Treatment of the primary tumor should always follow histologic assessment, necessitating penile biopsy. This message applies even when superficial noninvasive disease is suspected because invasive disease may exist in up to 20% of such cases [32]. Staged procedures are regularly employed, and invasive lymph node management conventionally follows treatment of the primary tumor. Treatment of inguinal and pelvic lymph nodes is determined by pathologic risk factors of the primary tumor such as presence of lymphovascular invasion, stage, and grade [33,34]. Surgical staging of lymph nodes is routinely indicated by the presence of palpable lymph nodes or adverse primary tumor histologic features. Disease cure can also be achieved surgically in regional lymph node disease [10].

With respect to the primary tumor, management has evolved from conventional surgical amputation (i.e., partial or total penectomy) to organ-preserving intervention (i.e., maintenance of penile function and length) when oncologically feasible. Today, a range of minimally invasive therapeutic options, including topical treatments, laser ablation, modified local excision, and radiation therapy, have been developed and can be employed. Treatment decisions for localized disease appropriately apply diagnostic clinical and pathologic information that defines the prognostic disease risk.

Primary Tumor of Low Adverse Prognostic Risk

Superficial noninvasive disease (Tis), particularly that involving the glans penis, is amenable to treatment using minimally invasive therapies. Topical chemotherapy with imiquimod or 5-fluorouracil (5-FU) offers first-line treatment [35]. These agents carry low toxicity effects and demonstrate a moderately successful 57% complete-response rate; however, the relatively modest durable response rate associated with this treatment implies that clinical follow up is appropriate, and failure of topical therapy should prompt timely alternative management. Laser ablation using a neodymium:yttrium-aluminum-garnet (Nd:YAG) or carbon dioxide (CO_2) laser [36] or alternatively total or partial glans resurfacing (i.e., removal of the glandular epithelium and skin grafting) [34] may also be used. Mohs micrographic surgery as a penis-preserving strategy has been used historically for small and noninvasive or minimally invasive tumors, although it is a tedious and highly specialized technique [37]. Recent studies suggest that this technique does not offer additional precision beyond surgical excision with intraoperative frozen section analysis of margin status [38]. Small Tis lesions of the prepuce or penile shaft skin may also be treated by wide local excision with little cosmetic detriment.

Expert opinion now supports the role of penis-preserving strategies for the management of small invasive lesions defined as Ta/T1a disease because of acceptable oncologic outcomes [10,11,13]. However, the risk of local recurrence for penis-sparing strategies is understood to be higher than that associated with partial penectomy 5–12% compared with 5%, respectively [39,40]. The treatment plan should well consider tumor size, histology, grade, location relative to the external urethral meatus, and patient preference based on informed counseling regarding the comparative risks. For tumors confined to the prepuce, circumcision is recommended. For tumors involving the glans penis, total glansectomy with reconstruction or skin grafting may be considered. In either scenario, the local recurrence rate is estimated to be low (approximately 2%) when achieving a 5-mm negative surgical margin [41,42]. The success of this strategy hinges on intraoperative assessment of surgical margin status by frozen section analysis to assess adequacy of surgical excision. Local recurrence rates are reportedly 0–4% for total or partial glans resurfacing [32,43] and 7v8% for glansectomy [42,44]. Laser ablation with visualization enhancement by photodynamic

techniques is also possible [45]. Local recurrence rates are reportedly 10–48% after Nd:YAG laser treatment and 14–23% after CO_2 laser treatment [46].

Primary Tumor of High Adverse Prognostic Risk

Definitive treatment of the invasive or high-grade primary tumor remains surgical amputation (i.e., partial or total penectomy with a 2-cm margin) because of the adverse risk of incomplete local disease removal by conservative management that may jeopardize cure [10,11]. This strategy is certainly appropriate for patients presenting with large and obviously invasive penile tumors extending into the corpus spongiosum or cavernosum or other local structures, with the objective at a minimum of obtaining local disease control. Suggested parameters include size greater than 4 cm, invasion deeply into subepithelial connective tissue or beyond, and presence of adverse pathology (i.e., poor differentiation, lymphovascular invasion) [47]. Disease control by surgical amputation is fairly good, with local recurrence rates ranging from 0% to 8% [39,40].

Radiation therapy in the forms of both external-beam radiation therapy and interstitial brachytherapy offers an option in the management of the primary tumor [48–50]. This therapeutic strategy is consistent with aims of penile preservation and is appropriate for patients who refuse surgery. It has also been used as primary therapy with the understanding that if treatment fails, salvage surgery may be applied with curative intent [51]. Five-year local control rates range from 70% to 88% for brachytherapy and from 44% to 70% for external-beam radiation therapy [48]. It is noteworthy that squamous cell carcinoma is characteristically radioresistant, and the dosage required to sterilize the tumor (i.e., 60 Gy) presents potential risks. Complications stemming from therapy may occur in as many as 45% of cases and include urethral fistula, urethral stricture or meatal stenosis, penile necrosis, pain, and edema

[50,52]. Circumcision is recommended preemptively when the lesion in beneath the prepuce to expose the lesion and to lessen the risk of tissue maceration and preputial edema. Management of serious complications may involve secondary penectomy [53]. Penile preservation rates of 50% to 65% and cause-specific survival rates of 58% to 86%, depending on primary tumor stage and lymph node status, are reported [48].

Regional Lymph Node Metastasis

It is well understood that the prognostic outcome of squamous penile cancer is dictated foremost by the presence of nodal metastasis to the inguinal region [1–3]. At the same time, it is recognized that 5-year cure rates with inguinal lymphadenectomy in the presence of nodal metastases may be as high as 80% [1,6,7]. Thus, proficiently practiced and timely management of possible inguinal lymph node progression is key to long-term patient survival. Radical inguinal lymphadenectomy is the mainstay of clinical practice and may be employed for clinically impalpable nodes, clinically node-positive disease, and when disease is predictably extensive warranting multimodal intervention with chemotherapy [10,11]. Alternative interventions for patients with clinically node-negative cancer include surveillance and inguinal radiotherapy, although overall survival is less for these options, 63% and 66%, respectively, when compared to surgery (74%) [54]. Laparoscopic and robot-assisted inguinal lymphadenectomy has been described, but it remains unclear whether these procedures are superior to open surgery [55,56]. Based on current surgical schemes assessing the risk of pelvic lymph node progression, pelvic lymphadenectomy may be performed concurrently or as a secondary procedure [4,8,15].

Patients presenting with intermediate- and high-risk disease and impalpable nodes may be offered two invasive diagnostic procedures: modified inguinal lymphadenectomy and dynamic sentinel node biopsy [10,11].

Modified inguinal lymphadenectomy has surpassed historically morbid standard dissection. The newer approach adheres to a limited template of dissection that preserves the dermis, Scarpa's fascia, and saphenous vein and may be staged based on intraoperative frozen section analysis indicating positive nodes into sequential superficial inguinal and deep ilioinguinal anatomic boundaries [57–59]. Dynamic sentinel node biopsy is performed with the presumption that the lymphatic drainage from penile cancer is unilateral, and although sensitivity rates of 90–94% have been reported [60,61], false-negative rates can be as high as 15% [62]. Although both techniques may miss micrometastatic disease, limited dissection offers more information and conceivably produces better disease control.

The morbidity of modified inguinal lymphadenectomy has been reduced significantly based on advances in surgical schemes (i.e., template dissection, staging), techniques (i.e., venous preservation, ligation and clips of lymphatic vessels), and postoperative measures (i.e., vacuum suction drains, inguinal/lower extremity pressure dressings) [63–65]. Accordingly, postoperative complication rates have been significantly reduced with contemporary reports describing these to be: wound infections (1.2–1.4%), skin necrosis (0.6–4.7%), lymphedema (5–13.9%), and lymphocele formation (2.1–4%) [65,66]. Pelvic lymphadenectomy generally adds little additional postoperative morbidity.

Surgical Procedures

The contemporary surgical management of penile cancer is characterized by a host of surgical interventions that has progressed beyond the historical centerpiece of penile amputation. Although partial or total penectomy is properly advised based on clinical and pathologic variables, these more emasculating or disfiguring procedures are not always required. Minimally invasive strategies offer the opportunity for disease control when possible while also achieving aims of quality of life preservation and sexual function maintenance. It is understood that the alternative less-invasive options carry higher risks of disease persistence and recurrence, such that careful patient selection, education, and follow-up protocols must be enacted. In the setting of uncontrolled disease, more aggressive management should be readily implemented. Furthermore, surgical management has evolved with regard to the preservation of sexual function rehabilitation even when major destructive surgeries are required. Surgical reconstructive techniques have been developed and are increasingly performed in the quest to restore form and function of the penis.

Partial and Total Penectomy

From a technical standpoint, plans for the removal of a portion or the entire penis should consider the extent of the lesion and the standard 2-cm margin proximal to the lesion that would then impact the patient's genitourinary functional status (i.e., voiding, sexual activity). If a significant portion of the penis must be removed and thus penile length is critically compromised, a perineal urethrostomy should become part of the surgical plan, whereby the patient may preferably evacuate urine although seated without the potential for urinary stream spraying and urine contacting skin and clothes when voiding through a penile stump.

Detailed descriptions of the procedure are provided elsewhere [67–69]. With consideration of surgical technique, several particular points merit highlighting. For urethral reconstruction with partial penectomy, it is noteworthy to create a length of the urethra of a distance 1–1.5 cm distally beyond the transected corporal bodies and spatulate the neomeatus, which facilitates a directed urinary stream and is less apt to stenose. For perineal urethrostomy, sufficient mobilization of the urethra transposition to the perineum without angulation, and wide neomeatal spatulation are critical principles. Release of the suspensory ligament and

dissection of the proximal corpora from the pubic arch may also be done to achieve maximal penile outward extension and length (both for possible voiding upright and sexual intercourse). When necessary, skin coverage may be additionally provided by local scrotal skin flaps, ventral penoscrotal junction phalloplasty techniques, or skin grafting [70].

Wide Local Excision

Local excision is possible in several ways for localized disease. Circumcision is readily performed for preputial involvement, and wide excision of penile shaft skin is employed for proximal lesions. Glansectomy has recently been described for disease located at the glans penis [71]. Technically, the procedure involves dissecting the glans off the distal ends of the corpora cavernosa using a surgical plane that is developed between the Buck's fascia and deep surface of the glans after making a circumferential subcoronal incision. This procedure may be combined with distal corporectomy depending on the local extent of disease as determined by intraoperative frozen section analysis [72]. Glans resurfacing distinctly involves excision of the epithelium and subepithelium of the entire glans with a less extensive surgical resection than glansectomy [32,73]. Primary closure is performed reproducing a glans penis-like conical shape or mobilizing a preputial skin flap to cover the surgical defect in instances when this defect is small [74]. Full-thickness penile skin graft or extragenital split-thickness skin graft are alternative options for skin coverage of the entire glans penis (e.g., total glans resurfacing) or significant surgical defects of the penile shaft [72]. It is technically important to consider applying skin grafts rather than advancing the penile shaft remnant to the neomeatus to prevent retraction of the residual penile shaft.

Neophalloplasty

For men whose penis has been extensively removed (i.e., total penectomy), phallic reconstruction is a possible option to create a male genital organ to serve for resumption of sexual activity. Tissue flap reconstruction most commonly involves the radial forearm, but alternative sources include the anterolateral thigh, the scapula/latissimus dorsi, fibula, and local rotational flaps from the abdomen, groin, and thigh [75]. Although penetrative intercourse is possible with the neophallus alone, implantation of a penile prosthesis within the neophallus optimally provides a mechanism for phallic rigidity [76,77]. The complexity of this further reconstruction demands an understanding of the anatomy of the native penile remnant and anatomical constraints of the neophallus to lessen adverse risks of prosthetic device erosion or infection.

References

1 Ravi R. Correlation between the extent of nodal involvement and survival following groin dissection for carcinoma of the penis. Br J Urol. 1993;72:817–9.

2 McDougal WS. Carcinoma of the penis: improved survival by early regional lymphadenectomy based on the histological grade and depth of invasion of the primary lesion. J Urol. 1995;154:1364–6.

3 Theodorescu D, Russo P, Zhang ZF, Morash C, Fair WR. Outcomes of initial surveillance of invasive squamous cell carcinoma of the penis and negative nodes. J Urol. 1996; 155:1626–31.

4 Pizzocaro G, Piva L, Bandieramonte G, Tana S. Up-to-date management of carcinoma of the penis. Eur Urol. 1997;32:5–15.

5 Slaton JW, Morgenstern N, Levy DA, Santos MW, Jr, Tamboli P, Ro JY, et al. Tumor stage, vascular invasion and the percentage of poorly differentiated cancer: Independent prognosticators for inguinal lymph node metastasis in penile squamous cancer. J Urol. 2001;165:1138–42.

6 Srinivas V, Morse MJ, Herr HW, Sogani PC, Whitmore WF, Jr. Penile cancer: Relation of extent of nodal metastasis to survival. J Urol. 1987;137:880–2.

7 Horenblas S, van Tinteren H. Squamous cell carcinoma of the penis. IV. Prognostic factors of survival: Analysis of tumor, nodes and metastasis classification system. J Urol. 1994;151:1239–43.

8 Lont AP, Kroon BK, Gallee MP, van Tinteren H, Moonen LM, Horenblas S. Pelvic lymph node dissection for penile carcinoma: Extent of inguinal lymph node involvement as an indicator for pelvic lymph node involvement and survival. J Urol. 2007;177:947–52; discussion 952.

9 Leijte JA, Kirrander P, Antonini N, Windahl T, Horenblas S. Recurrence patterns of squamous cell carcinoma of the penis: Recommendations for follow-up based on a two-centre analysis of 700 patients. Eur Urol. 2008;54:161–8.

10 Hakenberg OW, Comperat EM, Minhas S, Necchi A, Protzel C, Watkin N. EAU Guidelines on penile cancer: 2014 update. Eur Urol. 2015;67:142–50.

11 Clark PE, Spiess PE, Agarwal N, Biagioli MC, Eisenberger MA, Greenberg RE, et al. Penile cancer: clinical practice guidelines in oncology. J Natl Compr Canc Netw. 2013;11:594–615.

12 Hernandez BY, Barnholtz-Sloan J, German RR, Giuliano A, Goodman MT, King JB, et al. Burden of invasive squamous cell carcinoma of the penis in the United States, 1998–2003. Cancer 2008; 113(10 Suppl):2883–91.

13 Solsona E, Algaba F, Horenblas S, Pizzocaro G, Windahl T, European Association of Urology. EAU guidelines on penile cancer. Eur Urol. 2004;46:1–8.

14 Ficarra V, Zattoni F, Cunico SC, Galetti TP, Luciani L, Fandella A, et al. Lymphatic and vascular embolizations are independent predictive variables of inguinal lymph node involvement in patients with squamous cell carcinoma of the penis: Gruppo Uro-Oncologico del Nord Est Northeast

Uro-Oncological Group) penile cancer data base data. Cancer. 2005;103:2507–16.

15 Lont AP, Besnard AP, Gallee MP, van Tinteren H, Horenblas S. A comparison of physical examination and imaging in determining the extent of primary penile carcinoma. BJU Int. 2003;91:493–5.

16 Kayes O, Minhas S, Allen C, Hare C, Freeman A, Ralph D. The role of magnetic resonance imaging in the local staging of penile cancer. Eur Urol. 2007;51:1313–8; discussion 1318–9.

17 Horenblas S, Van Tinteren H, Delemarre JF, Moonen LM, Lustig V, Kroger R. Squamous cell carcinoma of the penis: Accuracy of tumor, nodes and metastasis classification system, and role of lymphangiography, computerized tomography scan and fine needle aspiration cytology. J Urol. 1991;146:1279–83.

18 Krishna RP, Sistla SC, Smile R, Krishnan R. Sonography: An underutilized diagnostic tool in the assessment of metastatic groin nodes. J Clin Ultrasound. 2008;36:212–7.

19 Leijte JA, Graafland NM, Valdes Olmos RA, van Boven HH, Hoefnagel CA, Horenblas S. Prospective evaluation of hybrid 18F-fluorodeoxyglucose positron emission tomography/computed tomography in staging clinically node-negative patients with penile carcinoma. BJU Int. 2009;104:640–4.

20 Schlenker B, Scher B, Tiling R, Siegert S, Hungerhuber E, Gratzke C, et al. Detection of inguinal lymph node involvement in penile squamous cell carcinoma by 18F-fluorodeoxyglucose PET/CT: A prospective single-center study. Urol Oncol. 2012;30:55–9.

21 Vapnek JM, Hricak H, Carroll PR. Recent advances in imaging studies for staging of penile and urethral carcinoma. Urol Clin North Am. 1992;19:257–66.

22 Tabatabaei S, Harisinghani M, McDougal WS. Regional lymph node staging using lymphotropic nanoparticle enhanced magnetic resonance imaging with ferumoxtran-10 in patients with penile cancer. J Urol. 2005;174:923–7; discussion 927.

23 Ornellas AA, Seixas AL, Marota A, Wisnescky A, Campos F, de Moraes JR. Surgical treatment of invasive squamous cell carcinoma of the penis: retrospective analysis of 350 cases. J Urol. 1994;151:1244–9.

24 Zhu Y, Zhang SL, Ye DW, Yao XD, Jiang ZX, Zhou XY. Predicting pelvic lymph node metastases in penile cancer patients: A comparison of computed tomography, Cloquet's node, and disease burden of inguinal lymph nodes. Onkologie. 2008;31:37–41.

25 Fraley EE, Zhang G, Manivel C, Niehans GA. The role of ilioinguinal lymphadenectomy and significance of histological differentiation in treatment of carcinoma of the penis. J Urol. 1989;142:1478–82.

26 Velazquez EF, Ayala G, Liu H, Chaux A, Zanotti M, Torres J, et al. Histologic grade and perineural invasion are more important than tumor thickness as predictor of nodal metastasis in penile squamous cell carcinoma invading 5 to 10 mm. Am J Surg Pathol. 2008;32:974–9.

27 Heyns CF, van Vollenhoven P, Steenkamp JW, Allen FJ, van Velden DJ. Carcinoma of the penis—appraisal of a modified tumour-staging system. Br J Urol. 1997;80:307–2.

28 Cubilla AL, Reuter V, Velazquez E, Piris A, Saito S, Young RH. Histologic classification of penile carcinoma and its relation to outcome in 61 patients with primary resection. Int J Surg Pathol. 2001;9:111–20.

29 Alves G, Heller A, Fiedler W, Campos MM, Claussen U, Ornellas AA, et al. Genetic imbalances in 26 cases of penile squamous cell carcinoma. Genes Chromosomes Cancer. 2001;31:48–53.

30 Kayes O, Ahmed HU, Arya M, Minhas S. Molecular and genetic pathways in penile cancer. Lancet Oncol. 2007;8:420–9.

31 Gunia S, Kakies C, Erbersdobler A, Hakenberg OW, Koch S, May M. Expression of p53, p21 and cyclin D1 in penile cancer: p53 predicts poor prognosis. J Clin Pathol. 2012;65:232–6.

32 Shabbir M, Muneer A, Kalsi J, Shukla CJ, Zacharakis E, Garaffa G, *et al.* Glans resurfacing for the treatment of carcinoma in situ of the penis: Surgical technique and outcomes. Eur Urol. 2011;59:142–7.

33 Graafland NM, Lam W, Leijte JA, Yap T, Gallee MP, Corbishley C, *et al.* Prognostic factors for occult inguinal lymph node involvement in penile carcinoma and assessment of the high-risk EAU subgroup: A two-institution analysis of 342 clinically node-negative patients. Eur Urol. 2010;58:742–7.

34 Alkatout I, Naumann CM, Hedderich J, Hegele A, Bolenz C, Junemann KP, *et al.* Squamous cell carcinoma of the penis: Predicting nodal metastases by histologic grade, pattern of invasion and clinical examination. Urol Oncol. 2011;29:774–81.

35 Alnajjar HM, Lam W, Bolgeri M, Rees RW, Perry MJ, Watkin NA. Treatment of carcinoma in situ of the glans penis with topical chemotherapy agents. Eur Urol. 2012;62:923–8.

36 Frimberger D, Hungerhuber E, Zaak D, Waidelich R, Hofstetter A, Schneede P. Penile carcinoma. Is Nd:YAG laser therapy radical enough? J Urol. 2002;168:2418–21; discussion 2421.

37 Mohs FE, Snow SN, Messing EM, Kuglitsch ME. Microscopically controlled surgery in the treatment of carcinoma of the penis. J Urol. 1985;133:961–6.

38 Shindel AW, Mann MW, Lev RY, Sengelmann R, Petersen J, Hruza GJ, *et al.* Mohs micrographic surgery for penile cancer: management and long-term followup. J Urol. 2007;178:1980–5.

39 McDougal WS, Kirchner FK, Jr, Edwards RH, Killion LT. Treatment of carcinoma of the penis: the case for primary lymphadenectomy. J Urol. 1986;136:38–41.

40 Horenblas S, van Tinteren H, Delemarre JF, Boon TA, Moonen LM, Lustig V. Squamous cell carcinoma of the penis. II. Treatment of the primary tumor. J Urol. 1992;147:1533–8.

41 Ornellas AA, Kinchin EW, Nobrega BL, Wisnescky A, Koifman N, Quirino R. Surgical treatment of invasive squamous cell carcinoma of the penis: Brazilian National Cancer Institute long-term experience. J Surg Oncol. 2008;97:487–95.

42 Philippou P, Shabbir M, Malone P, Nigam R, Muneer A, Ralph DJ, *et al.* Conservative surgery for squamous cell carcinoma of the penis: Resection margins and long-term oncological control. J Urol. 2012;188:803–8.

43 Hadway P, Corbishley CM, Watkin NA. Total glans resurfacing for premalignant lesions of the penis: initial outcome data. BJU Int. 2006;98:532–6.

44 Li J, Zhu Y, Zhang SL, Wang CF, Yao XD, Dai B, *et al.* Organ-sparing surgery for penile cancer: complications and outcomes. Urology. 2011;78:1121–4.

45 Frimberger D, Schneede P, Hungerhuber E, Sroka R, Zaak D, Siebels M, *et al.* Autofluorescence and 5-aminolevulinic acid induced fluorescence diagnosis of penile carcinoma —new techniques to monitor Nd:YAG laser therapy. Urol Res. 2002;30:295–300.

46 Meijer RP, Boon TA, van Venrooij GE, Wijburg CJ. Long-term follow-up after laser therapy for penile carcinoma. Urology. 2007;69:759–62.

47 Gotsadze D, Matveev B, Zak B, Mamaladze V. Is conservative organ-sparing treatment of penile carcinoma justified? Eur Urol. 2000;38:306–12.

48 Crook J, Ma C, Grimard L. Radiation therapy in the management of the primary penile tumor: an update. World J Urol. 2009;27:189–96.

49 Crook J, Jezioranski J, Cygler JE. Penile brachytherapy: technical aspects and postimplant issues. Brachytherapy. 2010;9:151–8.

50 de Crevoisier R, Slimane K, Sanfilippo N, Bossi A, Albano M, Dumas I, *et al.* Long-term results of brachytherapy for carcinoma of the penis confined to the glans (N- or NX). Int J Radiat Oncol Biol Phys. 2009;74:1150–6.

51 Azrif M, Logue JP, Swindell R, Cowan RA, Wylie JP, Livsey JE. External-beam

radiotherapy in T1-2 N0 penile carcinoma. Clin Oncol R Coll Radiol. 2006;18:320–5.

52 Kelley CD, Arthur K, Rogoff E, Grabstald H. Radiation therapy of penile cancer. Urology. 1974;4:571–3.

53 Duncan W, Jackson SM. The treatment of early cancer of the penis with megavoltage x-rays. Clin Radiol. 1972;23:246–8.

54 Kulkarni JN, Kamat MR. Prophylactic bilateral groin node dissection versus prophylactic radiotherapy and surveillance in patients with N0 and N1-2A carcinoma of the penis. Eur Urol. 1994;26:123–8.

55 Sotelo R, Sanchez-Salas R, Clavijo R. Endoscopic inguinal lymph node dissection for penile carcinoma: the developing of a novel technique. World J Urol. 2009;27:213–9.

56 Pahwa HS, Misra S, Kumar A, Kumar V, Agarwal A, Srivastava R. Video Endoscopic Inguinal Lymphadenectomy VEIL)—a prospective critical perioperative assessment of feasibility and morbidity with points of technique in penile carcinoma. World J Surg Oncol. 2013;11:42.

57 Catalona WJ. Modified inguinal lymphadenectomy for carcinoma of the penis with preservation of saphenous veins: Technique and preliminary results. J Urol. 1988;140:306–10.

58 Colberg JW, Andriole GL, Catalona WJ. Long-term follow-up of men undergoing modified inguinal lymphadenectomy for carcinoma of the penis. Br J Urol. 1997;79:54–57.

59 Nelson BA, Cookson MS, Smith JA, Jr, Chang SS. Complications of inguinal and pelvic lymphadenectomy for squamous cell carcinoma of the penis: a contemporary series. J Urol. 2004;172:494–7.

60 Leijte JA, Hughes B, Graafland NM, Kroon BK, Olmos RA, Nieweg OE, *et al.* Two-center evaluation of dynamic sentinel node biopsy for squamous cell carcinoma of the penis. J Clin Oncol. 2009;27:3325–9.

61 Lam W, Alnajjar HM, La-Touche S, Perry M, Sharma D, Corbishley C, *et al.* Dynamic sentinel lymph node biopsy in patients with invasive squamous cell carcinoma of the penis: A prospective study of the long-term outcome of 500 inguinal basins assessed at a single institution. Eur Urol. 2013;63:657–63.

62 Kirrander P, Andren O, Windahl T. Dynamic sentinel node biopsy in penile cancer: initial experiences at a Swedish referral centre. BJU Int. 2013;111:E48–53.

63 Margulis V, Sagalowsky AI. Penile cancer: Management of regional lymphatic drainage. Urol Clin North Am. 2010;37:411–9.

64 La-Touche S, Ayres B, Lam W, Alnajjar HM, Perry M, Watkin N. Trial of ligation versus coagulation of lymphatics in dynamic inguinal sentinel lymph node biopsy for staging of squamous cell carcinoma of the penis. Ann R Coll Surg Engl. 2012;94:344–6.

65 Koifman L, Hampl D, Koifman N, Vides AJ, Ornellas AA. Radical open inguinal lymphadenectomy for penile carcinoma: Surgical technique, early complications and late outcomes. J Urol. 2013;190:2086–92.

66 Yao K, Tu H, Li YH, Qin ZK, Liu ZW, Zhou FJ, *et al.* Modified technique of radical inguinal lymphadenectomy for penile carcinoma: Morbidity and outcome. J Urol. 2010;184:546–52.

67 Das S. Penile amputations for the management of primary carcinoma of the penis. Urol Clin North Am. 1992;19:277–82.

68 Loughlin KR. The rosebud technique for creation of a neomeatus after partial or total penectomy. Br J Urol. 1995;76:123–4.

69 Hegarty PK, Shabbir M, Hughes B, Minhas S, Perry M, Watkin N, *et al.* Penile preserving surgery and surgical strategies to maximize penile form and function in penile cancer: Recommendations from the United Kingdom experience. World J Urol. 2009;27:179–87.

70 Wallen JJ, Baumgarten AS, Kim T, Hakky TS, Carrion RE, Spiess PE. Optimizing penile length in patients undergoing partial penectomy for penile cancer: Novel application of the ventral phalloplasty oncoplastic technique. Int Braz J Urol. 2014;40:708–9.

71 Austoni E, Fenice O, Kartalas Goumas Y, Colombo F, Mantovani F, Pisani E. New trends in the surgical treatment of penile carcinoma. Arch Ital Urol Androl. 1996;68:163–8.

72 Pietrzak P, Corbishley C, Watkin N. Organ-sparing surgery for invasive penile cancer: Early follow-up data. BJU Int 2004;94:1253–7.

73 Palminteri E, Berdondini E, Lazzeri M, Mirri F, Barbagli G. Resurfacing and reconstruction of the glans penis. Eur Urol. 2007;52:893–8.

74 Ubrig B, Waldner M, Fallahi M, Roth S. Preputial flap for primary closure after excision of tumors on the glans penis. Urology. 2001;58:274–6.

75 Bluebond-Langner R, Redett RJ. Phalloplasty in complete aphallia and ambiguous genitalia. Semin Plast Surg. 2011;25:196–205.

76 Garaffa G, Raheem AA, Christopher NA, Ralph DJ. Total phallic reconstruction after penile amputation for carcinoma. BJU Int. 2009;104:852–6.

77 Segal RL, Massanyi EZ, Gupta AD, Gearhart JP, Redett RJ, Bivalacqua TJ, *et al.* Inflatable penile prosthesis technique and outcomes after radial forearm free flap neophalloplasty. Int J Impot Res 2015;27(2)49–53.

14

Testis Cancer: Testis-Sparing Cancer Surgery

Nilay M. Gandhi, MD,[1] and Pravin K. Rao, MD[2]

[1] *Department of Urology, Johns Hopkins University, Baltimore, MD, USA*
[2] *Department of Urology, Greater Baltimore Medical Center, Lutherville, MD, USA*

Introduction

Testicular cancer management is often touted as a model of success in multimodal and collaborative oncological care. However, this was not always the case; both the presentation and management of the disease have evolved remarkably over the last several decades.

Before the era of ultrasound imaging, almost all patients with testicular cancer presented with a palpable scrotal mass or symptoms of disseminated disease. Inguinal radical orchiectomy (RO) was the near universal first step in diagnosis and treatment because of the historically reported low prevalence of benign lesions (<1%) and the thought that intraoperative biopsies could lead to tumor progression and seeding [1]. In the early 1970s, before the development of cisplatin-based chemotherapy, survival with metastatic testicular cancer was around 5% [2]. Since then, combinations of surgery, chemotherapy, and radiation have led to 5-year relative survival rates around 98% [3]; overall survival rates with regional and distant metastases are now around 96% and 72%, respectively [4].

In the 1980s, studies found that the true proportion of benign testicular lesions was much higher than the 1% estimated by previous studies. In a study by Haas in 1986, 233 patients underwent inguinal exploration for suspicion of cancer and the authors calculated a 31% rate of benign tumors [5]. Another report 2 years later by Kressel *et al.* noted a 5% rate of benign lesions [6]. Over subsequent decades, widespread use of scrotal ultrasound for common conditions such as scrotal content pain, epididymo-orchitis, torsion, and hydrocele/spermatocele has also led to the detection of small, nonpalpable, or asymptomatic lesions of the testis. With this increased sensitivity for testicular lesions has come an increased incidence of benign testicular tumors.

Imaging of Testicular Tumors

The increased detection of benign tumors led to attempts to limit extirpative therapy for benign disease. As part of this effort, multiple studies have examined the ability of imaging characteristics to distinguish benign from malignant intratesticular lesions.

Wasnik *et al.* characterized common benign testicular lesions and their sonographic findings, which are summarized in Table 14.1 [7]. Carmignani *et al.* evaluated all urologic patients presenting with infertility, erectile dysfunction, or asymptomatic scrotal lesions over a 2-year period with duplex

Management of Urologic Cancer: Focal Therapy and Tissue Preservation, First Edition.
Edited by Mark P. Schoenberg and Kara L. Watts.

Table 14.1 Characteristic Ultrasound Findings of Benign Testicular Lesions.

Pathology	Ultrasound Findings
Simple cyst	Well-defined anechoic focus with thin imperceptible wall
Epidermoid cyst	Circumscribed, avascular intratesticular mass with lamellated configuration of alternating hyperechoic and hypoechoic rings
Testicular adrenal rest tumors	Bilateral, eccentrically located hypoechoic masses with variable vascularity
Hamartomas	Multiple hyperechoic avascular foci scattered bilaterally without parenchymal distortion
Leydig cell tumor	Peripheral hypervascularity in a hypoechoic testicular tumor

Summarized from Wasnik *et al.* [7]

ultrasonography. Of 1,320 patients, 27 (2%) focal testicular lesions were identified by ultrasound, of which 17 were palpable and 10 were nonpalpable. A benign lesion was diagnosed in 80% of the nonpalpable masses. The authors noted that ultrasound cannot differentiate benign from malignant lesions, and therefore surgical intervention is still warranted; however, imaging now allows improved prediction of candidacy for testis-sparing surgery [8]. Figure 14.1 shows ultrasound images of two incidentally detected hypoechoic intratesticular masses, both of which were found to be Leydig cell tumors.

Given the shortcomings of ultrasound in characterizing benign compared with malignant testicular masses, magnetic resonance imaging (MRI) has been investigated as a supplementary modality. Tsili *et al.* assessed the role of preoperative MRI in 33 patients with 36 ultrasound-proven testicular masses [9]. Criteria to suggest malignancy by MRI included the presence of a multinodular intratesticular lesion with low signal intensity or an inhomogenous mass with variable signal intensity on T2-imaging, heterogeneous contrast enhancement, coexistence of hemorrhage or necrosis, as well as demonstration of tumor extension. Following operative intervention, MRI findings were compared to the final pathologic specimen: 100% of malignant lesions were correctly classified by MRI, whereas 87.5% of benign lesions were correctly classified (one of eight benign lesions was predicted to be malignant

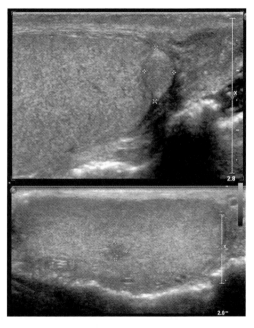

Figure 14.1 Two hypochoic intratesticular masses found incidentally on ultrasound. Both of these were found to be Leydig cell tumors on pathological review.

by MRI findings). The overall accuracy of MRI for detecting malignancy was 96.4%. The absence of contrast enhancement was the most sensitive sign for predicting the benign nature of a testicular mass. In another evaluation of 15 patients with testicular masses seen on ultrasound, the use of MRI diffusion-weighted imaging and signal intensity measurement was helpful for differentiating malignant neoplasms, which were noted to have significantly lower values than benign lesions [10]. Although much progress has been made on characterizing benign and malignant tumors on ultrasound and MRI, no imaging modality has been definitively shown to discern benign lesions with adequate specificity to forego surgical removal and pathological diagnosis.

Bilateral Tumors

Apart from patients with benign tumors, there is also interest in preserving functional testicular tissue in patients with bilateral tumors or tumors of a solitary testis. Two percent of patients with germ cell tumors develop bilateral lesions, with approximately 0.5% of these presenting synchronously. Because of this small but real risk, both testes require ultrasonic evaluation at the time of diagnosis. Approximately 1.5–5% of patients with a history of testicular cancer will develop a second primary in the contralateral testis [11]. In an evaluation of almost 2,500 patients over a 20-year span, investigators at MD Anderson Cancer Center identified 24 patients (1%) with a history of bilateral testicular germ cell tumors (20 metachronous). A statistically significant increase was noted in the incidence of bilateral tumors if the patient initially presented with seminoma rather than nonseminomatous germ cell tumor (NSGCT; p = 0.0053) and if the seminoma was first diagnosed at 30 years of age or younger (p = 0.000044). The majority of contralateral tumors (70%) presented within 5 years of the initial mass, and no correlation in histologic types was seen between the metachronous tumors (p = 0.06).

The Advent of Testis-Sparing Surgery

Testis-sparing surgery (TSS) carries the potential benefits of maximizing spermatogenesis and fertility, preserving Leydig cells to curb hypogonadism, and decreasing cosmetic and psychological impact of having just one or no testicles. The goals of TSS are closely paralleled by lumpectomy for breast cancer, in which organ-preservation techniques aim to reduce physical, functional, and psychological morbidity. Modern urologic oncology principles also incorporate organ preservation, namely seen with partial nephrectomy for renal cell carcinoma and focal therapy for prostate carcinoma. In contrast to other sites of malignancy, for testicular masses, inguinal RO has remained the gold standard for treatment and pathological diagnosis throughout the last four decades.

With increased detection of testicular tumors, increased rates of benign masses, and excellent cancer-specific survival rates, the focus for many patients with testicular tumors has now shifted toward functional, cosmetic, and psychological effects of management. Indeed, surveillance protocols with deferred adjuvant treatment have successfully limited the short- and long-term morbidity of adjuvant chemotherapy and radiation therapy in select patients after orchiectomy. However, in this new era, TSS has become a consideration for primary treatment of many small/bilateral testicular lesions or lesions of solitary testes.

Concerns about TSS

Many concerns exist regarding the oncological safety and the true benefit of TSS. We review these issues and their implications for patients considering organ preservation.

Presence of Intratubular Germ Cell Neoplasia or Multifocal Invasive Germ Cell Tumor

Carcinoma in situ of the testis, or intratubular germ cell neoplasia (ITGCN), is the common precursor for most germ cell tumors. Based on work from Skakkebaek in the 1970s, it is thought that approximately 50% of patients with ITGCN will progress to invasive germ cell tumors within 5 years [12]. Occurring as small foci of disease scattered within affected testes, ITGCN is thought to be present in nearly all testes harboring germ cell tumors and around 5% of contralateral testis [13,14]. This risk is thought to be higher in the presence of risk factors such as cryptorchidism and testicular atrophy (volume <12 mL) [15].

Because of the increased risk associated with ITGCN, biopsy of the contralateral testis should be considered in high-risk groups. In addition, multiple studies have demonstrated that low-dose radiotherapy (20 Gy) to the contralateral testis is oncologically effective while preserving testicular endocrine function [16,17]. This results from the relative radioresistance of Leydig cells compared to germinal epithelium. Of note, attempts at further dose reduction of radiotherapy have resulted in recurrent ITGCN so this is not recommended.

According to the European Consensus Conference regarding treatment of germ cell tumors, males with testicular volumes <12 mL and younger than 40 years of age have a 34% risk of ITGCN in the contralateral testis and represent the high-risk cohort for whom biopsy could most benefit [18]. Skakkebaek *et al.* defined a testicular dysgenesis syndrome (TDS) including factors such as hypospadias, undescended testis, low sperm count, testicular microlithiasis (TM) and inhomogenous ultrasound findings; these patients are at an increased risk of both germ cell tumors and contralateral ITGCN [19]. In patients with germ cell tumors found to have TM in the contralateral testis, the risk of concomitant ITGCN can be as high as 75%, suggesting that biopsy may be most beneficial in this specific cohort [20]. A biopsy should be performed at the time of orchiectomy.

In a study of RO specimens with germ cell tumors, 33% of patients were found to demonstrate multifocality; in addition to the ultrasound detected tumor(s), pathological evaluation showed separate tumor foci in 12% of patients, microinvasive tumor in 14%,

extratumor vascular invasion in 12%, and rete testis invasion in 1.4 % [21]. Of patients with multifocality, ITGCN was identified in 83.3%. Multifocality was noted to be more frequent in men with smaller tumors (<2 cm) and seminoma histology (p < 0.01). Despite this high incidence of multifocality, a low rate of recurrence has been reported in patients meeting these criteria undergoing TSS. However, this study's findings certainly reinforce the recommendation of performing RO when malignancy is detected on frozen section evaluation (FSE).

Accuracy of FSE

The accuracy of intraoperative pathological assessment is of critical importance for multiple reasons. First, the decision to proceed with organ preservation is often contingent on confirmation of a benign lesion. In addition, FSE of the tumor base helps minimize the chance of incomplete resection of a malignant tumor.

The increased accuracy of intraoperative FSE has been of increasing use in a manner that parallels the tumor bed biopsy in partial nephrectomy. A retrospective review of 354 patients who underwent RO from 1974 to 2000 assessed FSE findings and correlated them to the final pathologic diagnoses [22]. All malignant (317) and benign lesions (37) were accurately identified. An 8–10% misclassification rate was seen between seminoma and NSGCT. However this would not impact operative management in TSS because these patients would typically undergo RO or further biopsies of the resection bed to ensure negative margins. No recurrences were seen with a mean follow-up of 105 months. Another study investigated the accuracy of FSE in 10 patients with suspected testicular masses 2 cm or smaller and normal tumor markers between 2007 and 2011. RO was performed in all followed by ex vivo tumor excision and FSE evaluation. FSE correctly classified all four malignant lesions and all six benign lesions (and identified the correct histology in five out of six) when compared to the final orchiectomy specimen [23]. Subik *et al.* assessed intraoperative FSE for 45 testicular masses in a prospective manner between 1993 and 2010 and found 19 malignant tumors and 26 benign tumors by FSE. They concluded that FSE prevented unnecessary RO in 83.7% of cases and was useful for small, nonpalpable, incidental masses [24]. Given these findings, FSE by an experienced pathologist is thought to be satisfactory and necessary for intraoperative management decisions in testicular organ-sparing surgery.

Preexisting Infertility in Men with Germ Cell Tumors

Baseline semen analysis parameters can be abnormal in up to 60% of men diagnosed with testicular cancer. Findings are typically characterized by decreased total sperm counts with higher follicle-stimulating hormone (FSH) levels, suggesting a primary germ cell defect [25]. Indeed, the association between germ cell tumors and impaired spermatogenesis is fundamental to the TDS model. Many men remain infertile after TSS, so organ preservation for the purpose of fertility preservation is primarily considered most beneficial in men for whom RO would render them anorchid. Given the preexisting abnormalities of spermatogenesis and the extreme sensitivity of germinal epithelium to radiation and platinum-based chemotherapy, sperm banking is recommended before surgery for any patient interested in future paternity.

The Importance of Aesthetics

The true psychological distress experienced by the young patient with testis cancer is poorly understood [26]. With improved cancer survivorship in testis cancer, the psychological impact of orchiectomy and use of prosthetic testis insertion has recently been investigated. A questionnaire survey of 234 men found an approximate rate of 33% receiving a prosthetic implant following orchiectomy, a third declining, and a third never being offered one. More than 90% of men felt it was extremely important to merely be offered prosthesis regardless of decision [27]. Skoogh *et al.* conducted another questionnaire survey of 960 testicular cancer survivors (mean age of 30 years at diagnosis) focusing on uneasiness or shame following orchiectomy. Thirty-two percent of men reported a sense of loss, whereas 26% had feelings of uneasiness/shame; the majority of these sentiments occurred in patients who were never offered prosthesis (relative risk: 2.0, 95% confidence interval: 1.3–3.0). Although patients may decline prosthesis, the psychological impact of being offered one may alleviate the feelings of loss in some men [28]. Most importantly, this demonstrates that the psychological and cosmetic implications of orchiectomy are indeed substantial. With improving oncologic outcomes and survivorship for patients with testicular cancer, functional and psychosocial difficulties may indeed represent major long-term complications of therapy.

Development of Antisperm Antibodies

Following testicular surgery, there is concern for the development of antisperm antibodies (ASA). An increased baseline rate of ASA is noted in all patients with a diagnosis of testicular cancer, with higher percentages seen associated with higher-stage disease [29]. However, many other testicular conditions can predispose patients to elevated ASA levels [30]. Leonhartsberger *et al.* assessed 54 men from 2000 to 2005 undergoing operative intervention for testicular cancer (23 TSS, 31 RO). Serum samples were collected during follow-up visits for both groups and the ASA determined by enzyme-linked immunosorbent assay. The mean ASA levels were not statistically significant between patients undergoing TSS compared with RO (29 vs, 24.8 U/mL, $p > 0.3$) [31]. Although these data are reassuring, it should be interpreted in the broader context of overall impaired fertility in men with testicular tumors as discussed previously.

Indications for TSS

Criteria in Previous Studies and Guidelines

The role for TSS has evolved significantly in the past decade, and no consensus currently exists regarding its use. According to the European Association of Urology, TSS should be considered in patients with synchronous bilateral testicular tumors, metachronous contralateral tumors, or in a solitary testis tumor with normal endocrine function, provided that tumor volume is less than 30% of testicular volume [32]. Additionally, all patients are recommended to receive adjuvant radiotherapy (20 Gy) because of the elevated risk of ITGCN. The German Testicular Cancer Study Group reports TSS should be considered for testicular masses in a solitary testis or for patients with bilateral tumors 2 cm or smaller and normal preoperative endocrine function [33]. A growing body of evidence also supports the consideration of TSS for small tumors in the presence of a normal contralateral testis [18,23,34,35].

Preoperative Considerations and Surgical Technique

The physician should discuss the surgical, oncological, and functional risks and benefits of attempted organ preservation with the patient and informed consent should be obtained. A testicular oncologic work-up should be performed prior to the operation, including serum tumor markers (alfa fetoprotein [AFP], beta-human chorionic gonadotropin [β-HCG], lactate dehydrogenase [LDH]) with consideration of preoperative staging CT scan; evidence of metastasis might suggest malignancy and indicate immediate RO. Semen cryopreservation should be offered and patients informed of the potential impact of operative intervention on fertility.

At the time of the operation, preoperative antibiotics are administered, and the patient is induced under general anesthesia. The patient is positioned supine and is prepped and draped in standard fashion. The skin incision is made over the inferomedial aspect of the inguinal canal, long enough to deliver the testis atraumatically. The external inguinal ring is opened as the external oblique fascia is sharply incised. After dissecting and reflecting away the ilioinguinal nerve, the spermatic cord is mobilized and elevated. A rubber shod or Penrose drain tourniquet is optionally used to clamp the vessels of the cord, in which case ice can be applied to the testis for cold ischemia.

The testis is delivered through the incision, and a barrier drape or laparotomy pads are placed underneath the testis and over the surgical incision (Figure 14.2). The tunica vaginalis is opened longitudinally and the testis is exposed (Figure 14.3). For small tumors,

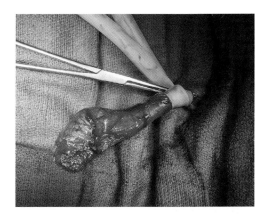

Figure 14.2 Mobilized testis and spermatic cord. Cord has been clamped using a Penrose drain as a tourniquet.

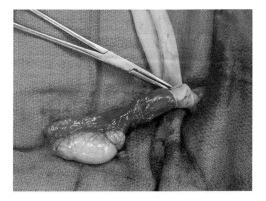

Figure 14.3 Tunica vaginalis has been opened, exposing that testicle.

the operating microscope (Figure 14.4) is brought into the surgical field, providing 5× to 25× optical magnification (optional for all tumors).

For palpable tumors, the tunica albuginea can be incised transversely overlying the tumor, avoiding subtunical vessels as possible. For nonpalpable tumors, intraoperative ultrasound is performed to localize the lesion and determine the optimal incision location. Needle or hook wire localization can optionally be performed (Figure 14.5). The tunica albuginea is then opened sharply or using cutting current with fine point cautery over a 16- to 18-gauge angiocatheter placed immediately under the tunica to protect the testicular parenchyma (Figure 14.6).

The divided tunica is gently spread with forceps, and the seminiferous tubules are bluntly dissected to facilitate exposure of the mass. Once the mass is located, sharp and blunt dissection are used to circumferentially mobilize and remove it (Figures 14.7, 14.8, and 14.9). Usually, a pseudocapsule enclosing

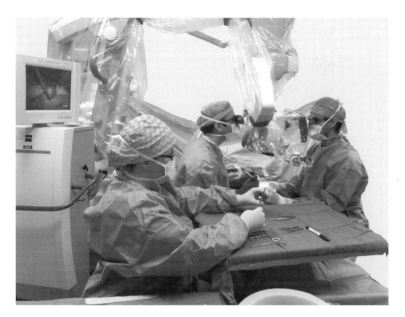

Figure 14.4 Setup for dual-head operating microscope.

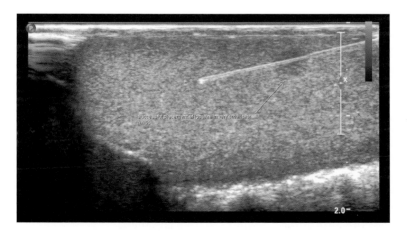

Figure 14.5 Ultrasound-guided needle localization of small intratesticular mass.

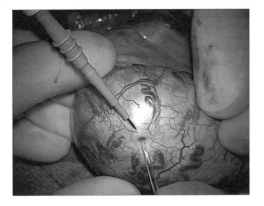

Figure 14.6 Use of fine-point cautery with cutting current to open the tunica albuginea over a 16-gauge angiocatheter.

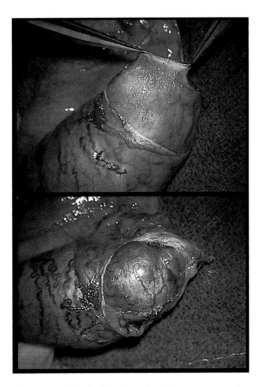

Figure 14.7 Testicular adrenal rest tumor exposed upon opening tunica albuginea.

the mass will be present. When surrounding seminiferous tubules are adherent to the mass or capsule, they are removed with the specimen to be included in the pathological evaluation. The mass, any suspicious regions, as well tubules from at least two sites at the

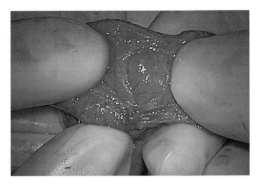

Figure 14.8 Exposure of deep intratesticular tumor.

base of the tumor are sent for frozen section pathological evaluation. The cord is unclamped to limit ischemia and to help identify bleeding intratesticular vessels.

When intraoperative pathological evaluation suggests germ cell tumor, ITGCN, or other malignancy, RO is typically performed for patients with a normal contralateral testis (or radiation therapy is used for ITGCN). In this case, the cord is dissected all the way to the internal ring and ligated in the retroperitoneum in standard fashion. For patients with a solitary testis or bilateral tumors, the decision between partial and complete orchiectomy is made based on preoperative discussion of the patient's preferences, priorities, and risk tolerance, in conjunction with intraoperative findings and pathological assessment. When margins are positive, further resection or orchiectomy must be performed as described previously.

Fine bipolar cautery is used to obtain hemostasis within the testis. The tunica albuginea (Figure 14.10) and vaginalis are closed with continuous 4-0 and 3-0 absorbable suture, respectively. The testis and cord are returned to their normal, untwisted position within the scrotum. The wound and scrotum are irrigated. The fascia is closed with a running 2-0 polyglactin suture, Scarpa's fascia and subcutaneous tissues are approximated with 3-0 polyglactin suture, and the skin is closed with 4-0 poliglecaprone suture. The wound is dressed as per surgeon's preference, supportive briefs are placed, and the patient is awaked from anesthesia.

Figure 14.9 Excision and removal of deep intratesticular tumor.

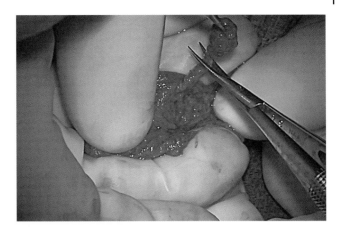

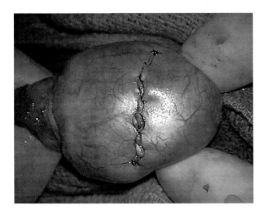

Figure 14.10 Completed continuous closure of tunica albuginea.

Postoperative Care and Follow-Up

Recovery instructions are similar to that for RO. In addition, patients are instructed to apply cold packs to the scrotum and wear tight-fitting underwear. Oral analgesic medications are typically used for 3 to 7 days. Patients are asked to refrain from heavy lifting and exercise for 4 to 6 weeks.

After partial orchiectomy in the setting of malignant tumor, adjuvant radiation treatment should be considered because of the increased risk of ITGCN. This carries the disadvantage of toxicity to germ cells and spermatogenesis, so the decision and timing of treatment should be individualized to each patient's preference and oncologic risk.

Most recommend clinic visit follow-up every 3 to 6 months for the first 3 years with physical examination, serum tumor markers, abdominal/scrotal ultrasound, annual chest X-ray, whereas those with a history of malignant pathology require an annual CT scan. Likely, a less rigorous schedule could be used for benign tumor types depending on individual histology.

Considerations Regarding Surgical Technique

The Impact of Cold/Warm Ischemia Compared with No Ischemia

Standard operative teaching recommends prompt clamping of the spermatic cord before mobilization of the testicle during RO but questions remain regarding cold versus warm ischemia when performing TSS. From 2003 to 2010, a prospective study compared 65 patients undergoing TSS (33 in 30 patients) in a nonischemic fashion to 35 patients who underwent standard RO [36]. No local/systemic recurrences occurred in any patient and all demonstrated no evidence of disease at median 52.5 month follow-up. Serum testosterone levels were within normal limits for all except two patients who underwent TSS (both with metachronous bilateral germ cell tumors); however, no testosterone supplementation was need. No tumor seeding or relapse was noted and the preservation of vessel integrity was hypothesized to have a potential effect on long-term fertility. Although no randomized controlled trial has been performed, similar results have been reported in patients undergoing TSS under cold ischemia, with only one patient having abnormal serum testosterone levels and all patients remaining free of disease at mean follow-up of 46.3 months [37]. Given these results, no consensus has been achieved and currently both approaches to vascular control are adequate pending further studies.

Use of Intraoperative Ultrasound

Stoll *et al.* were the first to suggest the utility of TSS by incorporating high-resolution intraoperative ultrasound to detect nonpalpable testicular tumors [38]. Intraoperative ultrasound allows for accurate and precise detection of testicular lesions to guide proper excision or enucleation. It has now become standard to use a high-resolution intraoperative ultrasound (8–13 MHz) when attempting TSS for nonpalpable tumors.

Use of Microsurgical Technique

The operative microscope has recently been incorporated as a method to increase surgical accuracy and to spare maximal healthy tissue in a manner similar to the role of surgical robotics in partial nephrectomy. A retrospective assessment investigating the impact of microsurgical TSS was conducted evaluating 23 patients from 2004 to 2011. Intraoperative ultrasound and FSE were used in each case and cold ischemia was also employed for two cases felt to be more complicated. RO was performed in cases where FSE suggested malignancy. All tumor resections were conducted within 30 minutes with a mean ischemic time of 18 minutes. All patients were free of disease at mean 35 months follow-up and no postoperative clinical hypogonadism was noted [39]. Currently, there is no consensus on the necessity for microsurgical dissection; likely, its use is tied to the size of the tumor and the appearance of the testicular parenchyma.

Hook Wire Localization and Enucleation

Additionally, one may choose to use a hook wire for tumor localization. A case report of a 20-year-old male with bilateral testicular mixed germ cell tumor (2.7 cm right and 1.3 cm left) describes the technique [40]. At 3 months follow-up, the patient had no evidence of disease recurrence and demonstrated normal tumor markers, testosterone, luteinizing hormone (LH) and follicle-stimulating hormone (FSH).

In this technique, ultrasound guidance is used for the insertion of a 20G × 9-cm introducer needle with hook wire. The needle is positioned beyond tumor margin and then the hook deployed. Hook wire allows accurate localization of tumor and excision, especially for nonpalpable masses. This novel technique may assist with more accurate localization of difficult nonpalpable masses. A needle without a hook wire can be used for tumor localization in a similar fashion.

Outcomes of TSS

Oncologic Outcomes

Outcomes are exceptionally favorable following TSS for benign lesions. A recent retrospective assessment of 37 patients undergoing TSS for benign testicular masses between 1999 and 2011 summarizes the improvements and efficiency involved in intraoperative FSE. All tumors were removed under ultrasound guidance and biopsies taken to ensure there was no ITGCN or positive margins. The patients ranged from 16 to 68 years of age, and no postoperative androgen supplementation was required. All patients were free of disease at mean follow-up of 63 months [41]. In another series of 47 benign lesions, 68% of patients were able to undergo TSS, and there was no evidence of recurrence after 7 years follow-up.

No randomized controlled trials currently exist comparing RO with TSS for benign or malignant disease. In a review across five academic centers from 1984 to 2013, long-term oncologic and functional outcomes were assessed in 25 patients undergoing TSS for bilateral tumors (11) or for a tumor in a solitary testis (14). For bilateral tumors, RO was performed for the larger tumor and TSS for the smaller. No patient with a preserved testicle required androgen supplementation and mean postoperative serum testosterone level was 400 ng/dL. Twenty of 25 tumors were malignant germ cell tumors, and overall survival was 100% at mean follow-up of 42.7 months. Three patients (15% of malignant tumors) developed ipsilateral recurrences in the same follow-up interval: two were deemed free of disease with RO and the third underwent repeat TSS with tumor bed resection [42].

The German Testicular Cancer Study Group reported on 73 patients with bilateral masses or solitary testis masses at eight centers from 1994 to 2000. TSS was performed for 52 metachronous, 17 synchronous, and 4 solitary testis tumors requiring enucleation. All operations used cold ischemia and biopsies were taken until negative margins were documented. ITGCN was present in 82% (46 patients), who then underwent local radiation with 18 Gy and demonstrated no relapse. After median follow-up of 91 months, 98.6% of patients were free of disease and one died of systemic progression. Local relapse was seen in 4 patients who were successfully treated with subsequent RO [18].

Fertility and Hypogonadism Outcomes

A literature review of TSS from 1999 to 2009 demonstrated that most patients do not require androgen supplementation following TSS and have satisfactory sexual function but remain infertile [43]. Ischemia to the testicle during spermatic cord clamping has been implicated as a possible source of damage for endocrine and exocrine function. Similar to testicular torsion, the contralateral testicle could be affected by a systemic cytokine response [44], autoimmunization against spermatogonia or Leydig cells [45], a reflex sympathetic response reducing contralateral testicular blood flow with ischemia-reperfusion injury, and the production of reactive oxygen species with excessive production of nitric oxide [46]. For TSS with FSE, it is recommended that the procedure be completed in less than 30 minutes clamp time, however at least one study has now prospectively assessed outcomes using a nonischemic technique [36]. Local adjuvant radiotherapy following TSS confers sterility.

Gentile *et al.* reported on a prospective study of 15 patients undergoing TSS from 2009 to 2013. Median age of patients was 38 years and cord clamping was performed in all but 1 patient (mean warm ischemia time of 18 minutes). FSE demonstrated 93% accuracy for histologic type and final pathologic analysis showed 6 patients without tumor, 7 with benign masses, and 2 with malignant lesions. All patients were free of disease after mean follow-up of 19.2 months. Hormonal profile and fertility assessments were normal postoperatively and no significant changes in serum testosterone were seen [47].

Summary

TSS is becoming a popular modality for the increasing numbers of benign testicular lesions and for some malignant tumors. As the cure rate for germ cell tumors continues to improve, much attention is directed toward quality of life regarding hormonal function, fertility, and aesthetic and psychological outcomes. TSS is a feasible option for patients with small, nonpalpable testicular masses (<2 cm), negative biopsies of the tumor bed, and the absence of ITGCN in the remaining testicular parenchyma. When ITGCN is identified, partial orchiectomy can still be performed however subsequent curative low-dose (18–20 Gy) radiotherapy should be employed. There is no current consensus regarding the need for surgical cord clamping (warm ischemia compared with cold ischemia or no ischemia), with all techniques demonstrating no long-term functional deficits. The true use of the operative microscope and hook wire localization require further study and follow-up. With the overall improvement in quality of life and lack of hormonal and fertility functional deficits, TSS should be considered in select patients in the management of all forms of testicular masses.

References

1 Heidenreich A, Bonfig R, Derschum W, von Vietsch H, Dilbert DM. A conservative approach to bilateral testicular germ cell tumors. J Urol. 1995;153:10–3.

2 Einhorn LH. Curing metastatic testicular cancer. Proc Natl Acad Sci USA. 2002; 99(7):4592–5.

3 Surveillance, Epidemiology, and End Results Program (http://seer.cancer.gov/statfacts/html/testis.html)

4 Giuliano CJ, Freemantle SJ, and Spinella MJ. Testicular germ cell tumors: A paradigm for the successful treatment of solid tumor stem cells. Curr Cancer Ther Rev. 2006;2(3): 255–70.

5 Haas GP, Shumaker BP, Cerny JC. The high incidence of benign testicular tumors. J Urol. 1986;136(6): 1219–20.

6 Kressel K, Schnell D, Thon WF, Heymer B, Hartmann M, Altwein JE. Benign testicular tumors: A case for testis preservation? Eur Urol. 1988;15(3–4): 200–4.

7 Wasnik AP, Maturen KE, Shah S, Pandya A, Rubin JM, Platt JF. Scrotal pearls and pitfalls: Ultrasound findings of benign scrotal lesions. Ultrasound Q. 2012;28(4):281–91.

8 Carmignani L, Gadda F, Gazzano G, Nerva F, Mancini M, Ferruti M, *et al.* High incidence of benign testicular neoplasms diagnosed by ultrasound. J Urol. 2003; 170:1783–6.

9 Tsili AC, Argyropoulou MI, Giannakis D, Sofitkitis N, Tsampoulas K. MRI in the characterization and local staging of testicular neoplasms. AJR Am J Roentgenol. 2010;194:682–9.

10 Sonmez G, Sivrioglu AK, Velioglu M, Incedayi M, Soydan H, Kara K, *et al.* Optimized imaging techniques for testicular masses: fast and with high accuracy. Wien Klin Wochenschr. 2012;124:704–8.

11 Che M, Tamboli P, Ro JY, Park DS, Ro JS, Amato RJ, *et al.* Bilateral testicular germ cell tumors: Twenty-year experience at M.D. Anderson Cancer Center. Cancer. 2002;95(6):1228–33.

12 Skakkebaek NE, Berthelsen JG. Carcinoma-in-situ of testis and orchiectomy. Lancet. 1978;2: 204–5.

13 Hoei-Hansen CE. Application of stem cell markers in search for neoplastic germ cells in dysgenetic gonads, extragonadal tumours, and in semen of infertile men. Cancer Treat Rev. 2008;34:348–67.

14 Dieckmann KP, Skakkebaek NE. Carcinoma in situ of the testis: review of biological and clinical features. Int J Cancer. 1999;83(6):815–22.

15 Dieckmann KP and Loy V. Prevalance of contralateral testicular intraepithelial neoplasia in patients with testicular germ cell neoplasia. J Clin Oncol.1996;14(12): 3126–32.

16 Heidenreich A, Weissbach L, Holtl W, Albers P, Kliesch S, Köhrmann KU, *et al.* Organ sparing surgery for malignant germ cell tumor of the testis. J Urol. 2001;166:2161–65.

17 Classen J, Dieckmann K, Bamberg M, *et al.* Radiotherapy with 16 Gy may fail to eradicate testicular intraepithelial neoplasia: Preliminary communication of a dose-reduction trial of the German Testicular Cancer Study Group. Br J Cancer. 2003;88(6):828–31.

18 Krege S, Beyer J, Souchon R, Albers P, Albrecht W, Algaba F, *et al.* European consensus conference on diagnosis and treatment of germ cell cancer: A report of

the second meeting of the European Germ Cell Consensus group (EGCCG): Part I. Eur Urol. 2008;53:478–96.

19 Skakkebaek NE. Testicular dysgenesis syndrome: new epidemiological evidence. Int J Androl. 2004;27(4):189–91.

20 Van Casteren NJ, Looijenga LH and Dohle GR. Testicular microlithiasis and carcinoma in situ overview and proposed clinical guideline. Int J Androl. 2009;32(4):279–87.

21 Ehrlich Y, Konichezky M, Yossepowitch O, Baniel J. Multifocality in testicular germ cell tumors. J Urol. 2009;181(3):1114–9.

22 Elert A, Olbert P, Hegele A, Barth P, Hofmann R, Heidenreich A. Accuracy of frozen section examination of testicular tumors of uncertain origin. Eur Urol. 2002;41(3):290–3.

23 Tuygen C, Ozturk U, Goktug H, Zengin K, Sener NC, Barkitas H. Evaluation of frozen section results in patients who have suspected testicular masses: A preliminary report. Urol J. 2014;11(1):1253–57.

24 Subik MK, Gordetsky J, Yao JL, di Sant'Agnese PA, Miyamoto H. Frozen section assessment in testicular and paratesticular lesions suspicious for malignancy: Its role in preventing unnecessary orchiectomy. Hum Pathol. 2012;43:1514–19.

25 Rives N, Perdrix A, Hennebicq S, Saïas-Magnan J, Melin MC, Berthaut I, *et al.* The semen quality of 1158 men with testicular cancer at the time of cryopreservation: Results of the French National CECOS Network. J Androl. 2012;33(6):1394–401.

26 Heidenreich A, Hofmann R. Quality-of-life issues in the treatment of testicular cancer. World J Urol. 1999;17(4):230–8.

27 Adshead J, Khoubehi B, Wood J, Rustin G. Testicular implants and patient satisfaction: A questionnaire-based study of men after orchidectomy for testicular cancer. BJU Int. 2001;88:559–62.

28 Skoogh J, Steineck G, Cavallin-Stahl E, Wilderäng U, Håkansson UK, Johansson B, Stierner U, *et al.* Feelings of loss and uneasiness or shame after removal of a testicle by orchidectomy: A population-based long-term follow-up of testicular cancer survivors. Int J Androl. 2011; 34:183–92.

29 Guazzieri S, Lembo A, Ferro G, Artibani W, Merlo F, Zanchetta R, *et al.* Sperm antibodies and infertility in patients with testicular cancer. Urology. 195;26 (2):139–42.

30 Lenzi A, Gandini L, Lombardo F, *et al.* Antisperm antibodies in young boys. Andrologia 1991;23(3):233–5.

31 Leonhartsberger N, Gozzi C, Akkad T, Springer-Stoehr B, Bartsch G, Steiner H. Organ-sparing surgery does not lead to greater antisperm antibody levels than orchidectomy. BJU Int. 2007;100(2):371–4.

32 Albers P, Albrecht W, Algaba F, Bokemeyer C, Cohn-Cedermark G, Fizazi K, *et al.* EAU guidelines on testicular Cancer. 2011 update. Eur Urol. 2011;60(2):304–19.

33 Heidenreich A, Albers P, Krege S. Management of bilateral testicular germ cell tumours—experience of the German Testicular Cancer Study Group (GTCSG), abstract 299. Eur Urol Suppl.2006;5:97.

34 Albers P. Management of stage I testis cancer. Eur Urol. 2007;51:34–43.

35 Hallak J, Cocuzza M, Sarkis AS, Athayde KS, Cerri GG, Srougi M. Organ-sparing microsurgical resection of incidental testicular tumors plus microdissection for sperm extraction and cryopreservation in azoospermic patients: Surgical aspects and technical refinements. Urology. 2009;73:887–91.

36 Leonhartsberger N, Pichler R, Stoehr B, *et al.* Organ preservation technique without ischemia in patients with testicular tumor. Urology. 2014;83(5):1107–11.

37 Steiner H, Holtl L, Maneschg C, Berger AP, Rogatsch H, Bartsch G, *et al.* Frozen section analysis-guided organ-sparing approach in testicular tumors: technique, feasibility, and long-term results. Urology. 2003;62:508–13.

38 Stoll S, Goldfinger M, Rothberg R, Buckspan MB, Fernandes BJ, Bain J. Incidental detection of impalpable

testicular neoplasm by sonography. AJR Am J Roentgenol. 1986;146(2):349–50.

39 Stefani S, Isgro G, Varca V, Pecchi A, Bianchi G, Carmignani G, *et al.* Microsurgical testis-sparing surgery in small testicular masses: Seven years retrospective management and results. Urology. 2012;79(4):858–62.

40 Ong T, Yaakup N, Sivalingam S, Razach AH. Hook wire localization for testis sparing surgery. Urology. 2013;81(4):904–8.

41 Leonhartsberger N, Pichler R, Stoehr B, Horninger W, Steiner H. Organ-sparing surgery is the treatment of choice in benign testicular tumors. World J Urol. 2014;32(4):1087–91.

42 Ferretti L, Sargos P, Gross-Goupil M, Izard V, Wallerand H, Huyghe E, *et al.* Testicular-sparing surgery for bilateral or monorchide testicular tumors: A multicenter study of long term oncological and functional results. BJU Int. 2014;114:860–4

43 Giannarini G, Dieckmann K, Albers P, *et al.* Organ-sparing surgery for adult testicular tumours: A systematic review of the literature. Eur Urol. 2010;57(5):780–90.

44 Visser AJ, Heyns CF. Testicular function after torsion of the spermatic cord. BJU Int. 2003;92(3):200–3.

45 Zanchetta R, Mastrogiacomo I, Graziotti P, Foresta C, Betterle C. Autoantibodies against Leydig cells in patients after spermatic cord torsion. Clin Exp Immunol. 1984;55(1):49–57.

46 Karaguzel E, Kadihasanoglu M, Kutlu O. Mechanisms of testicular torsion and potential protective agents. Nat Rev Urol. 2014;11:391–99.

47 Gentile G, Brunocilla E, Franceschelli A, Schiavina R, Pultrone C, Borghesi M, *et al.* Can testis-sparing surgery for small testicular masses be considered a valid alternative to radical orchiectomy? A prospective single-center study. Clin Genitourin Cancer. 2013;11(4):522–6.

15

Nanotechnology: An Evolution in Tissue Preservation and Focal-Targeted Oncologic Therapy

Kara L. Watts, MD, and Joshua M. Stern, MD

Department of Urology, Montefiore Medical Center, Albert Einstein College of Medicine, Bronx, NY, USA

Introduction

The treatment of urologic malignancies has witnessed an evolution toward minimally invasive surgical approaches commensurate with the demand for decreasing surgical morbidity and earlier detection of lower stage cancers. This is most notable in the development of treatments for renal and prostate cancers. More recently, there has been growing interest in developing therapeutics that optimize tissue preservation with a focal, targeted approach.

Before the era of radiologic imaging, the diagnosis of renal cancers was prompted by the classic presentation of a flank bulge, hematuria, and pain. The classic treatment for nonmetastasized lesions was an open radical nephrectomy with para-aortic lymph node dissection [1]. With the increasing use of computed tomography (CT) imaging, renal lesions have been detected at earlier stages and smaller sizes. In 1990, the trend toward minimally invasive surgery was pioneered by the introduction of laparoscopic radical nephrectomy as the standard treatment for lesions larger than 4 cm [2]. More recently, laparoscopic or robotic-assisted partial nephrectomy has been widely employed as a standard treatment for smaller lesions.

Similarly, the treatment of prostate cancer has shifted. Earlier detection of lower-stage lesions has been facilitated by the prevalent use of prostate-specific antigen (PSA) screening [3]. Indeed, nearly 90% of men diagnosed with prostate cancer present with clinically localized disease [4]. The original standard open retropubic radical prostatectomy, most common until the 1980s, has been largely replaced by minimally invasive approaches. Currently, more than 80% of all prostate cancers are treated by either laparoscopic or robotic-assisted laparoscopic radical prostatectomy [1].

Over the past decade, the concept of minimizing surgical invasiveness and morbidity has expanded to encompass a growing appreciation for the benefits of tissue preservation. For small renal masses, focal ablation using cryotherapy or radiofrequency has become more popular for the appropriate patient. Similarly, high-intensity focused ultrasound (HIFU) and cryotherapy have been employed for the treatment of focal, localized prostate neoplasms [5–14].

Management of Urologic Cancer: Focal Therapy and Tissue Preservation, First Edition.
Edited by Mark P. Schoenberg and Kara L. Watts.
© 2017 John Wiley & Sons Ltd. Published 2017 by John Wiley & Sons Ltd.

Introduction to Nanotechnology

The concept of nanoparticles was originally developed more than 50 years ago, although it was not fully realized for its application in modern oncologic therapy until the 1990s [15]. The increasing interest in developing tissue-sparing therapies for the treatment of localized cancers has prompted considerable biomedical investigation into the field of nanotechnology and nanoparticles. Therapeutic nanotechnology centers on the use of photothermal-based ablative energy, which is delivered to a lesion of interest through activation of various types of nanoparticles. Thermal ablative energy induces necrosis of the tissue of interest via temperatures high enough to cause focal cell death, while ideally sparing the surrounding healthy tissue.

Metal nanoshells consist of a spherical dielectric nanoparticle surrounded by a thin, conductive, metallic layer—typically silver or gold. Each metal shell has an intrinsic surface plasmon resonance (SPR) that can be tuned to interact with a range of light frequencies, which excite surface electrons, leading to collective oscillation. As the electrons relax to their ground state, the metal particles release thermal energy [16,17].

Varying the composition, core size, and shell thickness of a particular metal nanoshell results in alterations in its plasmon resonance, ranging from the visible to the near-infrared (NIR) regions of the spectrum. For biologic application, properties of nanoparticles are tuned to generate an optimal photothermal response to NIR light waves (650–900 nm). Light waves in this spectrum are transmitted through biologic tissue with very low scattering and minimal heating because waves in this frequency pass through water and chromophores with minimal absorption [16,18].

Phototherapy-induced thermal ablation attempts to induce a local temperature rise among targeted tissue. Temperatures from 45° to 60°C have been reported as the necessary threshold at which protein denaturation and cell death of cancer cells occur [19–22]. Early investigators into radiofrequency ablation (RFA) of renal tumors posited that heating tissues to 60°C routinely leads to desiccation and coagulative necrosis. In addition to the direct effects on cellular structure, supraphysiologic temperatures cause microvascular and arteriolar occlusion, resulting in ischemia at the target site. Similar to the concept of RFA for renal tumors, the goal is to concomitantly spare a lethal dose of heat energy to surrounding healthy tissue [23].

Several researchers have published their results on the use of various three-dimensional models and spherical-based bio-heat equations to optimize the radius of heat delivery to limit lethal doses of heat energy to less than 10% of surrounding healthy tissue [22,24]. Stern *et al.* demonstrated the concept of a strict zone of cell death, where a 1.6-mm zone of ablation correlated precisely to the laser spot size used to activate the nanoparticles in a PC-3 prostate cancer cell line (Figure 15.1) [25,26].

Types of Nanoparticles

There are a plethora of nanoparticles (NP), both in terms of their bulk metal constituents and their overall shape and composition (Figure 15.2). Nearly all nanoparticles derive their ablative potential through laser or magnetic activation and subsequent heat exchange. The first nanoparticle developed was a gold nanoshell (GNS), and many other gold-based nanoparticles have since been developed. Gold nanoparticles have been popular because gold is resistant to corrosion and oxidation, has a low toxicity profile, inert chemical properties, and conformational flexibility for use in a variety of structural applications [15]. It also has easily tunable optical absorption, with ordinary gold nanospheres and more complex gold-based shapes reaching plasmon resonance varying from 520 nm into the NIR range (800–1200 nm). Gold has also been shown to facilitate easy

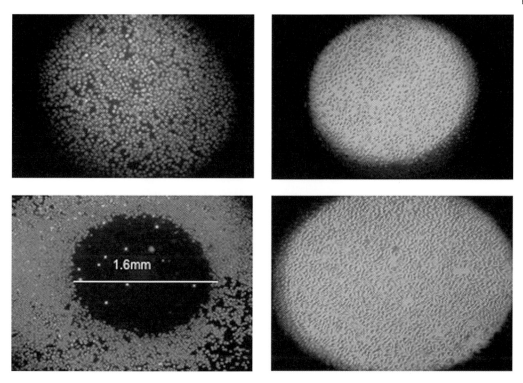

Figure 15.1 *Left,* Depicts a zone of nonviability/ablation in PC-3 cells after near-infrared laser ablation with gold nanoshells. The zone of nonviability (1.6 mm) correlates with laser spot size. *Right,* Dark field microscopy of PC-3 cells stained with Calcium AM 1 hour after laser activation. Despite loss of viability, cells maintain intact morphology, as seen under dark field microscope. Reprinted with permission from Stern JM, Stanfield J, Kabbani W, Hsieh JT, Cadeddu JA [26].

conjugation of proteins onto its surface and to support the addition of stealthing polymers (i.e., polyethylene glycol) to its surface to enhance biocompatibility and improve blood circulation times [27–29].

Currently, silica-based GNS comprise the most common structures used in photothermal therapeutics [16,30–35]. Silica-based GNS consist of a dielectric (silica) core with a gold metal shell [36,37]. Their use in urologic cancers will be discussed in more depth later. Gold nanorods (GNRs) are a structural variation of the GNS. Their anisotropic shape affords them two distinct SPR bands, which are tunable based on their aspect ratio (length/width). One peak occurs at 520 nm (similar to the GNS) and a second stronger peak occurs at NIR wavelengths (650–900 nm), making the latter most suitable for in-vivo applications [38–41].

Gold-gold sulfide (GGS) NPs replace the traditional silica core with a gold-sulfide core and pure gold shell. In comparison to silica-based gold nanoshells, GGS NPs have several advantages. First, they are significantly smaller particles—35-55 nm compared to 120–140 nm—which may facilitate their use in biologic applications. In addition, they witness a higher absorption efficiency at the NIR spectrum attributed to their higher absorption cross-sectional area ratio. GGS NPs have shown efficacy both in vivo and in vitro. In vitro, for example, they induced cell death by photothermal ablation when conjugated to HER2 and targeted to HER2 expressing breast cancer [16].

Other gold nanostructures have been developed, which include hollow gold nanoshells and gold nanocages. Hollow gold nanospheres have a core that is comprised of

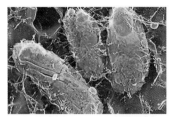

Escherichia coli (1 µM)

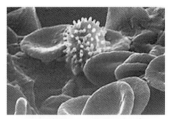

Red Blood Cell (7–8 µM)
White Blood Cell (12–15 µM)

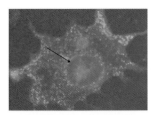

Cell Nucleus (4–7 µM)

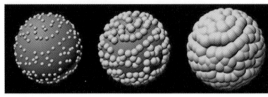

Gold Nanoshell (100 nM)

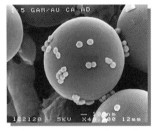

Gold Nanoparticle (10 nM)

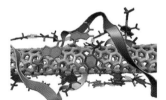

Carbon Nanotube (4–10 nM)

Figure 15.2 A comparison of the size of various nanoparticle structures to common cell types, cellular components, and bacterium.

the surrounding media, and varying the wall thickness adjusts the surface plasmon band absorption. Gold nanocages are characterized by hollow interiors and extremely thin, porous walls. They can be prepared in large quantities by a simple reaction, and the SPR of these structures is modifiable based on controlling the particle's size and wall thickness. They can create a lethal temperature when excited and have been shown to successfully ablate glioblastoma (GB) cells in mice subjected to laser treatment. GB cells without prior gold nanocage injection subjected to laser treatment did not reach a temperature greater than 37°C [42].

Nongold–based NPs have also shown considerable potential. Single- and multi-walled carbon nanotubes (SWNTs and MWNTs) have shown efficacy in vitro and in vivo. They are cylindrical structures ranging from a few to hundreds of nanometers, with lengths up to a few micrometers [43]. They are exceptionally photostable and demonstrate a strong optical absorption near the NIR region. When exposed to NIR light carbon nanotubs release vibrational energy that can create a heat lethal heat exchange [16,44–46]. In comparison to SWNTs, MWNTs absorb significantly more NIR radiation owing to their increased number of electrons per particle and greater number of metallic tubes. They also release substantial vibrational energy after exposure to NIR radiation [47–49]. Carbon nanotubes can also be functionalized by adding small molecular drugs, proteins, and even genes for delivery to a tissue [46,50]. Lastly, titanium oxide nanotubes (TiO-NTs) have also demonstrated a curative effect in cancers of the esophagus, gastrum, colon, skin, breast, and liver by using NIR laser–based photo-thermal energy [16,51].

A range of nanoparticles have also been developed for use in diagnostic assays. In the field of oncology, paramagnetic nanoparticles have been widely described to enhance the diagnostic use of magnetic resonance imaging (MRI). Investigational iron oxide particles (ferumoxtran-10, AMI-227, Combidex; Cambridge, MA, United States; Sinerem, Laboratoire Guerbet, Aulnay-sous-Bois, France) enjoyed a period of celebrity within the urology world based on their ability to enhance magnetic resonance detection of occult lymph node metastases from prostate cancer [52,53]. These particles measure between 30 and 50 nm and consist of an active iron oxide crystalline core surrounded by a low-molecular-weight dextran coating, which prolongs their time in circulation. They have been shown to facilitate detection of prostate cancer-containing lymph nodes as small as 2 mm and to have an overall positive predictive value of 95% for the detection of positive lymph nodes of any size [53–55].

Delivery and Use of Nanoparticles

A range of diagnostic modalities have employed nanoparticles to enhance their diagnostic accuracy. As discussed, MR lymphangiography (MRL) uses lymphotropic paramagnetic nanoparticles to enhance detection of occult or positive lymph nodes. These particles are injected intravenously after reconstitution with normal saline. Owing to their small size, they extravasate from blood vessels into the interstitium, both by direct transcapillary passage as well as nonselective endothelial transcytosis across permeable capillaries. From there, they are transported to lymph nodes. Macrophages within normal or benign lymph nodes phagocytose these particles, which are subsequently biodegraded within phagolysosomes. Nodes containing malignant cells lack functioning macrophages and will not uptake the nanoparticles and as such, malignant areas within the nodes retain their signal intensity and

remain bright on T2- and T2-weighted images (Figure 15.3) [52,53,56,57].

MRL has demonstrated an enhanced diagnostic capacity compared to standard CT or MRI for detecting positive lymph nodes. A meta-analysis of 12 studies evaluated the particles' efficacy across a range of malignancies, including prostate cancer, testicular cancer, seminoma, bladder cancer, and renal cancer. It revealed a pooled sensitivity of 82–100% and specificity of 80–100%, compared to 39% and 90%, respectively, for standard MRI [56,58].

In addition to their diagnostic potential, nanoparticles have been widely used in cancer therapeutics, both as a means to deliver thermal-based energy as well as to deliver targeted therapy to lesions. Particle delivery can be passive or targeted and can be delivered intravenously or injected directly into a tumor. Initial in-vivo studies used a direct injection of nanoshell suspensions into a tumor site, which was then subjected to a lethal dose of NIR-mediated thermal ablative energy. Given varied tumor types, some difficult to reach locations, and varied dispersion of particle within a tissue bed after direct tumor injection, this method has been of limited urologic use.

Intravenous passive particle delivery was subsequently developed. After injection, particles circulate and accumulate at the tumor site of interest based on the "enhanced permeability and retention" (EPR) effect. This states that as neoplastic tumors grow, they experience concomitant rapid angiogenesis which leads to a defect in the vascular architecture, causing "leaky vessels." Nanoparticles of a sufficiently small size extravasate out of the vasculature and accumulate within tumors. Particle retention is enhanced by the altered lymphatic drainage of tumors. Size is clearly of critical importance, with particles in the 60- to 400-nm range being ideal for passive tumor targeting [15,17].

Once the nanoparticles reach the tumor of interest, photothermal or photoacoustic energy is delivered by a variety of mechanisms: NIR lasers, magnetic hyperthermia, microwave and

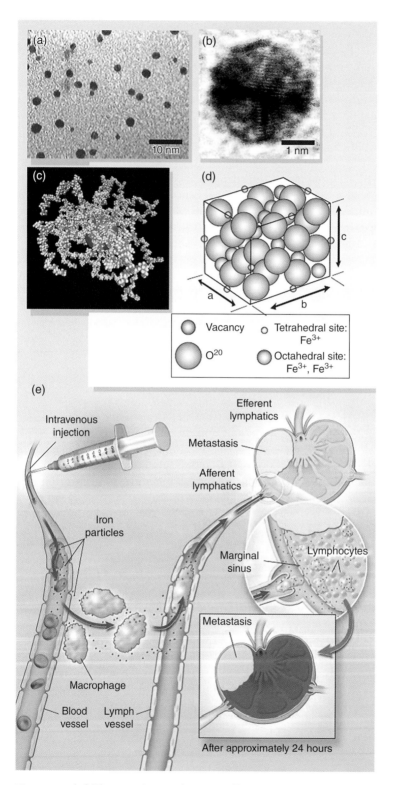

Figure 15.3 (a, b)Electron micrograph images of hexagonal lymphotropic superparamagnetic nanoparticles, which measure 2–3 mm. (c, d) Molecular model of packing iron oxide crystals. (e) Mechanism of action of lymphotropic superparamgnetic nanoparticles. Reprinted with permission from Clèment O, Guimaraes R, de Kerviler F, Frija G [57].

radiofrequency energy, and focused ultra-sound. They share a common goal of delivering a lethal dose of thermal energy to a prescribed volume of tissue, while sparing the surrounding healthy tissue. Although tissue necrosis is the ultimate goal, achieved at thermoablative temperatures of $45\,^{\circ}$C and above, mild temperature hyperthermia (40°–$45\,^{\circ}$C) also serves a utility. These slightly lower temperatures mediate antitumor effects via induction of apoptosis, activation of immunological processes, and induction of gene and protein synthesis. These factors can lead to greater efficacy of conventional treatment modalities, such as chemotherapy, immunotherapy, and radiation therapy [4,59–64].

Active tumor targeting has been widely studied in cell culture. The use of intravenous injection of a nanoparticle conjugated to a targeted ligand or antibody is an ongoing goal. The initial nanoparticle report of the ability to directly target tumor cells used adenovirus to deliver gold nanoshells to cervical and carcinoembryonic antigen (CEA)-expressive colon cancer cell lines [65]. Researchers were able to directly target CEA-expressing ligand on the tumor cell. Each vector delivered an astonishing 1,000 gold nanoparticles, which when activated by NIR light successfully ablated the targeted cells. Similarly, an in-vitro model using oral squamous cell carcinoma cells that overexpressed epidermal growth factor receptor (EGFR) were incubated with 40-nm GNS cells conjugated with an anti-EGFR monoclonal antibody and exposed to an argon laser at 514 nm. Complete cell death was achieved using a laser energy that alone, without the use of a nanoparticle, would be nonlethal [66].

Nanotechnology in Prostate Cancer

In urology, prostate cancer has received the most attention with regard to the use of nanotechnology for both diagnostic and therapeutic platforms. The prevalence of prostate cancer—affecting 1 in 6 men throughout their lifetime—and the marked trend toward using minimally invasive, tissue-sparing therapies have rendered it a target of considerable interest [4].

Imaging in Prostate Cancer

Iron oxide particles currently dominate the field of prostate cancer nanoparticle-based imaging. The first nanotechnology breakthrough in prostate cancer imaging was with Combivex, a monocrystalline iron oxide lymphotropic superparamagnetic nanoparticle (mentioned previously). In the authors' initial series, 80 patients had intravenous particle infusion subsequent preoperative MRI followed by radical prostatectomy with lymph node dissection. Pathologic and imaging characteristics were compared. On a patient to patient analysis, MRI was 100% sensitive and 96% specific for the detection of positive lymph nodes after nanoparticle injection. For lymph nodes with a diameter of 5–10 mm on the short axis, which would be considered normal on conventional MRI, the sensitivity of MRI with lymphotropic superparamagnetic nanoparticles was 96.4% [57].

Several studies since the incident study have looked at the diagnostic accuracy of MRL in comparison to nonenhanced-MRI for detection of occult lymph node metastases. MRL and standard MRI images were compared with the surgical pathology of resected lymph nodes at time of prostatectomy. The use of MRL with a 1.5-T MRI revealed an overall sensitivity and specificity of detecting cancer-containing lymph nodes at 82–100% and 87–99%, respectively [56,57,67,68]. The sensitivity of standard CT and MRI for suspicious lymph nodes, which is based on shape and size criteria, is a mere 39–42%. As such, this is a substantial improvement [69]. Figure 15.4 demonstrates the limitations of standard MRI and CT for detection of lymph node metastases in prostate cancer.

Recently, a prospective study compared the diagnostic accuracy of MRL to multidetector CT (MDCT) in 375 patients with prostate

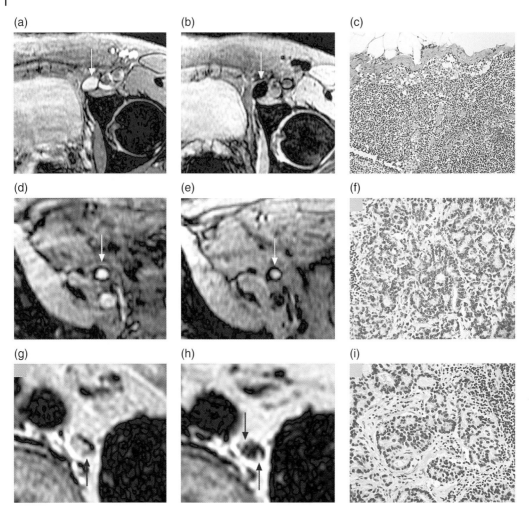

Figure 15.4 As compared with conventional MRI (Panel a), MRI obtained 24 hours after the administration of lymphotropic superparamagnetic nanoparticles (Panel b) shows a homogeneous decrease in signal intensity due to the accumulation of lymphotropic superparamagnetic nanoparticles in a normal lymph node in the left iliac region (arrow). Panel (c) shows the corresponding histologic findings (hematoxylin and eosin, ×125). Conventional MRI shows a high signal intensity in an unenlarged iliac lymph node completely replaced by tumor (arrow in Panel d). Nodal signal intensity remains high (arrow in Panel e). Panel F shows the corresponding histologic findings (hematoxylin and eosin, ×200). Conventional MRI shows high signal intensity in a retroperitoneal node with micrometastases (arrow in Panel g). MRI with lymphotropic superparamagnetic nanoparticles demonstrates two hyperintense foci (arrows in Panel h) within the node, corresponding to 2-mm metastases. Corresponding histologic analysis confirms the presence of adenocarcinoma within the node (Panel i, hematoxylin and eosin, ×200). Reprinted with permission from [60].

cancer with an intermediate or high risk of having lymph node metastases based on predictive nomograms. All patients were evaluated by both MRL and MDCT and underwent either pelvic lymph node dissection (PLND) or fine-needle aspiration biopsy. Imaging results were compared with histologic findings. Overall, the sensitivity and negative predictive value of MRL compared to MDCT were significantly higher, at 82% compared to 34% and 96% compared to 88%, respectively. The authors suggest that for patients with intermediate or high risk of having lymph node metastases, the posttest probability of having lymph node metastases after a negative MRL may be low enough to consider omitting the need for a PLND [67]. In an illustrative example of the power of MRL, Weidner *et al.*

used MRL to identify 5 cancer-containing lymph nodes in a patient who had undergone radical prostatectomy. This information was used to guide postsurgical intensity-modulated radiation therapy (IMRT). After his course of IMRT, a repeat MRL revealed no evidence of metastatic disease and a decrease in his PSA from 2.06 ng/mL before IMRT to 0.02 ng/mL after IMRT [70].

In addition to the enhanced sensitivity and specificity of MRL for detecting metastatic lymph nodes compared to standard CT and MRI, MRL appears to augment prediction of survival. Meijer *et al.* recently analyzed 138 patients with prostate cancer, with nonenlarged lymph nodes on CT, who underwent preoperative MRL using ferumoxtran-10 (iron oxide based) nanoparticles [71]. Histopathologic findings, obtained by either surgical lymph node dissection or CT-guided lymph node biopsy, were compared to preoperative imaging. They found that the 5-year overall survival for a negative MRL compared to a positive MRL was 96% and 57%, respectively. Five-year distant metastasis free survival was and 94% and 49%, respectively. Within the MRL positive group, a subgroup analysis of patients based on dimensions of positive lymph nodes was performed. The authors found that those patients with smaller positive lymph nodes (short axis of largest positive lymph nodes ≤8 mm) had a much better 5-year metastasis free (79% vs. 16%) and overall survival (81% vs. 36%) compared to those with larger positive lymph nodes (short axis of largest positive lymph nodes >8 mm). At the present time, ferumoxtran-10 is not approved by the Food and Drug Administration in the United States but is used in controlled trials in several European countries.

Beyond MRL, a recent in vitro study reported on the use of carbon nanotubes loaded with anti-PSA antibodies applied to an electrochemical immunosensor to detect differences in PSA concentration among normal prostate and prostate cancer cell lines. The authors reported that their immunoassay had a high sensitivity for detecting prostate-cancer containing cells and that it had good reproducibility and accuracy [72].

Therapeutics in Prostate Cancer

The first in-vivo study assessing the efficacy of nanoparticles for delivering thermal ablative energy to prostate cancer cells involved the direct tumor injection of paramagnetic nanoparticles into orthotopic Dunning R3327 prostate cancer-containing rats. The researchers demonstrated successful intraprostatic infiltration of the particles, excellent tolerability, and a stable lethal intratumoral temperature of 50°C when subjected to an alternating magnetic field [73]. A subsequent study by this group revealed that the combination of paramagnetic nanoparticles with radiation therapy (20 Gy) had the same therapeutic efficacy to that of a single radiation dose of 60 Gy, thus offering a potential adjunct to radiation therapy to reduce the overall radiation dose [74].

The first in-vivo study using passive intravenous injection of particles in a prostate cancer model used an orthotopic mouse model of human prostate cancer to assess the efficacy of gold nanoshells to thermally ablate prostate cancer. Stern *et al.* ablated 14 tumors with a 93% ablation rate reaching a maximum temperature within the tumor of 65.4°C [26]. Furthermore, the authors noted no ablative effect or local skin change from the application of NIR laser treatments at sites other than the PC-3 subcutaneous tumor in animals that received intravenous injection of GNS, suggesting success of passive targeted delivery of intravenous particles.

Ghosh *et al.* later investigated the in-vivo use of DNA-encased MWNTs to deliver a payload to PC3 xenograft tumors [75]. This study followed previous findings that DNA encasement of SWNTs increases their hydrophilicity [76]. The authors found that DNA encasement not only increased MWNT hydrophilicity and the ability to generate an aqueous solution for intratumoral injection, but it also generated heat with a linear dependence on laser power and irradiation time. DNA encasement yielded a threefold reduction in the total concentration of MWNTs needed to raise the temperature of the PC3 cells by 10 °C, demonstrating the malleable nature of nanoparticles. Furthermore, laser irradiation of the injected tumor cells resulted in complete eradication of tumor cells in all mice.

Evidence also supports the potential use of nanoparticles in suppressing tumor proliferation in metastatic prostate cancer. Prostate cancer nodules transplanted into the calvaria of male rats underwent intratumoral injection of paramagnetic nanoparticles conjugated to cationic liposomes. They were then subjected to alternating magnetic field irradiation. Results showed significant suppression of tumor proliferation in the bone microenvironment with induction of a necrotic mass around the magnetic particles in the tumor [77].

More recently, a number of studies have published their findings with regard to targeted therapy and nanoparticles. One group developed a dual-aptamer complex specific to prostate cancer cells to facilitate the delivery of Doxorubicin across the cell membrane. In vitro, Doxorubicin was loaded onto the complex and found to induce apoptosis of both prostate-specific membrane antigen (PSMA) (+) and (–) cells. In vivo, the aptamers were loaded onto superparamagnetic iron oxide nanoparticles and cultured with PSMA (+) and (–) prostate cancer cells, as well as with noncancer-containing cells. The authors demonstrated effective uptake by prostate cancer cells as well as apoptosis by histologic review in vivo [78].

Similarly, Yu *et al.* used a PSMA aptamer-conjugate thermally cross-linked to superparamagnetic iron oxide nanoparticles. As imaged by T2-weighted MRI, these particles demonstrated preferential binding toward prostate cancer cells both in vivo and in vitro. The molecules were then loaded with Doxorubicin, which showed selective drug delivery in the LNCaP xenograft mouse model, an example of the benefits of a targeted approach to nanoparticle delivery [79].

More recently, researchers have turned to the use of nanoparticles to enhance or modify Docetaxel (DTX) in the treatment of prostate cancer. DTX is one of the most important chemotherapeutic agents for castration resistant prostate cancer, but it is not without considerable side effects. Sato *et al.* investigated ways to limit the toxicity of chemotherapy. They found that conjugating Fe_3O_4 magnetic nanoparticles (MgNPs-Fe3O4) to DTX lowered the dose of DTX required to achieve a similar cytotoxic effect to that of a higher dose of free DTX. Specifically, 10 nM of DTX had an equivalent inhibitory effect as 1 nM of DTX combined with the nanoparticle. This shows promise for the use of MgNPs-Fe3O4 nanoparticles in combination with Docetaxel as a means of lowering the chemotherapeutic minimal effective dose and thereby reducing the adverse effects of this chemotherapeutic agent [80]. Similar findings were also reported by a Sanna *et al.* who reported on the in-vitro efficacy of Docetaxel-loaded polymeric nanoparticles [81].

Another recent study looked at the novel use of polymeric nanoparticles encapsulating trans-resveratrol (NP-RSV), an antiproliferative and chemopreventative phytoalexin derived from plants [82]. In prostate cancer cell lines, RSV has been shown to inhibit growth in a concentration-dependent manner, to induce apoptosis, and reduce oxidative stress and nitric oxide production in premalignant cells, thus slowing cellular growth [83–87]. The use of RSV alone is limited because of its poor solubility, low bioavailability, and instability. Sanna *et al.* loaded nanoparticles with RSV and tested them in vitro against three human prostate cancer cell lines: DU-145, PC3, and LNCaP. They found that the NP-RSV particle was readily internalized by the cells and subsequently controlled the release of RSV at a pH of 6.5 and 7.4, mimicking the tumoral acidic environment and physiologic conditions. Furthermore, NP-RSV compared to RSV alone resulted in a significant dose-dependent increase in cell growth inhibition.

Nanotechnology in Renal Cancer

Studies reporting the use of MRL for detection of renal cancer or metastases have received considerably less attention than that of prostate cancer. A pilot study evaluated the use of MRL for identifying nodal metastases in nine patients with primary renal masses. Both T2- and T2*-weighted MRI images were obtained for all patients before and after the administration of Combidex. All patients underwent radical nephrectomy, and lymph node dissection was performed for those with stage 2 renal cell carcinoma or transitional cell cancer. Pathologic comparison by two blinded pathologists in comparison with the MRL findings was performed. The sensitivity and specificity of MRL for detecting lymph node metastases was 100% and 95.7%, respectively. These results are promising but certainly warrant further, larger studies [88].

Similarly, there have been few studies reporting on the therapeutic effects of photothermal nanoparticle therapy. Bruners *et al.* employed CT-guided magnetic thermoablation of malignant renal tumors in a VX2 tumor rabbit model. CT-guided injection of superparamagnetic iron oxide particles into the tumor was performed. The tumors were then exposed to an alternating electromagnetic field. Hypovascular regions on posttherapy CT perfusion scans corresponded well to areas of tumor necrosis and to the zones containing the nanoparticle. These findings suggest that CT-guided magnetic thermoablation of renal malignancies is feasible in an animal model [89].

Pedro *et al.* used a 30-nm gold particle (CYT-6091, Cytimmune Sciences, Inc.) conjugated to tumor necrosis factor alpha to enhance the kill zone induced by RFA in renal tumors in New Zealand White rabbits. The rabbits were treated with either CYT-6091 alone, RFA alone, or CYT-6091 followed by RFA. Nanoparticles were delivered intravenously and accumulated at the tumor site passively. Posttherapy microscopic examination revealed that the combination of CYT-6091 and RFA had a larger zone of complete cell death compared to the RFA-alone group (Figure 15.5). Furthermore, the former group had a smaller zone of partially ablated tissue than the RFA-alone group. Augmenting existing technology is of a clear benefit, as seen previously with Docetaxel. This is an exciting early pilot study that warrants further study [90].

(a)

(b)

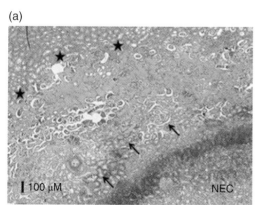 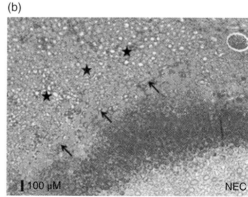

Figure 15.5 Microscopic images. (a) RFA only. (b) RFA and CYT-6091. Beginning of hemorrhagic rim and end of complete cell death zone indicated by arrow tips. The end of thermal injury is marked by the stars. Note the difference in diameter of zone of incomplete cell death between the two images. NEC, central necrotic area. Reprinted with permission from Wang TT, Hudson TS, Wang TC, Remsberg CM, Davies NM, Takahashi Y, *et al.* [90].

Nanotechnology in Other Urologic Cancers

The use of nanoparticles in other urologic malignancies has been reported to an even smaller degree. Regarding testis cancer, a prospective pilot study looked at the use of MRL to detect metastatic disease within retroperitoneal lymph nodes in patients with stage I testis cancer. Patients underwent a pelvic MRI both before and after injection of ferumoxtran-10. Lymph nodes were sampled by either CT-guided biopsy or laparoscopy and reviewed by a blinded pathologist. The authors demonstrated that MRL had a sensitivity of 88.2%, specificity of 92%, and accuracy of 90.4%. This was much improved compared to the sensitivity, specificity, and accuracy of unenhanced MRI or conventional CT based on nodal size criteria, at 70.5%, 68%, and 69%, respectively [91].

Similarly, the use of MRL for detection of regional lymph node metastases in penile cancer was evaluated. Seven patients with squamous cell carcinoma of the penis underwent MRL using ferumoxtran-10. All patients then underwent groin dissection and comparison of their nodal images with histologic review. MRL had a sensitivity of 100%, specificity of 97%, and negative predictive value of 100%. These findings suggest that MRL accurately predicts the pathologic status of regional lymph nodes in patients with cancer of the penis [92].

Urothelial carcinoma has received limited attention in regard to nanotechnology application. At present, patients with high-grade nonmuscle-invasive bladder cancer (NMIBC) that are treated with intravesical agents have a 50% chance of disease recurrence. A Phase I trial of nanoparticle albumin-bound paclitaxel for bacillus Calmette-Guérin (BCG)-refractory NMIBC was performed. The nanoparticle-bound paclitaxel was administered intravesically in a modified Fibonacci dose-escalation model until the maximum deliverable dose was achieved in 18 patients with recurrent NMIBC who failed at least two prior intravesical therapeutic agents. A review of adverse events revealed that 1 patient experienced systemic absorption after one treatment and 56% of patients experienced grade 1 local toxicity (i.e. dysuria). There were no reports of grade 2–4 toxicities. These findings support this particle as a tolerable agent for possible treatment of NMIBC [93].

In regard to platinum-refractory metastatic urothelial carcinoma, there is no standard treatment. Although taxanes and vinflunine are used, the local response is less than 20%. Furthermore, these treatments have shown no survival benefit. A recent Phase II trial evaluated the efficacy and tolerability of nanoparticle albumin-bound (nab) paclitaxel in 48 patients with platinum-refractory urothelial carcinoma. Overall, nab-paclitaxel was well tolerated. Furthermore, there was an overall response rate of 27.7%; 1 patient (2.1%) had a complete response and 12 patients (25.5%) had a partial response. These findings support further investigating into nab-paclitaxel as a potential second-line therapy for urothelial carcinoma [94].

Limitations of Nanoparticles

The use of nanotechnology in the treatment of urologic malignancies offers tremendous potential. Nonetheless human trials are badly needed and the technologies limitations require discussion. The first is that of toxicity of nanoparticles. The use of gold and iron oxide as bulk metals is accompanied by a familiar safety profile. As nanoparticles however, their unique formulations, properties, and size warrant continued systematic evaluation. The clinical use of monocrystalline iron oxide lymphotropic superparamagnetic nanoparticles has been under continued U.S. Food and Drug Administration (FDA) scrutiny. The investigational drug has been approved in some European countries for continued clinical investigation. In comparison, GNS have been widely tested in preclinical trials, and clinical trials are currently underway for further investigation. The Nanotechnology Characterization Laboratory, the National Institute of Standards and Technology (NIST), and the FDA facilitate current testing [4].

Another challenge is the biodistribution of particles within a tumor of interest. The spatial arrangement of nanoparticles within a tumor largely determines the distribution of heat when phototherapy is applied. Direct intratumoral injection of nanoparticles yields a nonuniform distribution and often requires multiple injections as compensation, further compounding uneven distribution [4].

Even more challenging is quantifying the distribution of particles within a tumor after systemic, or intravenous, injection. The accumulation of particles within the tumor is influenced by the particles' shape, surface charge, hydrodynamic diameter, and properties of the polyethylene glycol surface coating used to augment evasion from the reticuloendothelial system [95–97]. Although smaller particles (hydrodynamic diameter of 5.5 nm) typically evade the reticuloendothelial system, larger particles (20 nm) are generally captured by macrophages and may not reach the tumor of interest. Furthermore, nontargeted nanoparticles tend to accumulate—again, in a nonuniform manner—in the perivascular zone of a tumor because of leaky vascular fenestrations and immature vascular architecture. In the absence of targeting nanoparticles to tumor-specific biomarkers, the homogeneity of distribution is limited. Similarly, for some particles there is no effective means to confirm intravenous accumulation within a targeted tumor, hence limiting its clinical use.

An additional limitation of this technology is that of quantifying or visualizing particles after they have accumulated within a tumor. MRL, as discussed previously, uses iron oxide particles to detect a signal change in malignant lymph nodes. However, this modality is unable to quantify or visualize the number of particles in a tissue of interest. Quantification of particle concentration would assist in planning the thermal dose that could be achieved with laser or magnetic particle activation. One technique that is able to provide a rough estimate of the number of gold nanoparticles within tumors is diffuse optical spectroscopy (DOS). This technique delivers and collects light from a tissue by means of an optical fiber probe and indirectly measures gold concentration. It cannot, however, provide information about the spatial distribution of the particles [4].

Finally, consequent to the difficulties with mapping and quantifying the number of nanoparticles in a tissue of interest, the ability to generate a dosimetry model for a tissue of interest is limited. Although dosimetry formulations are used to guide radiation therapy, they are not directly applicable to photothermal therapy because of the uneven distribution of particles, as well as the effect of tissue physiology on thermal dosimetry (heat dissipation, tissue conductivity and perfusion, degree of vascularity). One study has used the technique of quantum dot (QD)–mediated fluorescence thermometry to monitor thermal energy in an in-vitro thermal ablation zone generated by laser-heated GNS in PC3 cells with promising results, although future work is needed [98].

Future Directions and Conclusions

Diagnostic imaging using nanoparticles largely centers around the use of MRL. Although original studies focused on iron oxide particles, recent studies have reported on ultrashort SWNTs encapsulating Gadolinium (Gd3 + n-ion clusters), or "gadonanotubes," as exceptional superparamagnetic molecular magnets. In comparison to standard Gd^{3+}-based contrast agent used for MRI, they have shown an efficacy 40–90 times greater. More recently, Hu *et al.* developed hybrid gold-gadolinium nanoclusters (NCs) [99,100]. These ultrasmall particles are stable, biocompatible, and suitable for triple-modal therapy using NIR fluorescence,

CT, and MRI imaging. They accumulate in tumor tissues and are easily cleared by the kidneys and have demonstrated to be promising probes for further research into cancer targeted imaging and diagnosis in vivo [101].

In future therapeutics, additional research into nanoparticles' capacity to enhance current therapies is needed. Nanoparticles have been used in combination with radiation therapy to enhance a focal dose of radiation preferentially within mice tumors, but human studies are currently lacking [102]. In addition, further development of nanoparticles loaded with a targeted agent to allow for both photothermal therapy as well as targeted therapy is predicted. Studies have already demonstrated promise for the use of Docetaxel-loaded nanoparticles for prostate cancer and tumor necrosis factor alpha-loaded nanoparticles in renal cell carcinoma, among others [81,90]. Further studies to standardize nanoparticle production and

loading of targeted agents, to evaluate the biocompatibility of functionalized nanoparticles, to standardize administration, and to improve distribution of particles within a tumor are needed.

In conclusion, the field of nanotechnology has exploded concomitant with an increasing interest in improving diagnostic accuracy in cancer therapeutics and trends toward tissue preservation. In urology, studies have demonstrated considerable promise for improved diagnostic accuracy of prostate cancer staging using MRL, as well as the potential for targeted and minimally invasive treatment. A smaller set of studies has also shown similar promise for renal cancer. As further clinical trials are conducted, the possibility of FDA approval follows. In turn, the evolution of nanotechnology holds remarkable potential for the future of cancer diagnostics and tissue-sparing therapy in urologic malignancies.

References

1 Rassweiler J, Rassweiler MC, Kenngott H, Frede T, Michel MS, Alken P, *et al.* The past, present and future of minimally invasive therapy in urology: A review and speculative outlook. Minim Invasive Ther Allied Technol. 2013;22(4):200–9.

2 Clayman RV, Kavoussi LR, Soper NR, Dierks SM, Meretyk S, Darcy MD, *et al.* Laparoscopic nephrectomy: Initial case report. J Urol. 1991;146(2):278–82.

3 Schroder FH. Screening, early detection, and treatment of prostate cancer: a European view. Urology. 1995;46(3 Suppl A):62–70.

4 Krishnan S, Diagaradjane P, Cho SH. Nanoparticle-mediated thermal therapy: evolving strategies for prostate cancer therapy. Int J Hyperthermia. 2010;26(8):775–89.

5 Komura K, Single session of high-intensity focused ultrasound for localized prostate cancer: Treatment outcomes and potential effect as a primary therapy. World J Urol. 2014;32(5):133–45.

6 Blana A, Walter B, Rogenhofer S, Wieland WF. High-intensity focused ultrasound for the treatment of localized prostate cancer: 5-year experience. Urology. 2004;63(2):297–300.

7 Cordeiro ER, Cathelineau X, Thüroff S, Marberger M, Crouzet S, de la Rosette JJ. High-intensity focused ultrasound (HIFU) for definitive treatment of prostate cancer. BJU Int. 2012;110(9):1228–42.

8 Akduman B, Barqawi AB, Crawford ED. Minimally invasive surgery in prostate cancer: Current and future perspectives. Cancer J. 2005;11(5):355–61.

9 Cohen JK, Miller RJ, Rooker FM, Shuman BA. Cryosurgical ablation of the prostate: Two-year prostate-specific antigen and biopsy results. Urology. 1996;47(3):395–401.

10 Park A, Anderson JK, Matsumoto ED, Lotan Y, Josephs S, Cadeddu JA. Radiofrequency ablation of renal tumors: Intermediate-term results. J Endourol. 2006;20(8):569–73.

11 Desai, MM, Aron M, Gill IS. Laparoscopic partial nephrectomy versus laparoscopic cryoablation for the small renal tumor. Urology. 2005.66(5 Suppl):23–8.

12 Singh PB, Anele C, Dalton E, Barbouti O, Stevens D, Gurgung P, *et al.* Prostate cancer tumour features on template prostate-mapping biopsies: Implications for focal therapy. Eur Urol. 2014;66(1):12–9

13 Valerio M, Ahmed HU, Emberton M, Lawrentschuk N, Lazzeri M, Montironi R, *et al.* The role of focal therapy in the management of localised prostate cancer: A systematic review. Eur Urol. 2014;66(4):732–51.

14 Bahn D, De Castro Abreu AL, Gill IS, Hung AJ, Silverman P, Gross ME, *et al.* Focal cryotherapy for clinically unilateral, low-intermediate risk prostate cancer in 73 men with a median follow-up of 3.7 years. Eur Urol. 2012;62(1):55–63.

15 Hirsch LR, Gobin AM, Lowery AR, Tam F, Drezek RA, Halas NJ, *et al.* Metal nanoshells. Ann Biomed Eng. 2006;34(1):15–22.

16 Young, JK, Figueroa ER, Drezek RA. Tunable nanostructures as photothermal theranostic agents. Ann Biomed Eng. 2012;40(2):438–59.

17 Stern JM, Cadeddu JA. Emerging use of nanoparticles for the therapeutic ablation of urologic malignancies. Urol Oncol. 2008;26(1):93–6.

18 Van de Broek B, Devoogdt N, D'Hollander A, Gijs HL, Jans K, Lagae L, *et al.* Specific cell targeting with nanobody conjugated branched gold nanoparticles for photothermal therapy. ACS Nano.2011;5(6):4319–28.

19 Hirsch LR, Stafford RJ, Bankson JA, Sershen SR, Rivera B, Price RE, *et al.* Nanoshell-mediated near-infrared thermal therapy of tumors under magnetic resonance guidance. Proc Natl Acad Sci USA. 2003;100(23):13549–54.

20 Pearce J, Giustini A, Stigliano R, Jack-Hoopes P. Magnetic heating of nanoparticles: The importance of particle clustering to achieve therapeutic

temperatures. J Nanotechnol Eng Med. 2013;4(1):110071–1100714.

21 Kobayashi T. Cancer hyperthermia using magnetic nanoparticles. Biotechnol J. 2011;6(11):1342–7.

22 Salloum M, Ma R, Zhu L. Enhancement in treatment planning for magnetic nanoparticle hyperthermia: Optimization of the heat absorption pattern. Int J Hyperthermia. 2009;25(4):309–21.

23 Margulis V, Matsumoto ED, Lindberg G, Tunc L, Taylor G, Sagalowsky AI, *et al.* Acute histologic effects of temperature-based radiofrequency ablation on renal tumor pathologic interpretation. Urology. 2004;64(4):660–3.

24 Golneshan AA, Lahonian M. The effect of magnetic nanoparticle dispersion on temperature distribution in a spherical tissue in magnetic fluid hyperthermia using the lattice Boltzmann method. Int J Hyperthermia. 2011;27(3):266–74.

25 Stern JM, Stanfield J, Lotan Y, Park S, Hsieh JT, Cadeddu JA. Efficacy of laser-activated gold nanoshells in ablating prostate cancer cells in vitro. J Endourol. 2007;21(8):939–43.

26 Stern JM, Stanfield J, Kabbani W, Hsieh JT, Cadeddu JA. Selective prostate cancer thermal ablation with laser activated gold nanoshells. J Urol. 2008;179(2):748–53.

27 Loo C, Lowery A, Halas N, West J, Drezek R. Immunotargeted nanoshells for integrated cancer imaging and therapy. Nano Lett. 2005;5(4):709–11.

28 O'Neal DP, Hirsch LR, Halas NJ, Payne JD, West JL. Photo-thermal tumor ablation in mice using near infrared-absorbing nanoparticles. Cancer Lett. 2004;209(2):171–6.

29 Li JL, Wang L, Liu XY, Zhang ZP, Guo HC, Liu WM, *et al.* In vitro cancer cell imaging and therapy using transferrin-conjugated gold nanoparticles. Cancer Lett. 2009;274(2):319–26.

30 Kirui DK, Rey DA, Batt CA. Gold hybrid nanoparticles for targeted phototherapy and cancer imaging. Nanotechnology. 2010;21(10):105105.

31 Choi J, Yang J, Jang E, Suh JS, Huh YM, Lee K, *et al.* Gold nanostructures as photothermal therapy agent for cancer. Anticancer Agents Med Chem. 2011;11(10):953–64.

32 Choi WI, Sahu A, Kim YH, Tae G. Photothermal cancer therapy and imaging based on gold nanorods. Ann Biomed Eng. 2012;40(2):534–46.

33 Dickerson EB, Dreaden EC, Huang X, El-Sayed IH, Chu H, Pushpanketh S, *et al.* Gold nanorod assisted near-infrared plasmonic photothermal therapy (PPTT) of squamous cell carcinoma in mice. Cancer Lett. 2008;269(1):57–66.

34 Huang X, Jain PK, El-Sayed IH, El-Sayed MA. Plasmonic photothermal therapy (PPTT) using gold nanoparticles. Lasers Med Sci. 2008;23(3):217–28.

35 Pissuwan D, Valenzuela SM, Cortie MB. Therapeutic possibilities of plasmonically heated gold nanoparticles. Trends Biotechnol. 2006;24(2):62–7.

36 Bickford LR, Agollah G, Drezek R, Yu TK. Silica-gold nanoshells as potential intraoperative molecular probes for HER2-overexpression in ex vivo breast tissue using near-infrared reflectance confocal microscopy. Breast Cancer Res Treat. 2010;120(3):547–55.

37 Bardhan R, Lal S, Joshi A, Halas NJ. Theranostic nanoshells: from probe design to imaging and treatment of cancer. Acc Chem Res. 2011;44(10):936–46.

38 Yasun E, Kang H, Erdal H, Cansiz S, Ocsoy I, Huang YF, *et al.* Cancer cell sensing and therapy using affinity tag-conjugated gold nanorods. Interface Focus. 2013;3(3):20130006.

39 Zhang Z, Wang J, Chen C. Gold nanorods based platforms for light-mediated theranostics. Theranostics. 2013;3(3):223–38.

40 Huang X, El-Sayed IH, El-Sayed MA. Applications of gold nanorods for cancer imaging and photothermal therapy. Methods Mol Biol. 2010;624:343–57.

41 Huang X, Jain PK, El-Sayed IH, El-Sayed MA. Gold nanoparticles: Interesting optical properties and recent applications in cancer diagnostics and therapy. Nanomedicine (Lond). 2007;2(5):681–93.

42 Skrabalak SE, Au L, Lu X, Li X, Xia Y. Gold nanocages for cancer detection and treatment. Nanomedicine (Lond). 2007;2(5):657–68.

43 Xia Y, Li W, Cobley CM, Chen J, Xia X, Zhang Q, *et al.* Gold nanocages: From synthesis to theranostic applications. Acc Chem Res. 2011;44(10):914–24.

44 Skrabalak SE, Chen J, Sun Y, Lu X, Au L, Cobley CM, *et al.* Gold nanocages: synthesis, properties, and applications. Acc Chem Res. 2008;41(12):1587–95.

45 Chen J, Glaus C, Laforest R, Zhang Q, Yang M, Gidding M, *et al.* Gold nanocages as photothermal transducers for cancer treatment. Small. 2010;6(7):811–7.

46 Zheng LX, O'Connell MJ, Doorn SK, Liao XZ, Zhao YH, Akhadov EA, *et al.* Ultralong single-wall carbon nanotubes. Nat Mater. 2004;3(10):673–6.

47 Mulvey JJ, Villa CH, McDevitt MR, Escorcia FE, Casey E, Scheinberg DA. Self-assembly of carbon nanotubes and antibodies on tumours for targeted amplified delivery. Nat Nanotechnol. 2013;8(10):763–71.

48 Carlson LJ, Krauss TD. Photophysics of individual single-walled carbon nanotubes. Acc Chem Res. 2008;41(2):235–43.

49 Lay CL, Liu J, Liu Y. Functionalized carbon nanotubes for anticancer drug delivery. Expert Rev Med Devices. 2011;8(5):561–6.

50 Burke A, Ding X, Singh R, Kraft RA, Levi-Polyachenko N, Rylander MN, *et al.* Long-term survival following a single treatment of kidney tumors with multiwalled carbon nanotubes and near-infrared radiation. Proc Natl Acad Sci USA. 2009;106(31):12897–902.

51 Burlaka A, Lukin S, Prylutska S, Remeniak O, Prylutskyy Y, Shuba M, *et al.* Hyperthermic effect of multi-walled carbon nanotubes stimulated with near infrared irradiation for anticancer therapy: In vitro studies. Exp Oncol. 2010;32(1):48–50.

52 Torti SV, Byrne F, Whelan O, Levi N, Ucer B, Schmid M, *et al.* Thermal ablation therapeutics based on CN(x) multi-walled nanotubes. Int J Nanomedicine. 2007;2(4):707–14.

53 Saito N, Usui Y, Aoki K, Narita N, Shimizu M, Hara K, *et al.* Carbon nanotubes: Biomaterial applications. Chem Soc Rev. 2009;38(7):1897–903.

54 Lee C, Hong K, Kim H, Kang J, Zheng HM. TiO2 nanotubes as a therapeutic agent for cancer thermotherapy. Photochem Photobiol. 2010;86(4):981–9.

55 Saokar A, Braschi M, Harisinghani, M. Lymphotrophic nanoparticle enhanced MR imaging (LNMRI) for lymph node imaging. Abdom Imaging. 2006;31(6):660–7.

56 Saksena, MA, Saokar A, Harisinghani MG. Lymphotropic nanoparticle enhanced MR imaging (LNMRI) technique for lymph node imaging. Eur J Radiol. 2006;58(3):367–74.

57 Clèment O, Guimaraes R, de Kerviler F, Frija G. Magnetic resonance lymphography. Enhancement patterns using superparamagnetic nanoparticles. Invest Radiol. 1994;29 Suppl 2:S226–8.

58 Guimaraes R, Clèment O, Bittoun J, Carnot F, Frija G. MR lymphography with superparamagnetic iron nanoparticles in rats: pathologic basis for contrast enhancement. AJR Am J Roentgenol. 1994;162(1):201–7.

59 Fortuin AS, Smeenk RJ, Meijer HJ, Witjes AJ, Barentsz JO. Lymphotropic nanoparticle-enhanced MRI in prostate cancer: Value and therapeutic potential. Curr Urol Rep. 2014;15(3):389.

60 Harisinghani MG, Barentsz J, Hahn PF, Deserno WM, Tabatabaei S, van de Kaa CH, *et al.* Noninvasive detection of clinically occult lymph-node metastases in prostate cancer. N Engl J Med. 2003;348(25):2491–9.

61 Will O, Purkayastha S, Chan C, Athanasiou T, Darzi AW, Gedroyc W, *et al.* Diagnostic precision of nanoparticle-enhanced MRI for lymph-node metastases: A meta-analysis. Lancet Oncol. 2006;7(1):52–60.

62 Horsman MR, Overgaard J. Can mild hyperthermia improve tumour oxygenation? Int J Hyperthermia. 1997;13(2):141–7.

63 Fuller KJ, Issels RD, Slosman DO, Guillet JG, Soussi T, Polla BS. Cancer and the heat shock response. Eur J Cancer. 1994;30A(12):1884–91.

64 Servadio C, Leib Z. Local hyperthermia for prostate cancer. Urology. 1991;38(4):307–9.

65 Zhang HG, Mehta K, Cohen P, Guha C. Hyperthermia on immune regulation: A temperature's story. Cancer Lett. 2008;271(2):191–204.

66 Kampinga HH, Dikomey E. Hyperthermic radiosensitization: Mode of action and clinical relevance. Int J Radiat Biol. 2001;77(4):399–408.

67 van der Zee J. Heating the patient: a promising approach? Ann Oncol. 2002;13(8):1173–84.

68 Everts M, Saini V, Leddon JL, Kok RJ, Stoff-Khalili M, Preuss MA, *et al.* Covalently linked Au nanoparticles to a viral vector: Potential for combined photothermal and gene cancer therapy. Nano Lett. 2006;6(4):587–91.

69 El-Sayed IH, Huang X, El-Sayed MA. Selective laser photo-thermal therapy of epithelial carcinoma using anti-EGFR antibody conjugated gold nanoparticles. Cancer Lett. 2006;239(1):129–35.

70 Heesakkers RA, Hövels AM, Jager GJ, van den Bosch HC, Witjes JA, Raat HP, *et al.* MRI with a lymph-node-specific contrast agent as an alternative to CT scan and lymph-node dissection in patients with prostate cancer: A prospective multicohort study. Lancet Oncol. 2008;9(9):850–6.

71 Harisinghani MG, Barentsz JO, Hahn PF, Deserno W, de la Rosette J, Saini S, *et al.* MR lymphangiography for detection of minimal nodal disease in patients with prostate cancer. Acad Radiol. 2002;9 Suppl 2:S312–3.

72 Hövels AM, Heesakkers RA, Adang EM, Jager GJ, Strum S, Hoogeveen YL, *et al.* The diagnostic accuracy of CT and MRI in the staging of pelvic lymph nodes in

patients with prostate cancer: A meta-analysis. Clin Radiol. 2008;63(4):387–95.

73 Weidner AM, van Lin EN, Dinter DJ, Rozema T, Schoenberg SO, Wenz F, *et al.* Ferumoxtran-10 MR lymphography for target definition and follow-up in a patient undergoing image-guided, dose-escalated radiotherapy of lymph nodes upon PSA relapse. Strahlenther Onkol. 2011;187(3):206–12.

74 Meijer HJ, Debats OA, van Lin EN, Witjes JA, Kaanders JH, Barentsz JO. A retrospective analysis of the prognosis of prostate cancer patients with lymph node involvement on MR lymphography: Who might be cured. Radiat Oncol. 2013;8(1):190.

75 Salimi A, Kavosi B, Fathi F, Hallaj R. Highly sensitive immunosensing of prostate-specific antigen based on ionic liquid-carbon nanotubes modified electrode: Application as cancer biomarker for prostate biopsies. Biosens Bioelectron. 2013;42:439–46.

76 Johannsen M, Jordan A, Scholz R, Koch M, Lein M, Deger S, *et al.* Evaluation of magnetic fluid hyperthermia in a standard rat model of prostate cancer. J Endourol. 2004;18(5):495–500.

77 Johannsen M, Thiesen B, Gneveckow U, Taymoorian K, Waldöfner N, Scholz R, *et al.* Thermotherapy using magnetic nanoparticles combined with external radiation in an orthotopic rat model of prostate cancer. Prostate. 2006;66(1):97–104.

78 Ghosh S, Dutta S, Gomes E, Carroll D, D'Agostino R Jr, Olson J, *et al.* Increased heating efficiency and selective thermal ablation of malignant tissue with DNA-encased multiwalled carbon nanotubes. ACS Nano. 2009;3(9):2667–73.

79 Zheng M, Jagota A, Semke ED, Diner BA, McLean RS, Lustig SR, *et al.* DNA-assisted dispersion and separation of carbon nanotubes. Nat Mater. 2003;2(5):338–42.

80 Kawai N, Futakuchi M, Yoshida T, Ito A, Sato S, Naiki T, *et al.* Effect of heat therapy using magnetic nanoparticles conjugated

with cationic liposomes on prostate tumor in bone. Prostate. 2008;68(7):784–92.

81 Min K, Jo H, Song K, Cho M, Chun YS, Jon S, *et al.* Dual-aptamer-based delivery vehicle of doxorubicin to both PSMA (+) and PSMA (-) prostate cancers. Biomaterials. 2011;32(8):2124–32.

82 Yu MK, Kim D, Lee IH, So JS, Jeong YY, Jon S. Image-guided prostate cancer therapy using aptamer-functionalized thermally cross-linked superparamagnetic iron oxide nanoparticles. Small. 2011;7(15):2241–9.

83 Sato A, Itcho N, Ishiguro H, Okamoto D, Kobayashi N, Kawai K, *et al.* Magnetic nanoparticles of Fe3O4 enhance docetaxel-induced prostate cancer cell death. Int J Nanomedicine. 2013;8:3151–60.

84 Sanna V, Roggio AM, Posadino AM, Cossu A, Marcedu S, Mariani A, *et al.* Novel docetaxel-loaded nanoparticles based on poly(lactide-co-caprolactone) and poly(lactide-co-glycolide-co-caprolactone) for prostate cancer treatment: formulation, characterization, and cytotoxicity studies. Nanoscale Res Lett. 2011;6(1):260.

85 Sanna V, Siddiqui IA, Sechi M, Mukhtar H. Resveratrol-loaded nanoparticles based on poly(epsilon-caprolactone) and poly(D,L-lactic-co-glycolic acid)-poly(ethylene glycol) blend for prostate cancer treatment. Mol Pharm. 2013;10(10):3871–81.

86 Hsieh TC, Wu JM. Differential effects on growth, cell cycle arrest, and induction of apoptosis by resveratrol in human prostate cancer cell lines. Exp Cell Res. 1999;249(1):109–15.

87 Shih A, Zhang S, Cao HJ, Boswell S, Wu YH, Tang HY, *et al.* Inhibitory effect of epidermal growth factor on resveratrol-induced apoptosis in prostate cancer cells is mediated by protein kinase C-alpha. Mol Cancer Ther. 2004;3(11):1355–64.

88 Ratan HL, Steward WP, Gescher AJ, Mellon JK. Resveratrol--a prostate cancer chemopreventive agent? Urol Oncol. 2002;7(6):223–7.

89 Seeni A, Takahashi S, Takeshita K, Tang M, Sugiura S, Sato SY, *et al.* Suppression of

prostate cancer growth by resveratrol in the transgenic rat for adenocarcinoma of prostate (TRAP) model. Asian Pac J Cancer Prev. 2008;9(1):7–14.

90 Wang TT, Hudson TS, Wang TC, Remsberg CM, Davies NM, Takahashi Y, *et al.* Differential effects of resveratrol on androgen-responsive LNCaP human prostate cancer cells in vitro and in vivo. Carcinogenesis. 2008;29(10):2001–10.

91 Guimaraes AR, Tabatabei S, Dahl D, McDougal WS, Weissleder R, Harisinghani MG. Pilot study evaluating use of lymphotrophic nanoparticle-enhanced magnetic resonance imaging for assessing lymph nodes in renal cell cancer. Urology. 2008;71(4):708–12.

92 Bruners P, Braunschweig T, Hodenius M, Pietsch H, Penzkofer T, Baumann M, *et al.* Thermoablation of malignant kidney tumors using magnetic nanoparticles: An in vivo feasibility study in a rabbit model. Cardiovasc Intervent Radiol. 2010;33(1):127–34.

93 Pedro RN, Thekke-Adiyat T, Goel R, Shenoi M, Slaton J, Schmechel S, *et al.* Use of tumor necrosis factor-alpha-coated gold nanoparticles to enhance radiofrequency ablation in a translational model of renal tumors. Urology. 2010;76(2):494–8.

94 Harisinghani MG, Saksena M, Ross RW, Tabatabaei S, Dahl D, McDougal S, *et al.* A pilot study of lymphotrophic nanoparticle-enhanced magnetic resonance imaging technique in early stage testicular cancer: A new method for noninvasive lymph node evaluation. Urology. 2005;66(5):1066–71.

95 Tabatabaei S, Harisinghani M, McDougal WS. Regional lymph node staging using lymphotropic nanoparticle enhanced magnetic resonance imaging with ferumoxtran-10 in patients with penile cancer. J Urol. 2005;174(3):923–7; discussion 927.

96 McKiernan JM, Barlow LJ, Laudano MA, Mann MJ, Petrylak DP, Benson MC. A phase I trial of intravesical nanoparticle albumin-bound paclitaxel in the treatment of bacillus Calmette-Guerin refractory nonmuscle invasive bladder cancer. J Urol. 2011;186(2):448–51.

97 Ko YJ, Canil CM, Mukherjee SD, Winquist E, Elser C, Eisen A, *et al.* Nanoparticle albumin-bound paclitaxel for second-line treatment of metastatic urothelial carcinoma: a single group, multicentre, phase 2 study. Lancet Oncol. 2013;14(8):769–76.

98 Choi HS, Liu W, Misra P, Tanaka E, Zimmer JP, Itty Ipe B, *et al.* Renal clearance of quantum dots. Nat Biotechnol. 2007;25(10):1165–70.

99 Akiyama Y, Mori T, Katayama Y, Niidome T. The effects of PEG grafting level and injection dose on gold nanorod biodistribution in the tumor-bearing mice. J Control Release. 2009;139(1):81–4.

100 Diagaradjane P, Orenstein-Cardona JM, Colón-Casasnovas NE, Deorukhkar A, Shentu S, Kuno N, *et al.* Imaging epidermal growth factor receptor expression in vivo: Pharmacokinetic and biodistribution characterization of a bioconjugated quantum dot nanoprobe. Clin Cancer Res. 2008;14(3):731–41.

101 Bensalah K, Tuncel A, Hanson W, Stern J, Han B, Cadeddu J. Monitoring of thermal dose during ablation therapy using quantum dot-mediated fluorescence thermometry. J Endourol. 2010;24(12):1903–8.

102 Sitharaman B, Kissell KR, Hartman KB, Tran LA, Baikalov A, Rusakova I, *et al.* Superparamagnetic gadonanotubes are high-performance MRI contrast agents. Chem Commun (Camb). 2005;(31):3915–7.

16

Trial Design Issues in the Study of Focal Therapy in Prostate and Kidney Cancer

John B. Eifler, MD,[1] and David F. Penson, MD, MPH[2]

[1] *Department of Urologic Surgery, Vanderbilt University, Nashville, TN, USA*
[2] *Department of Urology, Vanderbilt University Medical Center, Nashville, TN, USA*

The promise of focal therapy for localized prostate or kidney cancer lies in its potential ability to reduce the morbidity of more aggressive "definitive" therapies while maintaining equivalent oncologic outcomes. However, before endorsing widespread uptake of focal therapy for these common malignancies, it is critical that the scientific community generate well-designed studies that document that these novel therapeutic approaches truly fulfill this promise. Comparative effectiveness studies of "traditional" approaches to the treatment of localized prostate or kidney cancer, however, have proven difficult to complete for various reasons. It is, therefore, not surprising that there are few well-designed studies comparing the effectiveness of focal therapies to existing treatments in these malignancies. Specifically, there are no unequivocal observational or randomized clinical trials to guide clinicians regarding when to use focal therapy, when not to use it, and how best to follow patients after treatment.

Why is it so difficult to complete meaningful research in this space? Study design in these settings is hindered by a number of elements. First, the long natural history of prostate cancer [1,2], as well as that of small renal masses [3], renders the use of overall or cancer-specific mortality (CSM) as primary endpoints difficult and often makes studies unrealistically long and prohibitively expensive. To this end, focal therapy trials often rely on proxy endpoints. In the case of both prostate and kidney cancer, the validity of these outcomes has proven controversial. For example, the significance of a rise in serum prostate-specific antigen (PSA) levels after focal therapy for prostate cancer remains of unclear meaning. In fact, this is also true after radiotherapy and prostatectomy [4]. Simply put, the choice of endpoint in studies of the effectiveness of focal therapy is a challenge.

Even if one can identify proxy outcomes that are clinically meaningful and can be compared in short- or intermediate-term follow-up, there is still the issue of selection bias that is inherent in nonrandomized study designs around invasive interventions [5]. Specifically, observational studies that compare the effectiveness of focal therapy to more invasive whole-organ treatment are subject to confounding by indication. Patients who select focal therapy may be inherently different than those who select whole-organ treatment. Although there may be methods of risk adjustment that can account for this, at least in part, it is virtually impossible to completely eliminate this type of bias in observational studies.

The obvious solution to this problem is to perform a randomized clinical trial.

Management of Urologic Cancer: Focal Therapy and Tissue Preservation, First Edition.
Edited by Mark P. Schoenberg and Kara L. Watts.
© 2017 John Wiley & Sons Ltd. Published 2017 by John Wiley & Sons Ltd.

Unfortunately, this study design may also be problematic when assessing the effectiveness of focal therapy because patients tend to be reluctant to enroll in these studies, and it is extremely difficult to blind patients and clinicians to randomization in the setting of focal therapy, which may influence outcomes as well [6]. Acknowledging these issues, there is still a pressing need for better data on the effectiveness of focal therapy for prostate and renal cell cancers. In this chapter, we will discuss in greater detail some of the issues around clinical trial design for focal therapy in prostate and kidney cancer and identify potential ways to improve study design in the future.

Issues around Endpoints in Studies of Focal Therapy

Prostate Cancer

Numerous randomized [7,8] and observational studies [1,9,10] have demonstrated that the overall mortality and CSM remains low for many years following the diagnosis of prostate cancer, even in the absence of definitive therapy. For example, overall mortality and CSM in the placebo arm of the Prostate Intervention Versus Observation Trial (PIVOT) was only 49.9% and 8.4%, respectively, at a median follow-up of 10 years [8]. In the SPCG-4 randomized controlled trial (RCT) comparing radical prostatectomy to watchful waiting for men diagnosed with prostate cancer in Sweden, the cumulative incidence of death from prostate cancer at 18 years in the watchful waiting arm was 28.7% and only 14.0% for men with low risk prostate cancer [7]. Other population-based studies have demonstrated similarly low mortality for men with prostate cancer managed conservatively [1,2,9,10]. Given the low long-term overall mortality and CSM rates associated with prostate cancer, use of CSM as an endpoint would require a large number of patients with long-term follow-up. Sample power calculations, using

the CSM data from PIVOT and assuming equivalency between radical prostatectomy (RP) and focal cryotherapy at 10 years, are illustrative. If one designed a noninferiority study of RP compared with focal therapy using CSM as the primary endpoint, 472 men would need to be accrued to have 80% certainty that the difference in CSM rates between the two groups was less than 5% at 10 years. However, in the PIVOT study, the absolute reduction in CSM with RP was 3.0% compared to observation at 12 years [8]. In our sample power calculation, to capture an absolute difference in CSM of 3.0% or greater would require 1306 participants and at least 10 to 15 years of follow-up. Presuming that focal therapy improves CSM over surveillance, the number of participants would need to be even greater to accurately assess noninferiority at 12 years. The expense of following more than1300 patients for greater than 10 years would be enormous, prohibiting performance of such a study. To this end, alternative oncologic endpoints would have to be considered.

One possible proxy endpoint for use in studies of focal therapy in prostate cancer might be metastasis-free survival. However, metastasis typically occurs relatively late in the disease process and likely at rates not much greater than CSM [7,8]. In one study of men undergoing RP early in the PSA era, metastasis in only 18% of patients occurred and at a median of 8 years after biochemical recurrence in one study [4,11]. Thus, trials using metastasis-free survival as a primary endpoint would also take longer than a decade to complete, would require large sample size to be adequately powered, and would be prohibitively expensive.

PSA progression/biochemical recurrence (BCR) is another possible proxy endpoint. In one study, BCR following RP was defined as a PSA >0.2 ng/ml, and the median time to BCR was noted to be between 2 and 3 years [11]. This definition, however, could not reasonably used in the setting of focal therapy because viable benign prostate tissue will usually remain after treatment. In the case of radiation therapy, where viable prostate tissue also remains, the PSA may not nadir to zero even when the treatment is curative. To this end, various definitions of BCR exist for radiotherapy including the American Society for Therapeutic Radiology and Oncology (ASTRO) criteria (three consecutive rises in PSA, with the date of BCR backdated to the midpoint between the PSA nadir and the first date of increased PSA) [12] and the Phoenix criteria (nadir PSA + 2.0 ng/mL) [13]. One could argue that it would be appropriate to apply one of these definitions of BCR in the setting of focal therapy, as, in both whole-gland radiation and focal therapy, benign prostate tissue will remain and will produce PSA. It is important to acknowledge, however, that although the use of these definitions of BCR in focal therapy is based on sound clinical rationale, there are no published studies documenting their validity or identifying the optimal definition to use in focal therapy.

Regardless, all definitions of BCR require several PSA measurements over the course of months or even years with a rising PSA before they meet the definition of biochemical failure/PSA progression, compromising any time-to-event analysis. One analysis found men with detectable PSA after RP took more than 5 years to meet the Phoenix definition. As Nielsen *et al.* conclude "the standard definitions for each modality represent fundamentally different clinical scenarios" [14]. This certainly applies to focal therapy as well. Acknowledging these considerable limitations, BCR is likely the best short-term outcome for use in studies that compare focal therapy to whole-gland therapies in the treatment of localized prostate cancer, whereas CSM and overall mortality remain the gold standard over the long term.

Proponents of focal therapy will acknowledge that commonly accepted oncologic outcomes in prostate cancer such as overall mortality and CSM may not be feasible outcomes for focal therapy trials [15]. As such, they have proposed the use of other proxy endpoints, usually in the setting of single-arm studies. These include image changes on prostate magnetic resonance imaging (MRI) or pathological upgrading on repeat biopsy [16]. Although these endpoints have face validity, they have not yet been formally validated in this setting. In the case of pathological upgrading on follow-up biopsy, experience with this in active surveillance highlights the problems with using this as an endpoint in the study of focal therapy. Specifically, follow-up prostate biopsy likely has fairly low sensitivity because many men on active surveillance (57% in one AS series [17]) have negative repeat prostate biopsies despite having no treatment. The use of MRI in this context, however, has shown promise. In one study of biochemical recurrence after radiotherapy, MRI demonstrated local recurrence in 40 or 42 patients (confirmed by targeted biopsy) [18], possibly making MRI a reasonable modality to assess local control following focal therapy and potentially allowing comparison to patients undergoing active surveillance or radiotherapy. However, 21% of men with positive biopsy findings also had positive biopsies in areas without MRI-suspected recurrence. One objective of any focal therapy study should be to develop appropriate surrogate endpoints after nonextirpative treatments in prostate cancer.

Kidney Cancer: Small Renal Masses

As a result of the rising accuracy and availability of axial imaging, the incidence of renal masses has been increasing, particularly for masses less than 4 cm in maximal diameter (small renal mass [SRM]) [19]. As a result, active surveillance of these smaller lesions has gained popularity in intermediate- or poor-risk surgical candidates and is considered appropriate by the prominent guidelines panels [20,21]. Concurrently, focal ablative procedures such as cryoablation and radiofrequency ablation (RFA) destroy tissue via thermal energy, either via a percutaneous approach or laparoscopic approach, have also been suggested in these smaller lesions.

Like prostate cancer, the natural history of SRMs tends to be prolonged with minimal associated mortality. In a meta-analysis and systematic review of the literature, Chawla *et al.* identified 10 reports from nine single institutional series of untreated solid localized renal lesions [22]. Mean size at presentation was 2.6 cm with a mean growth rate of 0.28 cm per annum over a median follow-up of 32 months. Importantly, only 3 of 286 lesions (1%) ultimately resulted in metastatic disease and no deaths were reported. It is important, however, to remember that this is a selected population and that mortality may be higher in the general population, although it will likely still be quite low. Unlike the case of prostate cancer, however, there is no serum marker that can act as a proxy for tumor growth or volume in kidney cancer. To this end, there are fewer proxy endpoints for use in comparative clinical trials of focal therapy for renal masses.

In the setting of single-arm efficacy studies of focal therapy for SRMs, potential proxy endpoints include active disease on repeat biopsy and radiological progression on follow-up imaging. Given the relatively low metastatic potential (and ensuing mortality rates) of untreated SRMs, the significance of active cancer on follow-up biopsy is unclear. Certainly, the absence of viable malignancy on biopsy is a laudable goal and indicates that the focal treatment has "killed the cancer," but it is important to remember that renal mass biopsy does carry a considerable false-negative rate [23]. Furthermore, the finding of viable cancer does not necessarily mean that the patient will experience a clinically significant progression or ultimately succumb to the cancer [22]. To this end, active cancer on follow-up renal biopsy may not necessarily be a meaningful proxy endpoint for the study of focal therapy for SRMs.

Changes on follow-up imaging indicative of local recurrence or progression, however, may be serve as reasonable proxy outcomes for studies of focal therapy for SRMs. After focal ablation, absence of tumor growth or enhancement within the ablation region should be apparent by 6 weeks after treatment [24]. Given the experience using imaging to define local recurrence following partial nephrectomy, it may be reasonable to apply the same criteria in the setting of focal therapy to compare these modalities. That being said, limited studies have evaluated the long-term growth rate of renal masses in surveillance cohorts [22], and thresholds for definitive intervention have not been defined. Further research is needed to validate these radiographic endpoints in the setting of focal therapy.

Functional Outcomes

The *raison d'être* for focal therapy in prostate cancer is the belief that focal therapies will decrease that morbidity of RP and radiation therapy. However, no comparative trials of focal therapy and definitive therapy exist to validate this assumption. Furthermore, in the initial experience of focal therapy using high-intensity focused ultrasound (HIFU), functional outcomes following therapy have not been optimal, with significantly impaired erectile function and continence after focal HIFU [25]. Although excellent functional outcomes after focal cryotherapy have been reported [26], prospective comparative studies are needed to determine whether focal therapy delivers on the promise to decrease morbidity.

Comparative studies of focal therapy for prostate cancer and kidney cancer must include validated instruments to assess patient-reported outcomes and perioperative outcomes. Preferable instruments include the International Index of Erectile Function (IIEF) [27] and the International Prostate Symptom Score (IPSS) [28] for the measurement of functional outcomes and the Expanded Prostate Cancer Index Composite [29] for measurement of quality of life. Regarding assessment of urinary incontinence, use of pads should be measured. Perioperative adverse events should be recorded using the Clavien-Dindo classification system [30].

Issues around Defining the Study Population and the Control Arms of Comparative Studies in Focal Therapy

Prostate Cancer

There is a general perception by some proponents of focal therapy for localized prostate cancer that this treatment should be considered primarily as an alternative to active surveillance in low-risk patients. With the exception of low-risk patients who are absolutely insistent on having some form of active intervention, we do not feel that focal therapy should be considered in lieu of active surveillance. The rationale for active surveillance is firmly based on the notion that there is a considerable rate of overdiagnosis associated with PSA screening [31] and, as such, many men diagnosed at the time of screening have clinically indolent disease and do not require any therapy for their cancer. To this end, focal therapy should not be considered a replacement for active surveillance in patients with low-risk disease who likely will garner little or no benefit from any treatment, even one with fewer purported side effects (like focal therapy). These patients should be strongly encouraged to consider active surveillance.

Conversely, it would be ethically difficult to offer focal therapy to patients with high-risk disease because these patients are at greatest risk for dying of prostate cancer over the long term [9]. Without convincing "phase 2" data that focal therapy is truly effective in reducing prostate-cancer mortality in high-risk patients, we should not proceed with prospective studies comparing focal therapy to whole-gland treatments in this patient population. In our opinion, the optimal comparator arm for a study of focal therapy in localized prostate cancer are men with high-volume, low-risk disease or those with low-volume Gleason score, $3 + 4 = 7$ (effectively, intermediate-risk disease).

SRMs

The choice of both comparator arm and inclusion criteria for trials of focal therapy in kidney cancer is much less clear. Unlike the case of prostate cancer, radiation therapy is not effective for renal cell carcinoma (RCC), and in patients with larger lesions who are poor operative candidates, there are few alternatives currently to percutaneous ablation. For patients with larger lesions who are appropriate surgical candidates, focal cryotherapy may provide the same oncologic outcomes with decreased length of stay, decreased cost, and fewer complications [32]. However, the reported recurrence rate after focal ablative therapy has traditionally been higher than that for partial nephrectomy. A recent meta-analysis noted recurrence rates of 9.4% and 0.4% for laparoscopic cryoablation and laparoscopic partial nephrectomy, respectively [32]. Though some authors have reported recurrence rates less than 1% after percutaneous cryoablation [33], further research to select patients unlikely to recur is required before a randomized trial of focal therapy and robotic-assisted laparoscopic partial nephrectomy should be performed. As recent guidelines for SRM suggest [21], contemporary patients who are good surgical candidates should be recommended to undergo definitive surgical management.

Surveillance is likely a reasonable comparator in a comparative trial of focal therapy for the SRM. A common clinical dilemma is a SRM in an elderly patient with extensive comorbidities precluding surgical management. In this scenario, both focal therapy and active surveillance (AS) should be offered according to various guidelines [20,21]. An RCT comparing focal ablation and AS could answer this question and inform clinical management. One obstacle to performing this study is determining objective criteria to identify patients who are poor surgical candidates for inclusion [34]. The Charlson Comorbidity Index (CCI) has been shown to predict other cause mortality in an analysis of patients treated for kidney cancer in the SEER-Medicare data set [35]. The authors developed a nomogram for other-cause mortality incorporating age, CCI, tumor size, gender. and race. Men with CCI ≥ 3 and renal mass < 4 cm had a particularly high ratio of other-cause mortality to cancer-specific mortality. Of note, the majority of patients in the study received treatment for kidney cancer, and these results may not be applicable to patients on AS. Other analyses of SEER-Medicare have demonstrated high competing-cause mortality in patients older than 70 years of age [36], and those with high cardiovascular risk, each of which could be used as criteria for inclusion in a clinical trial of focal therapy [37].

Issues around Selecting the Optimal Study Design in Focal Therapy

RCTs for localized prostate cancer in which patients are randomized to RP or radiotherapy have historically suffered from low accrual because men (and their physicians) are unwilling to leave treatment choice to chance [38,39]. One of the reasons for the difficulty in accrual is that the treatments being compared were already widely diffused at the time of the study. Because focal therapy represents a new treatment strategy, patients may be more willing to undergo randomization.

In recent years, successful studies comparing RP and radiotherapy have employed a prospective, population-based observational cohort design, using extensive data collection and sophisticated statistical methods to minimize bias in treatment selection [40]. One advantage of this approach is that treatment decisions are left to patients and their physicians, partially alleviating the difficulty in accrual. Examples include PCOS [41], CaPSURE [42], and CEASAR [40]. This study design relies on periodic surveys to obtain clinical and patient-centered outcomes while linkages with the National Death Index can provide long-term mortality data. Because the participants are not randomly assigned to each cohort, statistical methods such as propensity scoring or instrumental variable analysis are used to account for the factors that determine a patient's propensity to receive a given treatment. Nonetheless, residual confounding from unmeasured factors remains a limitation of this type of study design. Still, this approach has great promise for testing the effectiveness of focal therapy.

In the case of SRM, data on AS are not sufficiently mature to recommend a RCT comparing focal therapy to AS. Similarly, long-term data demonstrating the efficacy of focal therapy for SRMs with low local recurrence rates are needed before patients that are surgical candidates should be routinely offered focal therapy, particularly as the surgical robot has made laparoscopic partial nephrectomy less morbid and easier to perform [43]. Thus, comparisons between focal therapy, partial nephrectomy, and AS are best made using observational data at the current time. Large administrative datasets such as SEER-Medicare are appropriate for this purpose. Ultimately, however, a RCT should be considered in this setting.

Conclusion

Focal therapy for prostate and kidney cancers may preserve the oncologic benefits of traditional therapies. For patients with RCC with SRM, comparative effectiveness research in large administrative data sets promise to identify which patients benefit most from focal therapy, active surveillance, or extirpative surgery. In prostate cancer, oncologic endpoints such as metastatic-free survival and CSM are difficult to evaluate in a clinical trial setting, and new surrogate endpoints need to be developed based on biopsy results and imaging studies to improve clinical trial design in the future. Imperative to both prostate cancer and kidney cancer is assessing the impact of focal therapies on functional outcomes in addition to oncologic outcomes. In the current environment of limited resources, optimizing clinical trial design is necessary to continue advancement in urologic oncology.

References

1 Chodak GW, Thisted RA, Gerber GS, Johansson JE, Adolfsson J, Jones GW, *et al.* Results of conservative management of clinically localized prostate cancer. N Engl J Med. 1994 Jan 27;330(4):242–8.

2 Lu-Yao GL, Albertsen PC, Moore DF, Shih W, Lin Y, DiPaola RS, *et al.* Outcomes of localized prostate cancer following conservative management. JAMA. 2009 ed. 2009 Sep 16;302(11):1202–9.

3 Crispen PL, Viterbo R, Boorjian SA, Greenberg RE, Chen DYT, Uzzo RG. Natural history, growth kinetics, and outcomes of untreated clinically localized renal tumors under active surveillance. Cancer. 2009 Jul 1;115(13):2844–52.

4 Freedland SJ, Humphreys EB, Mangold LA, Eisenberger M, Dorey FJ, Walsh, P.C., *et al.* Risk of prostate cancer-specific mortality following biochemical recurrence after radical prostatectomy. JAMA. 2005 Jul 27;294(4):433–9.

5 Stürmer T, Joshi M, Glynn RJ, Avorn J, Rothman KJ, Schneeweiss S. A review of the application of propensity score methods yielded increasing use, advantages in specific settings, but not substantially different estimates compared with conventional multivariable methods. J Clin Epidemiol. 2006 May;59(5):437–47.

6 Garas G, Ibrahim A, Ashrafian H, Ahmed K, Patel V, Okabayashi K, *et al.* Evidence-based surgery: Barriers, solutions, and the role of evidence synthesis. World J Surg. 2012 Aug;36(8):1723–31

7 Bill-Axelson A, Holmberg L, Garmo H, Rider JR, Taari K, Busch C, *et al.* Radical prostatectomy or watchful waiting in early prostate cancer. N Engl J Med. 2014 Mar 6;370(10):932–42.

8 Wilt TJ, Brawer MK, Jones KM, Barry MJ, Aronson WJ, Fox S, *et al.* Radical prostatectomy versus observation for localized prostate cancer. N Engl J Med. 2012 Jul 19;367(3):203–13.

9 Hoffman RM, Koyama T, Fan K-H, Albertsen PC, Barry MJ, Goodman M, *et al.* Mortality after radical prostatectomy or external beam radiotherapy for localized prostate cancer. J Natl Cancer Inst. 2013 May 15;105(10):711–8.

10 Cooperberg MR, Vickers AJ, Broering JM, Carroll PR. Comparative risk-adjusted mortality outcomes after primary surgery, radiotherapy, or androgen-deprivation therapy for localized prostate cancer. Cancer. 2010 Nov 15;116(22):5226–34.

11 Pound CR, Partin AW, Eisenberger MA, Chan DW, Pearson JD, Walsh, P.C. Natural history of progression after PSA elevation following radical prostatectomy [see comments]. JAMA. 1999;281(17):1591–7.

12 Consensus statement: guidelines for PSA following radiation therapy. American Society for Therapeutic Radiology and Oncology Consensus Panel. Int J Radiat Oncol Biol Phys. 1997 Mar 15; 37(5):1035–41.

13 Roach M, Hanks G, Thames H, Schellhammer P, Shipley WU, Sokol GH, *et al.* Defining biochemical failure following radiotherapy with or without hormonal therapy in men with clinically localized prostate cancer: Recommendations of the RTOG-ASTRO Phoenix Consensus Conference. 2006. pp. 965–74.

14 Nielsen ME, Makarov DV, Humphreys E, Mangold L, Partin AW, Walsh PC. Is it possible to compare PSA recurrence-free survival after surgery and radiotherapy using revised ASTRO criterion--"nadir + 2"? Urology. 2008 Aug;72(2):389–93– discussion 394–5.

15 Ahmed HU, Berge V, Bottomley D, Cross W, Heer R, Kaplan R, *et al.* Can we deliver randomized trials of focal therapy in prostate cancer? Nat Rev Clin Oncol. 2014 Aug;11(8):482–91.

16 van den Bos W, Muller BG, Ahmed H, Bangma CH, Barret E, Crouzet S, *et al.* Focal therapy in prostate cancer: international multidisciplinary consensus on trial design. Eur Urol. 2014 Jun;65(6):1078–83.

17 Tseng KS, Landis P, Epstein JI, Trock BJ, Carter HB. Risk stratification of men choosing surveillance for low risk prostate cancer. J Urol. 2010 May;183(5):1779–85.

18 Rud E, Baco E, Lien D, Klotz D, Eggesbø HB. Detection of radiorecurrent prostate cancer using diffusion-weighted imaging and targeted biopsies. Am J Roentgenol. 2014 Mar;202(3):W241–6.

19 Chow WH, Devesa SS, Warren JL, Fraumeni JF. Rising incidence of renal cell cancer in the United States. JAMA. 1999 May 5;281(17):1628–31.

20 Campbell SC, Novick AC, Belldegrun A, Blute ML, Chow GK, Derweesh IH, *et al.* Guideline for management of the clinical T1 renal mass. J Urol. 2009 ed. 2009 Oct;182(4):1271–9.

21 Motzer RJ, Jonasch E, Agarwal N, Beard C, Bhayani S, Bolger GB, *et al.* Kidney cancer, version 2.2014. Journal of the National Comprehensive Cancer Network : JNCCN. 2014. pp. 175–82.

22 Chawla SN, Crispen PL, Hanlon AL, Greenberg RE, Chen DYT, Uzzo RG. The natural history of observed enhancing renal masses: meta-analysis and review of the world literature. J Urol. 2006 Feb; 175(2):425–31.

23 Barocas DA, Rohan SM, Kao J, Gurevich RD, Del Pizzo JJ, Vaughan EDJ, *et al.* Diagnosis of renal tumors on needle biopsy specimens by histological and molecular analysis. J Urol. 2006 Nov;176(5): 1957–62.

24 Donat SM, Diaz M, Bishoff JT, Coleman JA, Dahm P, Derweesh IH, *et al.* Follow-up for Clinically Localized Renal Neoplasms: AUA Guideline. J Urol. 2013. pp. 407–16.

25 Ahmed HU, Hindley RG, Dickinson L, Freeman A, Kirkham AP, Sahu M, *et al.* Focal therapy for localised unifocal and multifocal prostate cancer: A prospective development study. Lancet Oncol. 2012 Jun;13(6):622–32.

26 Barqawi AB, Stoimenova D, Krughoff K, Eid K, O'Donnell C, Phillips JM, *et al.* Targeted focal therapy for the management of organ confined prostate cancer. J Urol. 2014 Sep;192(3):749–53.

27 Cappelleri JC, Rosen RC. A comparison of the International Index of Erectile Function and erectile dysfunction studies. BJU Int. 2003 Oct;92(6):654.

28 Barry MJ, Fowler FJJ, MP OL, Bruskewitz RC, Holtgrewe HL, Mebust WK. Correlation of the American Urological Association symptom index with self-administered versions of the Madsen-Iversen, Boyarsky and Maine Medical Assessment Program symptom indexes. Measurement Committee of the American Urological Association. J Urol. 1992;148(5):1558–63, discussion 1564.

29 Wei JT, Dunn RL, Litwin MS, Sandler HM, Sanda MG. Development and validation of the expanded prostate cancer index composite (EPIC) for comprehensive assessment of health-related quality of life in men with prostate cancer. Urology. 2000;56(6):899–905.

30 Dindo D, Demartines N, Clavien P-A. Classification of surgical complications: a new proposal with evaluation in a cohort of 6336 patients and results of a survey. Ann Surg. 2004 Aug;240(2):205–13.

31 Etzioni R, Penson DF, Legler JM, di Tommaso D, Boer R, Gann PH, *et al.* Overdiagnosis due to prostate-specific antigen screening: Lessons from U.S. prostate cancer incidence trends. J Natl Cancer Inst. 2002 Jul 3;94(13):981–90.

32 Klatte T, Shariat SF, Remzi M. Systematic review and meta-analysis of perioperative and oncologic outcomes of laparoscopic cryoablation versus laparoscopic partial nephrectomy for the treatment of small renal tumors. J Urol. 2014 May; 191(5):1209–17.

33 Breen DJ, Bryant TJ, Abbas A, Shepherd B, McGill N, Anderson JA, *et al.* Percutaneous cryoablation of renal tumours: outcomes from 171 tumours in 147 patients. BJU Int. 2013 Oct;112(6):758–65.

34 Pierorazio PM, Hyams ES, Mullins JK, Allaf ME. Active surveillance for small renal masses. Rev Urol. 2012;14(1-2):13–9.

35 Kutikov A, Egleston BL, Canter D, Smaldone MC, Wong Y-N, Uzzo RG. Competing risks of death in patients with

localized renal cell carcinoma: a comorbidity based model. J Urol. 2012 Dec;188(6):2077–83.

36 Hollingsworth JM, Miller DC, Daignault S, Hollenbeck BK. Five-year survival after surgical treatment for kidney cancer: a population-based competing risk analysis. Cancer. 2007 May 1; 109(9):1763–8.

37 Patel HD, Kates M, Pierorazio PM, Allaf ME. Balancing cardiovascular (CV) and cancer death among patients with small renal masses: Modification by CV risk. BJU Int. 2015 Jan; 115(1):58–64

38 Crook JM, Gomez-Iturriaga A, Wallace K, Ma C, Fung S, Alibhai S, *et al.* Comparison of health-related quality of life 5 years after SPIRIT: Surgical Prostatectomy Versus Interstitial Radiation Intervention Trial. J Clin Oncol. Am Soc Clin Oncol; 2011 Feb 1;29(4):362–8.

39 Hoffman RM, Penson DF, Zietman AL, Barry MJ. Comparative effectiveness research in localized prostate cancer treatment. J Comp Eff Res. 2013 Nov;2(6):583–93.

40 Barocas DA, Chen V, Cooperberg M, Goodman M, Graff JJ, Greenfield S, *et al.* Using a population-based observational cohort study to address difficult comparative effectiveness research questions: The CEASAR study. J Comp Eff Res. Future Medicine Ltd London, UK; 2013 Jul;2(4):445–60.

41 Potosky AL, Harlan LC, Stanford JL, Gilliland FD, Hamilton AS, Albertsen PC, *et al.* Prostate cancer practice patterns and quality of life: The Prostate Cancer Outcomes Study. J Natl Cancer Inst. 1999 Oct 20;91(20):1719–24.

42 Lubeck DP, Litwin MS, Henning JM, Stier DM, Mazonson P, Fisk R, *et al.* The CaPSURE database: A methodology for clinical practice and research in prostate cancer. CaPSURE Research Panel. Cancer of the Prostate Strategic Urologic Research Endeavor. Urology. 1996;48(5):773–7.

43 Emara AM, Kommu SS, Hindley RG, Barber NJ. Robot-assisted partial nephrectomy vs laparoscopic cryoablation for the small renal mass: Redefining the minimally invasive 'gold standard'. BJU Int. 2014 Jan;113(1):92–9.

Index

Note: Page references in *italics* refer to Figures; those in **bold** refer to Tables

Management of Urologic Cancer: Focal Therapy and Tissue Preservation, First Edition.
Edited by Mark P. Schoenberg and Kara L. Watts.
© 2017 John Wiley & Sons Ltd. Published 2017 by John Wiley & Sons Ltd.